Praise for

Today Is the First Day

Today Is the First Day will draw the reader to God and His Word and bring balance and renewal to heart and body. Don't miss it!

Cheri Fuller
Founder, Families Pray USA
Author, *When Mothers Pray*

Until I read *Today Is the First Day* I had no idea how much the Bible says about guilt, temptation, our bodies, sweets and bread—all issues for each person whose daily intake is out of control. Whether you eat too much or too little, this book of devotions will give you daily bread that has no calories.

Florence Littauer
Speaker and Author, *Personality Plus* and *Silver Boxes*

The best help we can acquire as we're striving to eat as God would lead us is found right in His Word and through prayer. Carole Lewis has provided that help for us in daily doses through *Today Is the First Day,* which provides a Scripture focus, inspiring testimony, prayer and journaling ideas for every day of the year. This wonderful guide will help anyone who wants to put God first to find victory every single day.

Janet Holm McHenry
Author, *PrayerWalk: Becoming a Woman of Prayer, Strength and Discipline* and *PrayerWalk: Meditations for a Deeper Prayer Life*

Carole Lewis and dozens of others have started down the road to health and vitality by putting Christ in first place. Reading their stories every day will help the rest of us stay on course and travel that awesome way of obedience, blessing and victory.

Karen Porter
Author and Speaker

TODAY *is the* FIRST DAY

CAROLE LEWIS
GENERAL EDITOR

Regal

From Gospel Light
Ventura, California, U.S.A.

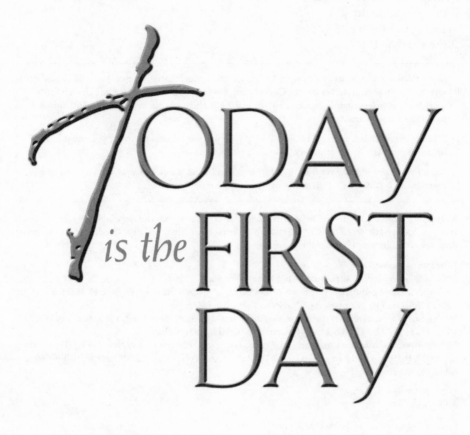

Published by Regal Books
From Gospel Light
Ventura, California, U.S.A.
Printed in the U.S.A.

Regal Books is a ministry of Gospel Light, an evangelical Christian publisher dedicated to serving the local church. We believe God's vision for Gospel Light is to provide church leaders with biblical, user-friendly materials that will help them evangelize, disciple and minister to children, youth and families.

It is our prayer that this Regal book will help you discover biblical truth for your own life and help you meet the needs of others. May God richly bless you.

For a free catalog of resources from Regal Books/Gospel Light, please call your Christian supplier or contact us at 1-800-4-GOSPEL *or* www.regalbooks.com.

Cover design by Samantha A. Hsu
Interior design by Rob Williams
Edited by David Hazard and Deena Davis

Rights for publishing this book in other languages are contracted by Gospel Light Worldwide, the international nonprofit ministry of Gospel Light. Gospel Light Worldwide also provides publishing and technical assistance to international publishers dedicated to producing Sunday School and Vacation Bible School curricula and books in the languages of the world. For additional information, visit www.gospellightworldwide.org; write to Gospel Light Worldwide, P.O. Box 3875, Ventura, CA 93006; or send an e-mail to info@gospellightworldwide.org.

Contents

FOREWORD

What good food is to the daily maintenance of the body, the Word of God is to the daily maintenance of the soul. In our media-driven culture, we are invited to binge on everything but what our souls crave the most, while our true famine remains undiagnosed. No amount of food, relationships, money or luxuries can fill the black hole of our need for God.

To live a safe life calls for wise moderation in many categories, but within each of us is an insatiable need to give way to a ravenous appetite in some area of our lives. Beloved, you can have all of God, all of His Spirit (see Luke 11:13; John 3:34!), and all the meat and gravy of His Word that you could possibly want. "Open wide your mouth," Psalm 81:10 says, "and [He] will fill it"!

I love the words in Psalm 63:5, spoken by the man God said was "a man after my own heart" (Acts 13:22). David said, "My soul will be satisfied as with the richest of foods; with singing lips my mouth will praise you." When our souls are deeply satisfied with the richest of spiritual foods, the cravings of our flesh are far more likely to subside. Dear one, each of us was born with a need to have *a lot* of something. That something is God. So take your fill!

Nothing in the believer's experience can replace a daily personal encounter with God through prayer and Scripture. No amount of tireless service and noble effort can suffice. In John 15:8, Christ said, "This is to my Father's glory, that you bear much fruit, showing yourselves to be my disciples." Grasp this, beloved one: Your Father's desire is for *you* to bear *much fruit.* You don't have to wonder if great effectiveness is God's will for your life; your life was set apart to be tremendously productive in the Body of Christ. He requires our cooperation, however, because fruit can only be produced from the inside out. The fruit that hangs on the end of a branch or vine has come from the nutrition of the tree itself. Christ explained that the fruit of which He spoke comes from His words *abiding* in us (see John 15:7).

That's what this devotional book is all about. The wonderful folks at First Place have learned from personal experience that victory eludes any believer who ignores prayer and Bible study and so misses an opportunity to have a deeper, ongoing relationship with God. Within these pages First Place members offer you a guide to help you seek God and find Him on a daily basis. Certainly any of us could simply open the Bible and start reading, but most of us are greatly helped by a daily devotional guide. Though I love reading the Word of God all by itself and do so often, I almost always use a devotional guide of some kind in the morning.

I am a firm believer in becoming a student of many *(sound!)* teachers, as endless stacks of devotional guides on my shelves suggest. Following only one human teacher is dangerous. In your pursuit of sound material, look for a number of teachers who closely (albeit imperfectly) follow the one true rabboni, Jesus Christ Himself. I'm delighted that First Place has provided us with another opportunity to receive a fresh, spontaneous meditation from God's Word and His servants. These are sound people, ones you can trust.

One other thing is certain: Every entry you will find within this cover is from the heart. My good friend Carole Lewis, the national director of First Place, penned many of the pages during a time of harrowing loss and great desperation for God. God was Jehovah Shammah to her—the God who is *there*. You will quickly discover proof of what you hope by faith—that He is there for you too, dear one—day in and day out, 24/7. He is in your den or breakfast room, waiting every single morning to start your day. He is beside your desk throughout the day. He is at your bedside at night, waiting to tuck you in. Give Him those opportunities! Even with a sink full of dirty dishes and a table piled high with clean clothes, Jesus can turn your house into the Holy of Holies. Grab your Bible and this devotional book and let Him be Jehovah Shammah to you!

—Beth Moore
Author of *Praying God's Word* and *Breaking Free*

Preface

I was very excited when our publisher suggested a devotional book written by friends of the First Place program. I must admit, though, that collecting devotionals from so many men and women was a little like trying to herd beautiful butterflies. I'm glad I didn't know the full extent of this project, its magnitude, because I might have missed the tremendous blessing of reading all the wonderful devotionals about how God has used the First Place memory verses in the lives of First Place members.

Creating this book has been a joy and also one of the great challenges of my life.

Challenge—and Grace

To begin with, First Place members, leaders and friends submitted several devotionals based on each of our 80 memory verses. My job was to oversee the project and to write at least one devotional based on each of the 80 verses as well. As you read the amazing stories of how God has used His Word to teach and inspire, I believe you will be as blessed by them as I have been.

Then there was the *real* challenge. Throughout the fall of last year, I felt confident the book was progressing well as I reviewed the work of others. With a deadline of January 20, I thought I could easily write my devotionals during my Christmas vacation. But as many of you know, Shari, my 39-year-old daughter, was standing in the driveway of her in-laws' home on Thanksgiving night, when an 18-year-old girl who was driving drunk lost control of her car. Shari was killed.

Needless to say, I didn't do much writing during the Thanksgiving or Christmas holidays. I came back to work January 7 with just a little anxiety about my part in this project. The devotionals of all the other folks had continued to come in regularly, and I was reasonably sure we could meet our deadline–if only I could accomplish my part.

Things did not go as planned. The first week back at work I didn't write one devotional. After being out for six weeks, I was overwhelmed with work. I began to pray for God's help. I knew He understood my dilemma and would help me. Our mighty God came through, and from my mind spilled every story I had ever shared as I quickly typed them onto the flow of paper. I can truthfully say that God's grace has been with me.

God's Sufficiency

I have always heard that writers tend to write from their lives and speak from their hearts about the things they are presently walking out. I don't know whether or not this is a universally true statement. I can tell you for sure that what I have been able to write about from this challenging time is God and His sufficiency.

Yes, to a great degree my family and I are still in shock and reeling from the death of our precious Shari. You will see that I share some stories about Shari's death in the devotionals I wrote for the section "Everyday Victory for Everyday People." This tragedy brought home in a forceful and new way the sufficiency of God that I had already discovered during my husband's health struggle. I also mention our four-year journey through cancer in the devotionals I wrote for "Life Under Control" and "Life That Wins." These sections include devotionals about some of my best friends who are also winners on our First Place staff.

Balance Through God's Word

Finally, I would like for you, the reader of this book, to know this: The balance I have learned in First Place during the last 20 years is the reason this book was finished on time. I have learned through my study of God's Word that He is able, even when I am not. When we make ourselves available to God, even at our weakest moment, His strength is able to give us the balance we need to accomplish anything He has called us to face or to do.

If this book blesses you, stop and give thanks to the One who made it possible—our Lord Jesus Christ.

Always remember: *When you can't, that's when He does His best work.*

"I can do everything through him who gives me strength" (Phil. 4:13).

—Carole Lewis
First Place National Director

How to Use This Book

This 365-day devotional book has been designed for use by anyone seeking inspiration and growth in a daily time of fellowship with God.

The book is divided into eight sections, one section for each of the first eight Bible studies released by First Place—and consists of writings based around 80 key Scripture verses—10 within each section. To help you absorb and meditate on each verse before moving to a new one, several devotionals are built around a single verse, exploring it from different angles. The verses have been carefully selected to encourage and inspire a closer walk with the Lord, especially when the verses are committed to memory. Each new verse is identified by an open Bible icon.

If you're not participating in a First Place group but would like additional help with Scripture memorization, each First Place Bible study includes its own CD with the Scriptures set to music.

If you are a member of a First Place group, you may want to start reading in this devotional in the Bible study section you are currently using. This will help you in several ways:

- Using the devotionals that correspond to the memory verse you are memorizing will help impress the truths of that particular verse in your mind.
- Since there are four or five devotionals for each verse, you will be able to meditate on that verse each day as you pray and as you journal.
- The verses will take on a fresh new meaning as you read personal accounts of how God has used the verses in the lives of First Place members.

If you are not a member of a First Place group, you will still benefit from the wisdom and encouragement found in this devotional. *Today Is the First Day* is for anyone wishing to gain inspiration and strength in the following areas:

- Weight loss
- Prayer
- Journaling

You will notice throughout the devotional that contributors mention terms that may be unfamiliar—such as "Commitment Record," "Live-It plan," etc. These are labels that describe some of the nine commitments of First Place. The purpose of these commitments is to help people draw closer to the Lord and to become stronger and healthier in every area of life—mental, physical, emotional and spiritual. For those of you who are not participants in a First Place group, here is a complete list of the nine commitments:

Attendance—Choosing to show up
Encouragement—Choosing to reach out to others
Prayer—Choosing to pray
Bible reading—Choosing to read God's Word
Scripture memory verse—Choosing to memorize God's Word
Bible study—Choosing to study the Bible
Live-It plan—Choosing to eat right
Commitment Record—Choosing to be accountable
Exercise—Choosing to exercise

Many blessings to you, reader, as you allow the scriptural principles contained in this book to strengthen you—and as you allow the words of personal wisdom gained from God's Word and His Holy Spirit to inspire you. Today is the first day of the rest of your life!

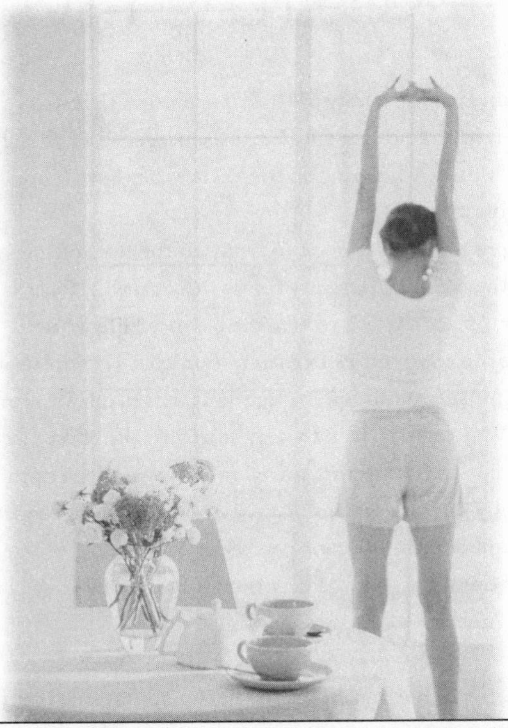

Giving Christ First Place

Section One

INTRODUCTION

After we are born again into the family of God, it is natural that we begin to grow. Some people grow spiritually at a rapid rate. Others, it seems, get stuck in the "baby" stage. It's important to note that those who grow do so because they have found a balance in their lives, a balance that fosters growth.

The First Place program is designed to bring to the lives of men and women who follow its principles the balance necessary for healthy growth, for it is only as we learn how to give Christ first place that we receive the balanced life we need.

God wants to do amazing things in each of our lives. He tells us in Jeremiah 29:11 that His plans are to prosper us and not to harm us. His plans for us include a wonderful hope and future. Why then wouldn't we want to give Him first place in everything?

The devotionals in this first section are all taken from the Scripture memory verses found in the Bible study *Giving Christ First Place*. To help give you adequate time to absorb these scriptural principles from different perspectives, several devotionals are presented about each verse. It is our hope that the devotionals written by First Place members and leaders from all over America will inspire and motivate you to give Christ first place in your life.

As you begin this section of the book, my personal prayer is that you will each day be obedient to meet God in a time of devotion and with an attitude of prayer. If you will do this, I believe your life will become *fresh again* because of the Spirit's work in and around you. If we do not take the time to be alone with God each day, we become dry, lifeless and stale.

Oswald Chambers says in his classic book *My Utmost for His Highest* that "staleness is an indication of something out of joint with God—'I must do this thing or it will never be done.'"[1]

Chambers goes on to explain a basic principle of the spiritual life that we need to learn: When we jump into our day before we connect with God in spirit, giving into the pressure "to do," we deplete our spirits. We become more and more busy, and busyness becomes the source and the sign of our spiritually stale condition.[2]

I wholly agree with Chambers when he asks in conclusion, "Are we freshly born this minute or are we stale, raking in our minds for something to do? Freshness does not come from obedience, but from the Holy Spirit; obedience keeps us in the light as God is in the light."[3]

—Carole Lewis

JANUARY 1

NEW YEAR, NEW LIFE

But seek first his kingdom and his righteousness, and all these things will be given to you as well.

MATTHEW 6:33

I love the fact that God is a God of new beginnings. What this means to me is that God created us so that we can always start over.

This grace—the ability to begin again—was built into things when God created the world. Think about it. His design included the first day of each *year,* the first day of each *month,* the first day of each *week,* the first hour of each *day,* the first minute of each *hour,* the first second of each *minute!*

Too often we give in to a defeated mind-set, instead of seeing each moment as hope filled. We stay stuck in the past, instead of living in vital fellowship with the God who is the God of new beginnings.

I have learned in First Place that I *need* to give God the first part of each day by spending time with Him, reading His Word, listening to His voice and praying. New beginnings come whenever I seek Him. On those days when I don't seek Him first, I get stuck. On my own, I resort to old habits, and my life goes out of control again. But when I realize what I'm doing, He always allows me to start over.

As we begin this New Year, let's take time to remember the word "first." Let's ask ourselves, *Who is in first place in my life today?*

If God is in His rightful spot—taking first place in my life—then I become obedient to Him, and I know what's right for me to eat, to say, to do and to be.

PRAYER

Help me learn to put You in first place in my life in everything I say and do.
Help me remember that You are in first place today, not me.

Journal: Confess areas in which God is not in first place in your life. Thank Him for giving you the opportunity to start fresh.

—Carole Lewis

JANUARY 2

WHOM DOES GOD LOVE?

But seek first his kingdom and his righteousness, and all these things will be given to you as well.

MATTHEW 6:33

Today is my birthday. The thing I always love best about my birthday is that for one entire day *I am special.*

Friends will call and ask to take me to lunch. My family will give me presents and fix my favorite dinner. Sometimes I receive a surprise bouquet of flowers. As for me, it doesn't really matter how much or what is done for me on this day. What is important is that I just know it's my special day.

Since my birthday comes so soon after Christmas—just one week—it must not have been easy for my parents to make my birthday special. My parents must have been tired of hoopla and celebrations and shopping for just the right presents. Yet they loved me so much that they took care to see that my birthday was always a special time, and they helped me know that I had a special place in their hearts.

When we give God first place in our lives, we treat Him as if every day is His birthday. We give God the place of special importance He deserves. Our thoughts center around what would make Him happy today, and we set about doing those things that please Him.

Giving God first place means finding out whom He loves and loving them too. It means finding out where He loves to go and going there too. How do we learn all these things about God? By reading, studying and memorizing His Word.

As we seek to know God in His Word, each day offers us the fresh start we need, because the more we learn about who He is, the more we learn how to give Him first place in our lives.

PRAYER

Dear Lord, help me learn everything about You so that I can please You with my life. I want my life to be a present that only I can give to You.

Journal: Consider how you can make your life a present for God today. What specific things will you do to make today His day all day?

—Carole Lewis

JANUARY 3

All These Things

But seek first his kingdom and his righteousness, and all these things will be given to you as well.

MATTHEW 6:33

What are "all these things" that God offers to give us when we seek first His kingdom and His righteousness?

The apostle Paul tells us that God will give us the fruit of the Spirit, which is "love, joy, peace, patience, kindness, goodness, faithfulness, gentleness and self control" (Gal. 5:22-23). If my life possesses all these spiritual qualities, then I truly have "all these things" because my life is richly blessed and in balance.

As wonderful as spiritual fruit is, these are not the only things God gives His children. There is much more.

As we give God first place, He will also make us into better spouses and parents, children and siblings. By giving Him first place, He restores even the most broken relationships. He will also meet our financial needs. As we give Him first place, He restores financial stability and well-being, even for people who have been teetering on the edge of ruin. I've had the blessed privilege of watching God turn a variety of seemingly hopeless situations into fruitful experiences of abundance and peace.

When we give God first place in our lives, He takes care of "all these things" that we want and need. That's because by giving God top priority we remove ourselves from the decision-making process. We stop demanding and insisting that things be done our way and instead learn to ask what He wants, what He thinks and what He would do in a specific situation.

As we learn to do this, we finally allow Him to give us *all things,* including the blessed, peaceful, ordered lives we have always wanted.

PRAYER

Dear Father, help me today to quit worrying about all the things in my life that need fixing and help me trust You to fix them. Help me to seek You first in everything I say and do.

Journal: Tell God the "things" you need in your life. Confess the places where you have had little success trying to fix these things. Tell Him specifically how you will give Him first place today.

—Carole Lewis

JANUARY 4

EYES OFF THE SCALES

But seek first his kingdom and his righteousness, and all these things will be given to you as well.

MATTHEW 6:33

Shortly after I became a new believer, I gave birth to my fourth child. I was already overweight from a lifetime of food problems and several pregnancies that came quickly one after another.

Of course I had made attempts to lose weight. But the programs I tried caused me to focus on myself and on the weight I had to lose. Oddly enough, I found that the more I focused on the numbers on the scale, the heavier I became. I came to believe that it wasn't going to be possible for me to lose weight. And I felt hopeless.

When a friend told me about the First Place Bible study, I attended with her for one reason: I wanted to lose weight. Little did I know what God had in store for me. Not only did I lose weight, but I also gained far more than I could ever imagine: I gained a personal relationship with the Lord Jesus Christ.

What made the difference? First Place taught me to set my primary focus on Jesus. As I practiced the principles of the First Place program, I realized that God is the One—the only One—who can meet all my needs. My weight was still an important issue—but only of secondary importance. Now my relationship with the Lord was put in its rightful place: first place.

Today I can say that the more I have grown in Jesus Christ, the less I have actually come to weigh on the scale. I have maintained my weight loss for seven years now.

God did this in my life. He can do it in your life too.

PRAYER

Lord, forgive me for all the things I place ahead of You. Help me to get my focus right and put You in Your rightful place. When You are first in my life, then You will give me victory with my weight and with other life issues.

Journal: What holds first place in your life? In what ways have you tried to achieve weight loss before and failed? What would it mean to you to give Jesus first place?

—Roberta Wasserman

JANUARY 5

GOD'S DESIRES

But seek first his kingdom and his righteousness, and all these things will be given to you as well.

MATTHEW 6:33

"Seek first his kingdom and his righteousness." I know why God impressed this Scripture verse on the founders of the First Place ministry to make it their first key verse. God has continually brought this foundational truth back to my mind to teach me the one important lesson He wants all of us to know. We can read, study, go to seminars and conferences, and earn degrees; but the most important lesson God wants us to learn in our Christian walk is this: We only grow in spirit as we learn how to live daily in a consistent and loving relationship with the God who created us and the whole universe.

I must confess: It is still beyond my comprehension that the King of kings and Lord of lords is interested in every detail of my life. It's amazing that He desires a personal love relationship with me—*but I know that He does!* And it pleases me that every time I get just a little too far away from Him, my loving Father gently corrects, convicts and draws me back to Himself.

As a believer, I often tried to resolve my struggles and fill my needs my way. Today I know that when I look to my Lord *first* for all my help, He will show me what He wants. As I obey, His desires become my desires—that's when everything else in my life falls into place. He gives me the desires of my heart—because they are *His* desires.

PRAYER

Lord, help me to keep my eyes on You. Always turn my eyes back to You, seeking You first for help in every area of my life. May my desires be Your desires.

Journal: What is the most important thing or person in your life? How could you truly seek to give God first place in every area of your life?

—Janet Kirkhart

FAITH TO EMBRACE HIS PROMISES

If you believe, you will receive whatever you ask for in prayer.

MATTHEW 21:22

Whatever I believe in, I am passionate about. What's more, if I know God is also passionate about the same thing, then I can pray passionately about it. Belief, passion, faith—these three things go together.

I have faith, for instance, that God wants to answer my prayers. This comes from my passionate belief that He is interested in everything that lifts Him to the position of first place in my life. Therefore, I can be passionate about prayer, rather than coming at it half-heartedly—which is often how we pray when we don't really believe that God hears or when we really don't have the faith that He will answer.

I also have a passion to see First Place utilized in the lives of people all over the world. I pray boldly for this every day, having faith that God will hear and answer.

In order to believe that God will hear and answer our prayers we must ask ourselves some questions: *Is my prayer in line with what God's Word teaches? Will the answer to my prayer honor and glorify Christ? Will people come to know Christ personally through the answer to my prayer?*

Praying in faith, boldly, is not always easy though, is it? I know this only too well. We at First Place experienced two very difficult years during our transition from one publisher to another. We didn't have tangible proof that First Place had a bright future. But we prayed, believing that God would do mighty things with His First Place program. Why? Because First Place is not built on a personality but on giving Christ His rightful position in our lives. And sure enough, during those rough two years, people continued to have their lives transformed when they learned how to give Christ first place.

If your prayer life lacks passion, then it's time to reexamine your beliefs and priorities and ask God for increased faith to believe His promises.

PRAYER

Dear Lord, help me to always keep Your priorities mine. May my faith today be equal to Your power to answer my prayers.

Journal: List your current prayer requests and compare them with the three questions above. How do they match up?

—Carole Lewis

JANUARY 7

If You Believe, You Will Receive

If you believe, you will receive whatever you ask for in prayer.

MATTHEW 21:22

There I was, racing to the hospital with my husband gasping for breath beside me. His lips were turning blue. Fervently I prayed for God to get us to the emergency room safely—and in time.

When we arrived, the nurses and a doctor looked at each other. "Heart," the doctor said. "Get him started on oxygen." I watched my husband's gurney disappear into an examining room while I was left to answer questions about insurance.

Then came more delay as I was left to sit in the waiting area. *What was going on?* My thoughts raced anxiously. But as I sat there, words from a Scripture verse I had memorized during the study *Giving Christ First Place* came up from the depths of my spirit: "If you believe, you will receive."

The peace of God rose within me. Anxiety slowed and then drained from me. I could think. I could believe. My husband would be all right.

Shortly after this, our two older sons arrived to be with me. Our oldest, Bailey, paced back and forth. Finally he asked, "How can you sit there so calmly? Aren't you afraid of what's happening with Dad back in the emergency room?"

"Yes," I replied quietly. "But I know God is in control. I know Dad will be okay because of God's promise."

Bailey looked puzzled. "What promise?"

I smiled and repeated from God's wonderful, sure Word, "If you believe."

Rex, my husband, survived the heart attack. Later he underwent successful bypass surgery and has now made a full recovery. How thankful I am not only for his life but also for the fact that God walked with me through the crisis, giving me peace from His Word.

PRAYER

Dear God, help me to claim Your promises every day in every situation.
Help me to believe You will hear and answer my prayers.

Journal: When God answers a prayer, write it in your journal, noting the date and time of the answer. Then write a word of praise and thanksgiving to Him.

—Martha Rogers

JANUARY 8

You Are Not a Failure

If you believe, you will receive whatever you ask for in prayer.

MATTHEW 21:22

Before I began the First Place program, I didn't believe God was interested in my need to lose weight. Not that God's ability to help was an issue. Far from it! I just didn't believe God would care about such a comparatively small issue as my weight problem.

Because of this fundamental mistake, I had actually set myself up for failure. In fact, a number of previous attempts to lose weight by other methods had failed. Truthfully, I was so discouraged that I didn't have much hope for success when I began the First Place program. This is one of the negative results of dieting to lose weight. We focus too much on weight loss. Sure, we set out with the very best intentions. But when we meet failures and setbacks, we tend to believe we are failures *in ourselves.* Without a proper focus and a foundation of faith, we may also come to believe that God doesn't care about something as "small" as helping us lose weight. Or worse, we may think He just doesn't care about *us.*

First Place taught me that in order to achieve success, I had to be willing to do something more profound and wonderful than just "go on a diet." I had to be willing to let God change my lifestyle. The First Place program helped me to develop life-changing habits to achieve victory and gain success.

With this changed perspective, I came to believe that God does care about me and my whole life—including my weight. I was able to ask Him for help and to believe that He would answer my prayers. And He did. I have maintained my weight loss and my growing relationship with God for seven years now.

PRAYER

Lord, I thank You that You want to change more than my appearance. I know now that You want to change my whole life and make it full of the blessing that comes from living close to You. Thank You for caring about all my concerns, including my weight issues.

Journal: Do you doubt God's care for you? Have you been trying to reach your goals without His help? Tell God about it and ask Him to lead you to victory.

—Roberta Wasserman

JANUARY 9

IN GOD'S SKILLFUL HANDS

If you believe, you will receive whatever you ask for in prayer.

MATTHEW 21:22

My prayer was a simple one. I was 14—old enough to be beyond asking for bicycles and toys. Since my walk with Jesus Christ began when I was a child, I had matured in faith, surrendered to serving God in the area of missions and knew God wanted to do something special with my life. Therefore, I boldly asked to be healed.

A year before, when I was 13, I'd had back surgery to correct the severe curvature in my spine, the result of scoliosis. The surgeon had done his best but had only been able to repair about 60 percent of the problem. My spine remained crooked and, worse, the surgeon had cautioned my parents to prepare me for the fact that childbirth might be impossible.

At 14, of course, being unable to bear children wasn't my immediate problem. I was, however, in distress about my future. How could God possibly use me with a crooked back?

God had something better in mind than repairing my back. The Spirit guided my every step as I studied His Word, participated in great church programs and mostly walked obediently with Him. He wove together a beautiful pattern in my life, rich with godly people and amazing events. In God's skillful hands, my wounded spirit was lifted and made whole.

My back is still crooked; but because God is faithful, I have received much more than I asked for in prayer as a 14-year-old. To date, I have spent two years in the mission field. I married my precious husband, who is a minister. Together with him, I have found full involvement in Christian ministry.

And, oh yes, I gave birth to two wonderful children. And they have given me three grandchildren who are the delight of my life.

PRAYER

Lord, help me never to believe that my prayers to You go unanswered. Guard my mind to be quick to see when I am choosing not to believe You. Give me patience and perspective because You and I have eternity together.

Journal: List three actions you can take today that will break through the mind-set of limiting God in how He answers your prayers. Then ask Him to show you His purposes for your life.

—Nan Olmsted

JANUARY 10

ASKING FORGIVENESS, GAINING PEACE

Whoever has my commands and obeys them, he is the one who loves me. He who loves me will be loved by my Father, and I too will love him and show myself to him.

JOHN 14:21

The greatest thrill of my life is when God shows Himself to me. I "see" God with the eyes of my soul—that is, I sense His presence when I listen to His commands and obey them.

How well I remember the distress I experienced during a time when I let a negative frame of mind take over, which resulted in my wanting to see a coworker lose her job.

The woman I was fretting over wasn't under my supervision or even in my department, but I had influence in the department where she worked. One morning, as I was running, I thought about what I was going to say to this woman's supervisor. Suddenly, a clear message came into my mind. I knew God was speaking: "Carole, do you know that I love her as much as I love you?"

I was so astounded that I argued with God for almost a mile! But in the end I knew what I had to do.

When I got to the office, I immediately went down the hall to the restroom. I knew I would find this woman there. She was always at least 20 minutes late; and on top of that, the restroom, where she put on her makeup, was always her first stop. When I walked in, she turned from the mirror, and I said, "I need you to forgive me if I've hurt you in any way."

Her eyes filled with tears. "Oh, Carole, I thought you hated me."

From that day on, we had a new and different relationship—one that honored Christ. By allowing God to work in her life and by my not taking matters into my own hands, I was able to see the worth of every individual in His eyes.

PRAYER

Father, I want to obey You today. Help me to be as loving and forgiving today as You have been to me. My prayer for today is that You would show Yourself to me.

Journal: Confess to God one specific area in which you are refusing to obey. Ask Him to help you obey His commands.

—Carole Lewis

JANUARY 11

MERCIES BEYOND MEASURE

Whoever has my commands and obeys them, he is the one who loves me. He who loves me will be loved by my Father, and I too will love him and show myself to him.

JOHN 14:21

I drive to work each morning on one of the most heavily traveled freeways in Texas. One morning I left home later than usual and the traffic was very heavy. Things only got worse from there.

Within just a few miles, I was involved in a small accident, for which I was at fault. As I waited for the highway patrolman to complete his investigation, I was hoping for mercy. When I saw the policeman walk toward me with that familiar piece of paper in his hand, I knew there would be no leniency for me that day.

While driving to work in the days that followed, I pleaded my case before the Lord. I argued that I am a rule follower. I drive the speed limit and obey the traffic laws. As other drivers flew by me on the highway, I would interrupt my self-defense arguments and complain about "these lawbreakers"—and also about the people who were driving illegally in a newly completed traffic lane for high-occupancy vehicles. They were not following the rules. They were creating large traffic jams. When I saw someone pulled over, I felt a sense of satisfaction when the officer handed the driver a ticket for their offense.

And then the Lord spoke to my spirit. "You want justice for others. But you want mercy for yourself."

I blushed. It was true. I repented and thanked the Lord for revealing this truth about myself to me.

Today as I drive to work, people still speed by me. People still drive illegally in the new lane. I continue to obey the rules, doing what is right. And as I drive, I ask the Lord to show mercy to others.

PRAYER

Thank You, Lord, for Your mercies that are new every morning and for loving us and showing Yourself to us. Help us to extend mercy to others as You have abundantly poured out Your love and mercy on us.

Journal: Is there someone you think deserves justice rather than mercy? Are you willing to forgive them and ask God to show them mercy?

—Pat Lewis

JANUARY 12

CHOOSING THE OBEDIENT PATH

Whoever has my commands and obeys them, he is the one who loves me. He who loves me will be loved by my Father, and I too will love him and show myself to him.

JOHN 14:21

When the year began, I asked the Lord to help me over the next 12 months to grow in obedience. He has honored that request through several venues. One of them was First Place.

One day during the First Place study time, I found myself thinking about how compliant I had been as a child. Because I was obedient, my parents were able to teach me some great habits that have helped me throughout my life.

During the First Place study, however, I began asking myself, *If you were obedient to your parents and that obedience taught you good habits, why are you so often disobedient to God?*

That realization was embarrassing—but also eye-opening. If my earthly parents had many good things to teach me, how much more blessed would my life be if I listened more often to the instructions of my heavenly Father?

Clearly, I was hearing a call for repentance.

In the year that followed, I gradually lost almost 15 pounds. And while weight loss is not the only area in which I need to grow in obedience, it is an easily measured one. Yet I pray that I might continue to grow in obedience to the Lord in all the areas of my life.

PRAYER

Lord, what choices am I making today that are not in accord with Your demand for obedience? I pray that I might be willing to surrender my will to Yours. Help me grow in obedience.

Journal: What choices did you make today that led to obedience? What choices led to disobedience? How could you begin to make more compliant, obedient choices?

—Helen McCormack

JANUARY 13

"OBEDIENCE" IS A VERB

Whoever has my commands and obeys them, he is the one who loves me. He who loves me will be loved by my Father, and I too will love him and show myself to him.

JOHN 14:21

"The person who knows my commandments and keeps them, that's who loves me. And the person who loves me will be loved by my Father, and I will love him and make myself plain to him." This is the way John 14:21 reads in *The Message*.

Loving anyone, especially God, is not so much a matter of feelings but of *decision*. When we base love on feelings, in any relationship, we're on unsteady ground. Even if Prince Charming were to ride up on his white charger, sooner or later you would notice things about him that were unlovable. And if love were based only on feelings, you would fall out of love with him.

Jesus tells us plainly that it's not just knowing God's commandments but also obeying them that proves our love for God. If you know I hate liver and you fix it for me anyway, that's pretty clear evidence that you don't care about my wishes. Too many times, I've fixed liver for God, instead of seeking His will and His plan. "Love" is an action word and can only live and grow in our lives if we actively pursue a relationship with God.

And what a promise is associated with obeying God's commands! God the Father will love us and show Himself to us.

PRAYER

I love You, Lord, and I want to love You more! Forgive me for the times I've ignored Your plans for my life and "fixed liver" for You.

Journal: Have you studied God's commands and plans for you? What does He want for your life?

—June-Marie Avery

JANUARY 14

BECOMING A "BRISCO" FOR GOD

Whoever has my commands and obeys them, he is the one who loves me. He who loves me will be loved by my Father, and I too will love him and show myself to him.

JOHN 14:21

"Obeying God" is another term for "staying in His will." Sometimes the idea of staying obedient to God, remaining in His will, can seem confining. I knew something was wrong with the way I was looking at obedience, so I asked God to teach me a new way of seeing things. His lesson came in a very scruffy form—with four feet.

Brisco is our Beagle-Jack Russell terrier. She's very active, and we are her third home. We had been told she just couldn't be trained to obey. At first this was a concern because we own two acres surrounded by a muddy creek and have a neighbor who definitely doesn't want dogs on his property.

It has taken some work, but Brisco is "getting it." While she stays inside the perimeter, she is free to go wherever she chooses. She is fed wonderful table scraps and bones and receives lots of love and attention. Here she finds warm shelter. This is doggie heaven!

If she goes too near the fenced perimeter, however, she has learned that she will receive an unpleasant correction. When she gets too close to the fence, her collar beeps as a warning that she's getting too close to danger.

Every time I look at Brisco I, too, "get it." There is such peace in obeying God's commands. It's when I allow something that is outside of His will to distract me that I suffer unpleasant consequences. And make no mistake: God will correct His children and give them boundaries.

PRAYER

Father, when I am tucked into the comfort of doing Your will, thank You for a peace that passes all understanding. Thank You, too, for my conscience and the "Holy Reminder" who causes me to not be so busy that I disregard that still small voice.

Journal: Do you have a growing desire to know God's will for your life? What, if anything, is keeping your heart from joy today?

—Denise Peters

THAT SWEET, CLEAN-INSIDE FEELING

You know my folly, O God; my guilt is not hidden from you.

PSALM 69:5

When I write in my prayer journal and get to the place where I need to confess sin, I usually stop writing. It's like reaching a roadblock.

The various excuses for not writing down my sin range from not wanting anyone to read about what a bad person I am to feeling like my sin is somehow justified because there are so many people whose sins are worse than mine. I've found that if I will just sit quietly before the Lord, the Holy Spirit will pinpoint the sin for me. Then I have a decision to make: I can either argue with God or confess what He and I already know to be true. There's not much of an alternative. Only if I confess and agree with God can He cleanse my heart and renew fellowship with me. When fellowship is restored, that sweet, clean-inside sense returns.

Do you remember how you felt when you first accepted Jesus? I felt clean all over, and the feeling remained with me—until I sinned. Then the good feeling of closeness to God vanished.

I remember a time, in fact, when a backlog of sins piled up so high I had to set aside a few hours and write out every sin I remembered. It was disheartening. But as I asked God to forgive each one, I felt movement and change inside. After I finished, I destroyed the sheet of paper. The clean feeling returned.

From that time on, I have tried to keep a relatively short list with God. Now I try to relate to God as a child whose father longs for her to confess so that we might restore our close relationship once again.

PRAYER

O Lord, help me today to confess those things in my life that are creating a wall between You and me. Thank You for the miracle of forgiveness.

Journal: Write down your sins of commission; then write down your sins of omission.

—Carole Lewis

JANUARY 16

DROPPING THE DOUGHNUT

You know my folly, O God; my guilt is not hidden from you.

PSALM 69:5

As I meditated on this verse, images of the various "follies" I had committed during the previous week ran before my eyes. My heart was pierced.

Among the list of follies were many poor food choices, and now I had to face facts. Keeping my Commitment Record had not been difficult as long as I wrote food down as I ate it. When I chose healthy food and portions, I enjoyed filling out the Commitment Record. On days that I made foolish choices, I "forgot" to record them, thinking that if they weren't written down, somehow God wouldn't know about them.

Together, the psalmist and the Spirit were now reminding me that God not only knew about the invisible record of what I'd consumed in the last week, but He also knew I *intended* to eat all those unhealthy foods. I had neglected to ask God for help in resisting temptation because, deep inside, I wanted to eat whatever I wanted.

At the time, if I'd thought anything at all, it probably ran along the lines of that terrible old adage "It's easier to ask forgiveness than permission."

Now I faced up to the fact that this attitude doesn't belong in a Christian's thinking. God would certainly have said no to the doughnuts and candy bars and would have provided me with healthy alternatives and a desire to obey. I would have escaped the rebellious attitude and subsequent guilt trip, *and* I would not have gained a bit of weight. Today I let this verse from God's Word do its good work in me. I bring it to mind *before* I raise the doughnut or candy to my lips.

Yes, it is comforting to know God forgives a truly repentant heart. But what's better is to experience God at work in you, giving you strength, helping you choose the path that leads out of temptation.

PRAYER

Thank You, God, for being all-knowing and for the conviction of Your Holy Spirit. I want to live an honest and open life before You.

Journal: Is there something in your life that you are trying to hide from God?

—June Chapko

JANUARY 17

FINDING STRENGTH THROUGH WEAKNESS

You know my folly, O God; my guilt is not hidden from you.

PSALM 69:5

Have you ever eaten something and not wanted to write it on the Commitment Record because you didn't want anyone to know? Have you ever been walking on the treadmill and left it running while you answered the phone, counting all the time as exercise?

I've done these things. And these are the kinds of actions that can only be called "folly." Why? Because no one who really matters was fooled. Sure, the First Place leader may have given me great words of encouragement for the fabulous week I'd had—but God knew the truth, and so did I.

The apostle Paul tells us to do whatever we do heartily as unto the Lord and not men, knowing that it's the Lord alone who gives us our reward (see Col. 3:23-24).

Trying to hide our behavior by doctoring our Commitment Records may bring kudos from other people, but it feels so much better to write it all down just as it happened. I can tell you this from the times I've been purely honest and faced up to my failures, for it is then that God can work with our weakness and show us the way to strength and obedience. God is the only One who can turn shame and embarrassment into victory.

My advice? Don't hide your sins and mistakes. Be honest. There *is* glory in a clear conscience.

PRAYER

Lord, thank You for allowing me the opportunity to come to You with my guilt and confess it. You already know what I've done, but acknowledging my sin and agreeing with You about it frees me and affords me the privilege of having a right relationship with You.

Journal: Guilt weighs you down. Let go of hiding, pretense, deceit and sin. Confess any folly and walk free and clear with the Savior.

—Diana Robinson

January 18

Cheating at Solitaire

You know my folly, O God; my guilt is not hidden from you.

Psalm 69:5

As a young child, I would often play solitaire with a deck of cards. Of course, I always wanted to win. And so I sometimes rearranged the cards to my benefit.

This is called cheating, but who wanted to look at it that way? My mother would remind me, "If you cheat at solitaire, you are only cheating yourself." But it was hard not to give in to that craving to win, even if it meant taking the easy route.

Later, I learned the hard way that what Mother had told me was right. Most especially, I found her principle to be true with regard to weight loss. In times past, I would start a weight-loss program and eventually give in to temptation. It seemed so much easier to give in to those cravings by sneaking a favorite binge food item, as if my sneaking would keep it from counting.

The truth was that both God and I knew exactly what I was doing. And of course my body knew what I was doing. My folly brought overwhelming guilt that was a natural consequence of my behavior. Then the guilt would make me feel bad. To get rid of the bad feeling I would binge even more. Eventually I would throw out my eating plan entirely.

First Place helped break this habit with the Commitment Records that required me to record all the food I eat, even if it isn't on my food plan. By bringing the facts out into the open, I was able to face my sinful habit of cheating and deal with food honestly.

First Place has helped me to do what is best for me, which is walking in God's Spirit and truth.

Prayer

Lord, forgive me for the times that I choose sin over honesty. Forgive me for the times that I purposefully go off my food plan, thinking it won't count.

Journal: What foolish tricks do you play with your mind? What forbidden foods do you eat, pretending they won't count? Ask God to help you be more honest, for His glory.

—Roberta Wasserman

JANUARY 19

SHE WHO HESITATES . . .

No temptation has seized you except what is common to man. And God is faithful; he will not let you be tempted beyond what you can bear. But when you are tempted, he will also provide a way out so that you can stand up under it.

1 CORINTHIANS 10:13

I've heard it said that temptation has three stages: temptation, hesitation and participation.

The first stage happens to every one of us. No harm is brought to us simply by being tempted. It is when we hesitate and begin to think about the temptation that we find ourselves in the participation stage before we know what has happened.

Thankfully, God's faithfulness is never more evident than when we take a temptation to Him. We will always find that His desire is to help us overcome.

In First Place, we talk a lot about overeating, but we don't talk a lot about overspending. We can get ourselves in a real mess financially if we buy things every time we are tempted. When you find the temptations are nearly more than you can bear, it's time to walk away and pray before making a decision to purchase. Get a cup of coffee, sit down, pray and wait a little while. The temptation will usually pass. This also works for food temptations. Try this, and I promise that God will answer, if you will only ask.

Just the other day I was in a store that had the most beautiful gift items. I was tempted to buy things I absolutely didn't need. I asked God to help me. He might have helped me pick up one foot after the other and march out of the store, but instead He suddenly reminded me of a friend who needed encouragement. With her in mind I picked up a small item, purchased it and left the store. I felt so much better than if I had purchased for myself something I didn't need.

If you ask Him, He will always show you a way out of temptation. The secret is, when He shows you the way out, be sure to take it!

PRAYER

Father, today when I am tempted, help me to ask You for the way out.

Journal: Tell God about your greatest areas of temptation and ask for His help.

—Carole Lewis

The Excuse Buster

No temptation has seized you except what is common to man. And God is faithful; he will not let you be tempted beyond what you can bear. But when you are tempted, he will also provide a way out so that you can stand up under it.

1 CORINTHIANS 10:13

Temptation comes in many forms. For many us, our most common temptation relates to food. We ask the Lord for deliverance from candy and cookies. We think if He could create the world by merely speaking it into existence, then surely He could make carrot cake a vegetable!

In reality, when temptation comes knocking, it's often disguised in activities that don't *seem* harmful. Have you ever gone to the mall and engaged in a little retail therapy? How about the appointments on your calendar? Is your quiet time a thing of the past? Are others stressing you out, so you've turned to watching a movie, rather than exercising?

The Lord allows temptations to come our way as opportunities to put this verse from 1 Corinthians into practice. I like to refer to this verse as "the excuse-buster." It is a reminder that whenever we choose to yield to temptation, it's because we wanted *it*—whatever *it* may be—more than we want the joy of obedience.

PRAYER

Lord, thank You for making a way of escape from the temptations I face. Please let my feet, mouth, head and heart all choose to follow the path of victory that awaits me on the other side of the exit door.

Journal: Make a list of the things that repeatedly tempt you. Choose one to pray about and ask God to break the stronghold of this temptation.

—Diana Robinson

JANUARY 21

MORE THAN ABLE

No temptation has seized you except what is common to man. And God is faithful; he will not let you be tempted beyond what you can bear. But when you are tempted, he will also provide a way out so that you can stand up under it.

1 CORINTHIANS 10:13

Sweet, sticky, gooey, crunchy temptations! My mind can always imagine foods that bring on the "hungries." Each delicious desire takes on a voice of its own. Together these many voices become like the Israelites of the Old Testament—arguing with Moses, craving the foods they ate in captivity. If I listen to these voices, they can make me like those Israelites in their on-again, off-again obedience to God.

We can tell ourselves that God is in control of our lives. But in fact, God is in control when we allow Him control. When we allow our lusts to get out of His control, we eat that cookie or candy bar, those chips, that fried chicken or double-stuffed potato.

Daily we must determine to be like Moses and Joshua who allowed God to guide them in leading His people.

God is able, and He desires to direct us in how to tame and silence the voices of our "hungries." When Moses' time was up, God commissioned Joshua with these words: "Be strong and courageous, because you will lead these people to inherit the land I swore to their forefathers to give them . . . for the LORD your God will be with you" (Josh. 1:6,9).

God has promised to provide us with a way out of temptation's grasp. He showers us with blessings too numerous to count. How many blessings do we miss because we aren't looking? How often do we miss His way out of the snare because we are too preoccupied with our lusts? Don't miss God's faithfulness in giving you an opportunity to escape.

PRAYER

Lord, thank You for Your faithfulness and Your promise to monitor temptations in my life. Make me mindful of tempting situations so that I can look for the way out that You have arranged for me.

Journal: What was your most recent temptation, and what way out did God provide? Did you see it? What can you do to be more mindful of the exit when you are faced with temptation?

—Judy Marshall

JANUARY 22

GIVING THE BATTLE TO GOD

No temptation has seized you except what is common to man. And God is faithful; he will not let you be tempted beyond what you can bear. But when you are tempted, he will also provide a way out so that you can stand up under it.

1 CORINTHIANS 10:13

"I just couldn't help myself. It was just too tempting!"

How often have I thought or said these words? Too many times, I'm afraid.

Last summer, I was part of a First Place Bible study. We reviewed the lessons and then went over our memory verses. This verse from 1 Corinthians came to mind frequently—often when I least expected it. Sometimes when I didn't want it. This "involuntary" meditation brought not only conviction but also encouragement.

Conviction came in the realization that I assumed I was helpless to resist sin. In essence, I was saying that the Lord was insufficient, that He was unfaithful to His Word. Of course, the Lord is most sufficient—the only other option was that I chose disobedience.

This verse also exploded the myth that my struggle was unique. I would try to excuse my failure to obey. Again, the Word with its sharp edges told me temptation wasn't unique and that it was common to all. I was reminded that the temptation or struggle is not the central issue; what matters is what I do with the commands of Christ—a very common and human problem.

Victory over sin and conforming my life to Christ are not about me but about Christ. By that, I mean it's all about His constancy, His power, His intimate involvement in my life and also about His fathomless love for me.

Now when I sense temptation, I remember the wonderful promise that God is in control and that He is absolutely sufficient for all my needs, including resisting temptation. By God's grace and power, I will daily become more consistent in obedience. To God be the glory!

PRAYER

Lord, please help me each day to look to You for victory and not to myself. Be glorified in my obedience, for I can only obey by Your grace.

Journal: In what areas of your life do you try to excuse sin? What will you give over to God's control today?

—Bonnie Ler

ALWAYS A WAY OUT

No temptation has seized you except what is common to man. And God is faithful; he will not let you be tempted beyond what you can bear. But when you are tempted, he will also provide a way out so that you can stand up under it.

1 CORINTHIANS 10:13

Oh, Lord, I need Your help, I prayed. *I need a way out tonight.*

The tables in the church fellowship hall were set up and full of food that was definitely not on a First Place menu!

Please, Lord. Don't let this be a setup for me to fail. I need You to provide a way out and open my eyes to see it! This was my desperate plea as I rushed out the door after the evening worship service. Actually, my husband and I had a plan. We would be the first in line, choose only the healthy food and get out as quickly as possible.

As we entered the fellowship hall, it was obvious that no one had been assigned to serve the people. We got busy filling cups with ice. We became frantic servants—wrapping food and putting out paper plates and napkins. After everyone had been served, I went to the table to prepare my plate. No food! It had all been wiped out. No temptation!

There we stood, laughing and thanking God for the way out.

Church socials used to be a setup for wrong food choices. But not anymore. I have learned to busy myself by focusing and feasting on serving people rather than focusing and feasting on food. God is so faithful, and I am learning that truth more and more through First Place.

Where is your focus when you are faced with a tempting feast? Ask God to show you a way out. Believe me—He will!

PRAYER

Father, help me today to turn to You when I am tempted.
Thank You for providing a way out for me.

Journal: Share with God your plans for today and ask Him to alert you before you give in to temptation.

—Kathy Runion

JANUARY 24

OUR ONLY TRUE COMFORT

Man does not live on bread alone, but on every word that comes from the mouth of God.

MATTHEW 4:4

I awakened early on Thanksgiving morning of 2001. The knowledge that it would be a hectic day with 22 family members coming to eat dinner caused me to open my Bible to receive God's marching orders for the day.

My reading for that day was the first chapter of James. My eyes lit upon one of the first directives: "Consider it pure joy, my brothers, whenever you face trials of many kinds, because you know that the testing of your faith develops perseverance" (vv. 2-3).

Little did I know that at the close of that day I would face the greatest trial of my life: My daughter would be killed by a drunk teenaged driver.

In the days immediately following Shari's death, the greatest consolation any of my family received was the truths found in the Bible. My son-in-law held on to the words of Psalm 18:1-2. My thoughts centered on Psalm 139:7-16. Over time, Matthew 4:4 became very real to me.

One of the things I learned through our terrible trial is this: Food is only a temporary fix for a spiritual need. God's Word is our only true comfort when we face life's ordeals.

It is so important that we read and memorize the Bible during good times. If we have first hidden His Word in our hearts, God will bring back to us the eternal truths we need for our soul when we go through every fiery trial this world throws at us. Count on it.

PRAYER

Lord, give me a hunger and thirst for Your Word. It is the only thing that satisfies in times of distress.

Journal: Ask God to help you want to study and memorize His Word. Ask Him every day until you start doing it.

—Carole Lewis

JANUARY 25

FILLED BY HIS WORD

Man does not live on bread alone, but on every word that comes from the mouth of God.

MATTHEW 4:4

Soon after beginning the First Place weight-loss program, I realized that behind my lifetime struggle with food and weight was something deeper than poor eating habits or my appetite. It took awhile, but in time core issues were revealed.

Excess weight was only the surface problem. Inside I had a hole in my soul that no amount of food could ever fill. I vividly remember the day this revelation came to mind.

I had been grazing. You know—wandering through the kitchen looking for that something that would satisfy the gnawing inside. Only vaguely was I aware that the gnawing I felt was not stomach hunger but something deeper—a love hunger. As I stood in front of my pantry door—restless, dissatisfied—nothing looked appealing. I realized for the very first time that no amount of food would satisfy me. A thousand bites would never be enough. I was looking in the wrong place.

After that day, I turned to my First Place Bible study and began to feast on the Word of God. The more of God's Word I tasted, the less excess food tempted me. God was showing me how to really live in Him and His love. Meeting with Him became my favorite and most satisfying meal of the day.

PRAYER

Lord, forgive me for seeking satisfaction in that which does not satisfy the hunger in my heart. Help me to feast on Your holy Word every day. May that be my most important meal of the day, tasting Your Word.

Journal: What else have you looked to, besides food, to fill your heart? If you don't yet have a daily quiet time and meal with the Lord, tell Him that He is invited to your table.

—Roberta Wasserman

JANUARY 26

FINDING YOUR BALANCE

Man does not live on bread alone, but on every word that comes from the mouth of God.

MATTHEW 4:4

If ever there was a Scripture for which I wanted a loophole, Matthew 4:4 is it!

While other First Place members were struggling with sugary food, I struggled with wanting more *bread*. It seemed like all my food choices involved bread!

My dinners were colorful yet full of starch. It wouldn't be uncommon for me to serve corn, peas, rolls and meat with gravy. I thought that a variety of colors on the plate signified balance. Boy, was I wrong! Menu planning was frustrating, and the more I tried to reduce my bread intake, the more tempted I became. I noticed that whenever I was tired or struggled with a negative emotion, bread was my comfort.

What's true in the physical sense is also true spiritually. Dealing with temptation requires that I know who God is and that I know Him personally. Corporate worship is wonderful and necessary; but to know the words that come from the mouth of God, I must spend time in His Word—reading, studying, praying and memorizing Scripture.

Today I can say that balanced food choices give me the energy I need to face physical demands. But a balanced relationship with my Savior is what I need to give me spiritual strength to grow past my temptations and become whole in spirit.

PRAYER

Thank You, Lord, for Your example. It was brilliant of You to quote Scripture in order to foil Satan's attacks. May I not be satisfied with bread alone but rather with the fullness that comes from Your Word.

Journal: Review your Scripture memory verses to date. For each of the verses, ask God to give you a person to pray for—or a need. Praying specifically and using the Scriptures to do it aid memorization.

—Diana Robinson

January 27

I Finally Got It

Man does not live on bread alone, but on every word that comes from the mouth of God.

Matthew 4:4

For most of my adult life I've had this hang-up with memorizing Bible verses. I just didn't get it. It didn't make sense to me that I should spend time memorizing sentences and ideas when I could pick up the Bible and read it almost anytime. After all, I reasoned, you will eventually forget part or all of it—right?

Then something happened in First Place to cause me to change my mind about memorizing Bible verses. For that week our memory verse was Matthew 4:4. I had never really understood the real meaning of this verse until that day in First Place. Our Bible study leader explained that this Bible verse tells us it is God's will for us to have a steady stream of words from His mouth by memorizing Bible verses.

Then I understood: God wants us to continually be nourished by His Word so that we will be able to tell others about His kingdom and righteousness.

Prayer

Father, You are all that I need. Your almighty and precious holy Words are the way, the truth and the life for all who call You Father. In the name of Your Son, Christ Jesus, I pray. Amen.

Journal: Are you having a difficult time when you try to memorize a Bible verse? Ask God to help you understand His Words today.

—Ben Steelman

JANUARY 28

FINDING HIS FRUIT

Man does not live on bread alone, but on every word that comes from the mouth of God.

MATTHEW 4:4

I *love* bread!

Jesus liked bread too. It's the food the enemy used to tempt Him after His 40-day fast. Notice that the enemy did not offer Jesus fruit like he did to Eve in the garden. No, I am pretty sure Jesus liked bread a lot for the temptation to be so appealing.

After looking back over my Commitment Records (CR) for the past few months, it is *very* apparent that I suffer from "bread bondage." I really struggle to keep my daily bread from having dominion over my CR. I remember the shock I felt when I first read the food plan and realized green peas, corn and potatoes have to be counted as bread exchanges instead of vegetables! Many times I have had to write Matthew 4:4 on my CR to remind myself to keep a balance.

When I joined First Place, I had a longing deep within my soul that could not be satisfied. I used sports and food to quench that longing. Surrendering my food plan to Christ was the first of many areas He reclaimed in my heart. The Bible studies helped me get a glimpse of how precious I am to God. His love and faithfulness have brought complete satisfaction.

These days I have a new longing deep within my soul. I *long* to know Christ in all His glory in a personal and intimate relationship.

PRAYER

My Lord Jesus, help me to really know You. Give me a deeper understanding of how much You love me and how special I am to You. You told us that You are "the bread of life" (John 6:35). You promised that if we come to You, we will never go hungry. Daily fill my heart and mind with Your Word until my spiritual hunger is satisfied.

Journal: What do you really hunger for? Are there areas in your life that you have not surrendered to God? Tell Him about it.

—Becky Sirt

JANUARY 29

FINDING HIS PATH

Do not conform any longer to the pattern of this world, but be transformed by the renewing of your mind. Then you will be able to test and approve what God's will is—his good, pleasing and perfect will.

ROMANS 12:2

I have heard it said God's will is never contrary to His Word. I remember a time when I was counseling a woman who wanted to leave her husband for another man. She rationalized that because God wanted her to be happy and because this man was more spiritual than her husband—it must be God's will.

The pattern of this world says that marriage is designed to make us happy and if that isn't happening, then end the marriage. God's Word says that He hates divorce. God's will is for us to stay married to our first husband or wife. This doesn't mean that God won't forgive us when we go against His perfect will for us, only that our lives will work out far better if we leave our circumstances in His hands.

Unfortunately, the lady I was counseling left her husband and married the other man. He proved to be quite different from who she had thought he was, because she was "following the pattern of this world." The sad truth is that her second marriage ended in divorce just like the first.

God's Word is the key to renewing our minds and living lives of stability. If we search His Word to find the answers to the dilemmas of this life, we can be assured that He will lead us in paths of righteousness, not paths of destruction.

PRAYER

Lord, renew my mind so that I may know Your good, pleasing and perfect will for my life.

Journal: Be honest with God about any area of your life in which you are following the pattern of this world through what you read or watch or what you do. Ask Him to help you desire His will in everything that concerns you.

—Carole Lewis

JANUARY 30

WHAT ARE YOU WORTH?

Do not conform any longer to the pattern of this world, but be transformed by the renewing of your mind. Then you will be able to test and approve what God's will is—his good, pleasing and perfect will.

ROMANS 12:2

As I entered the First Place weight-loss program, the thought pattern I had inherited from the world was that "thin was in." I was willing to go to any lengths to get thin.

Before First Place I had used many self-destructive weight-loss methods. These methods had been taught to me by the world, and all followed the standards the magazine covers displayed. My value, or measure of worth, was based on the number on the scale and what the mirror displayed. I didn't realize that the weight-loss industry had become a multimillion-dollar industry based on people's weaknesses and failures. The success rate of weight-loss programs is very poor. My success with weight-loss programs was poor also. As a result, I felt like a failure.

In First Place, God began to renew my mind. I learned what His will was for me. I learned to look into His holy Word for a true measure of my worth. I learned that developing my relationship with Him through a discipline of prayer, Bible study and Scripture memorization is the solution to disciplined eating. I was not a failure, but the programs and patterns of this world had failed me.

Jesus Christ never fails. I experienced success at losing weight loss and have maintained a healthy weight for seven years.

PRAYER

Lord, forgive me for following the pattern of this world. Thank You for renewing my mind each day. Thank You for showing me Your perfect will.

Journal: What pattern of the world do you follow? How can you allow God to renew your mind? Are you on your last diet?

—Roberta Wasserman

JANUARY 31

CREATED—WITH PURPOSE

Do not conform any longer to the pattern of this world, but be transformed by the renewing of your mind. Then you will be able to test and approve what God's will is—his good, pleasing and perfect will.

ROMANS 12:2

For the first 50-plus years of my life I allowed others to tell me what I should be in order to meet their needs. I pretended to be happy with this arrangement.

The study of personalities in the First Place program (and the prodding of a sweet lady I'll call "Carole") helped me to discover I had been wearing a mask. Later, at home, I filled out the study form *again*—truthfully this time. I also promised that I would pray for three days, asking God to help me remove the mask and discover the person He had created *before* I put pen to paper.

After I had finished the form, I saw that God had made me to be a sanguine/choleric personality. It was the first time I had gotten a glimpse of who I really was. A weight lifted from my shoulders. I no longer needed to be molded to someone else's needs. I knew who God had created me to be!

To be honest, I met opposition from some of my family, and it did take some time for them to get used to the "new me." My husband was heard to say on several occasions, "Life is never dull or boring in our house!" Just before his death, he told a friend that he knew beyond a shadow of a doubt that because of my confidence in who I was and my faith in God, he could go home knowing I was going to be all right.

PRAYER

Father, I thank You for the lessons on our personalities and for the prompting of "Carole," who refused to let me wear a mask any longer. Thank You for Your good, pleasing and perfect will.

Journal: Spend time in prayer asking God to reveal to you the person He made you to be. What thoughts did He bring to mind?

—Betha Jean Cunningham

FEBRUARY 1

ENTERING GOD'S COCOON

Do not conform any longer to the pattern of this world, but be transformed by the renewing of your mind. Then you will be able to test and approve what God's will is—his good, pleasing and perfect will.

ROMANS 12:2

Sometimes we worry more about what people think about us than what God thinks about us, don't we?! We want to change but find ourselves more and more trapped in the "sin that so easily entangles" (Heb. 12:1). This Scripture shows us how to really change.

The *New Living Translation* of Romans 12:2 makes our path of change particularly clear: "Let God transform you into a new person by changing the way you think." To get to the place where God can change us, we must stop following the world's plans.

Then to make the change you crave, you must realize that you can't make the change yourself. You can't even change what you think about! You can only change by allowing God to transform you. The word translated as "transform" is the Greek word *metamorphosis*, which describes what happens to a butterfly in the cocoon. The only part of the metamorphosis the caterpillar can control is entering the cocoon. In the same way, we must let God transform us by changing the way we think. That's the only way we can ever really please Him and ourselves.

PRAYER

Okay, Father, I'm crawling into my cocoon. Transform me, please!

Journal: Are you more concerned about what people think about you than what God thinks about you? Talk to God about it.

—June-Marie Avery

ACHIEVING BEAUTIFUL BALANCE

Do you not know that your body is a temple of the Holy Spirit, who is in you, whom you have received from God? You are not your own; you were bought at a price. Therefore honor God with your body.

1 CORINTHIANS 6:19-20

When I purchase something, it belongs to me. I own it. Did you ever apply this thought of ownership to the fact that God purchased our redemption through the blood sacrifice of His Son, Jesus? When we accept Jesus' sacrifice on the cross and ask Him to come in and control our lives, we belong to God.

Sometimes, though, I treat my body as if it still belonged to me. I eat what I want and I don't exercise. I don't read my Bible or pray. These actions always bring negative consequences.

But when I choose to honor God with my body by eating healthy foods, exercising, and reading and studying my Bible, I find that my life takes on a beautiful balance. Zig Ziglar said it like this: "It is easier to act your way into a new way of feeling, than to feel your way into a new way of acting."[4]

Each day we make choices that ultimately determine the people we will become. What choices have you made today?

PRAYER

O God, help me today to act like my body belongs to You, because it does. Remind me of this every time I take control as though I still own it.

Journal: Ask God to show you areas of your life in which you still retain ownership of your body. Ask God to make you willing to give up ownership to Him.

—Carole Lewis

FEBRUARY 3

THE TREASURE GOD MADE

Do you not know that your body is a temple of the Holy Spirit, who is in you, whom you have received from God? You are not your own; you were bought at a price. Therefore honor God with your body.

1 CORINTHIANS 6:19-20

Before First Place, I had spent a lifetime alternating between feeding my body with junk food and following self-destructive weight-loss methods. I had often stuffed my body with too much food. I didn't exercise it or take care of it. My body was starving for nutritious foods and a healthy way of life.

First Place taught me that my body is *not* mine to do with as I wished. I learned from the Word of God that I was created by the Master Artist. There has been no other person like me since the beginning of time. I am a treasure bought at a great price, by a great King. Not only has He created me to live inside my heart, but He has also paid to live there too.

It was then that I realized I wasn't treasuring this temple where God dwells, nor was I honoring Him for the great price He paid for me. I decided to learn how to start serving Him with my whole self—including my body.

I began to think about the most nutritious foods I could eat. My mind was renewed, and I didn't feel deprived of the junk food. In fact, I delighted in my healthy meals. Eventually, I lost weight and became a walking testimony for the Lord Jesus Christ.

It's an awesome and humbling thought to know that the Lord of heaven dwells within us!

PRAYER

Lord, forgive me for not honoring Your dwelling place. Show me today what food You would have me prepare for this temple. How may I glorify You in me?

Journal: How do you feel about your body? What does it mean to you that Jesus bought you with His life?

—Roberta Wasserman

FEBRUARY 4

My Body, His Temple

Do you not know that your body is a temple of the Holy Spirit, who is in you, whom you have received from God? You are not your own; you were bought at a price. Therefore honor God with your body.

1 CORINTHIANS 6:19-20

I initially joined First Place because I had tried many other diet plans and none of them worked for very long. As soon as I stopped dieting, the weight would return. Back then, my reason for dieting grew from a desire to be thinner, not healthier.

The first Bible study I attended in First Place included 1 Corinthians 6:19-20 in its memory verses. The week these verses appeared, we had been in session four weeks and I had lost 10 pounds. How proud I was to have accomplished this. When I read these verses, however, I immediately realized I had not been honoring God with my body. My goal had been for my clothes to fit better and to look more attractive. God helped me see that I had my focus on the wrong goal.

That day my attitude changed. My goal also changed. I wanted to please God and honor Him in every area of my life, especially with a healthy body.

After I reached my goal of losing 40 pounds, I honored God by taking on the leadership of a First Place class so that I could be a testimony of what He had done in my life. This body is His temple, and I worship Him each day in it.

PRAYER

Father, may I never forget that I am Your dwelling place.

Journal: Examine your reasons for wanting to lose weight and list them. Do your reasons honor God? Pray and make any changes that are necessary to follow God's command to honor what is His.

—Martha Rogers

FOUR-SIDED BLESSING

Do you not know that your body is a temple of the Holy Spirit, who is in you, whom you have received from God? You are not your own; you were bought at a price. Therefore honor God with your body.

1 CORINTHIANS 6:19-20

These verses are the ones God used to bring me to First Place nine years ago. As I study them now in teaching *Giving Christ First Place* in my home church, they have taken on a whole new meaning for me.

God has done so many amazing things in my life through First Place that it would take a book to list them all. I must mention a couple of the most important miracles God has done. If He never does another thing in my life, He has done more than enough.

First, God has blessed me in spirit. He has taught me how to have a daily quiet time early in the morning. He has drawn me into a personal love relationship with Him that is simply amazing.

Second, He has blessed me physically. As I learned to eat right, God healed my colitis, which was so severe that I had to go on disability leave from work. I was taking four different medications. I do not have to take any now and have not had an attack of colitis in about five years.

Third, God has blessed me emotionally. He has worked in my marriage and made me fall in love again with my husband.

Fourth, He has blessed me mentally. Even though the circumstances in my life and around me are still here and at times very difficult, the peace of God that surpasses all understanding is so real. I can only thank Him and praise His holy name.

PRAYER

Dear heavenly Father, I thank You that Your Holy Spirit lives within me. Lord, I pray that in all four areas of my life I will bring glory to You.

Journal: Begin to give thanks to God every day for all the circumstances of your life and then record what He accomplishes in you spiritually, mentally, emotionally and physically.

—Janet Kirkhart

FEBRUARY 6

HORSES, THEN CARTS

Do you not know that your body is a temple of the Holy Spirit, who is in you, whom you have received from God? You are not your own; you were bought at a price. Therefore honor God with your body.

1 CORINTHIANS 6:19-20

As I teach aerobics and work closely with First Place leaders, I see how easy it is to "put the cart before the horse." We may be faithful to do our Bible studies, but if we're not careful, our focus can subtly shift until we have our eyes off the Lord and only on losing the weight.

After struggling with excess weight—which is what brought me to First Place—I was finally able to lose weight. But then I gained some back. Feeling frustrated, I took my brokenness to the Father and asked Him to give me a proper attitude toward my physical self, especially my weight.

God began to reveal to me that the scale and my body were my "gods." (Anything that distracts us from the one true living God will become a god to us.)

After much time in prayer, I began to take to heart that my body was a temple. What is the use of a temple? Pure and simple—*it houses worship!* Then I had to ask myself some tough questions: *At the size I am today, am I willing to worship Him? And if my body never changes, can I love Him and thank Him for the physical temple He gave me?*

I can tell you honestly that my weight is no longer a burden. My health is critical, but I focus more on the interior wellness than the exterior weight. And it is working!

The number on the scale had such bondage over my heart and vision, but the freedom I experience now feels so good. Thank You, Lord!

PRAYER

Lord, am I using my temple the way You have called me to do? Are there parts of my body that are distracting me and keeping me from using it for worship? If at the size I am today I am holding back from serving You, then change me, Lord, and bring me to freedom in this awesome creation You made just for me.

Journal: Are you a slave to your body or is your body a slave to you? Are you worshiping the Creator or the creation?

—Denise Peters

BRING ON THE SANDPAPER!

Commit to the LORD whatever you do, and your plans will succeed.

PROVERBS 16:3

When you fail to plan, you plan to fail.

This is a great statement for those teaching time management, but it's not always appropriate for God's timetable. By committing whatever I do to God, I am saying to Him that His plans are more important than anything I might plan to do today.

This means that I need to rearrange the way I see things. In particular, I have to learn to see interruptions as divine appointments. It also means I need to see petty annoyances as God's divine sandpaper that smooths off rough edges and makes me more like Christ. And I need to see that pain and suffering help me become stronger, if I will lean *into* the pain, instead of running *from* it.

Some days when I have planned everything I want to accomplish, it seems like I have nothing but interruptions. If I give all these interruptions to God and ask Him to use me, I always find at the end of the day that everything I needed to do was accomplished. This is a miracle that I don't understand but joyfully accept.

My walk with Christ is a journey that He has planned down to the tiniest detail. But I can miss wonderful stops along the way by insisting on my own way or adhering to my own plans. God gives me the wonderful freedom to choose His plans or my own. If I follow His plans, I am often surprised but never disappointed.

PRAYER

O God, help me today to see every interruption as part of Your plan for my life. Use me today for Your glory.

Journal: Bring God into your plans for today and tell Him that you are willing for Him to readjust your schedule if necessary.

—Carole Lewis

FEBRUARY 8

GOD, MY BAKER

Commit to the LORD whatever you do, and your plans will succeed.

PROVERBS 16:3

As a longtime Christian, I faithfully read my Bible, went to church, prayed and, in general, lived "the Christian life." I discovered, however, that these disciplines were fragmented and compartmentalized and that I performed them in a shallow, sporadic style. I was unable to balance it all to give my spiritual life meaning—until I began First Place.

Then I coined a new name for God and the way He works in my life—*God, my Baker.* Let me explain.

All the right ingredients were somewhere on a shelf in my life—reading the Bible; prayer; knowledge of healthy foods and exercise benefits; responsibilities at home, church and work. Through First Place I have learned to allow God to select, mix and stir the necessary ingredients of my spiritual, emotional, mental and physical self to keep my life in balance.

During my five years in First Place, God has "baked" me in His oven with care and His perfect timing. So many blessings and positive changes have occurred in all areas of life. I have become constant in prayer and consistent in Bible reading and study; I lost 70 pounds and have improved relationships; and now I lead two First Place groups. God can be pleased with the sweet aroma He's creating as long as I am doing my part, keeping the nine commitments to bring balance to my life.

As for me—well, I'll be done only when He's ready to take me to His house for His bountiful banquet. The table is set. See you there!

PRAYER

Lord, today I commit to You all that I am and all that I do. My desire is for Your plans to become my plans so that You will be glorified. May the scent of Your presence rise from my actions today.

Journal: What have you planned for today that you need to speak to God about?

—Judy Marshall

FEBRUARY 9

AN ACT OF FAITH

Commit to the LORD whatever you do, and your plans will succeed.

PROVERBS 16:3

"Commit to the LORD . . . and your plans will succeed." What a promise! What a new concept! Who doesn't want success in weight loss? I sure did.

An opportunity was now available to me. Would I take it? Honestly, I had never considered God in my efforts to control my weight. In fact, I wanted to do things my way most of the time. Ideally, I wanted to eat whatever I wanted, whenever I wanted and as much as I wanted—*and* be thin. Of course that was not possible. It goes against the natural order God has created.

When the First Place program introduced me to this Scripture, this new concept, I was encouraged by the possibility of true success. If I made a commitment to God to follow this plan, I would succeed. That was His promise. For me, this was not just an attitude of positive thinking but also an act of faith that His promise would be true for me.

Commitment involves follow-through. I had to do my part and also allow God to do His. As I committed my program to God, He was faithful.

Now I have enjoyed seven years of victory in regard to my weight. I maintain a healthy weight today; but more important than anything else, my relationship with God grows more intimate each day. I have discovered that He is trustworthy.

PRAYER

Lord, forgive me for all the times I tried to follow my own plans, my own way. Forgive me for not considering Your plans first and obeying them. Thank You for granting me success in this area of my life.

Journal: Have you ever considered totally and completely committing your weight-loss program to God? Tell Him what you believe about His promises to you.

—Roberta Wasserman

FEBRUARY 10

COMMITTED FOR SUCCESS

Commit to the LORD whatever you do, and your plans will succeed.

PROVERBS 16:3

Although I learned this verse a number of years ago when I first began participating in a First Place class, it didn't have a serious impact on my thinking until recently.

Writing had been a love of mine since my teen years, but I had experienced very little success with it. Two years ago, Carole Lewis offered me the wonderful opportunity to revise and update the First Place Bible studies and other materials related to the program. I approached the project with fear, excitement and a resolve to write what God laid on my heart.

Shortly after I began the project, Proverbs 16:3 appeared as the memory verse. I prayed this verse of Scripture and committed the entire project to His glory and honor. From that day on, the writing began to flow. He gave me new Scriptures to use, new questions, new insights and a new love for First Place.

Now, anytime I have an assignment, project or event, I commit the plans to Him. When our Texas Christian Writer's Conference was in the planning stages, I committed the meeting to Him and prayed for at least 50 people to attend the conference. At final count, we had 63 attend, and the conference was one of the best we ever had!

Commit your plans to Him—and they *will* succeed.

PRAYER

Lord, today I commit my plans to You. Give me the patience to wait for Your direction and to not run ahead of You.

Journal: Make a list of your plans for the day and then commit them to Him during your prayer time.

—Martha Rogers

SUBMITTED FOR APPROVAL

Commit to the LORD whatever you do, and your plans will succeed.

PROVERBS 16:3

Wait! Do you mean that my plans won't be blessed unless they are preapproved by the Lord?

That is exactly what Proverbs 16:3 is saying.

Unfortunately, I—like so many Christians—often make decisions based on what I want or what feels or tastes good to me. I tend to picture God's blessing like seasoning added to an already prepared meal. Often, I ask Him to spread His blessings over my meal choices without first consulting Him about His menu for my life.

Through the First Place Bible studies, I am discovering how crucial it is that I daily bow before my Savior and ask Him what he has planned for me. Through prayer and His Word, we are able to gain a better understanding of His will for our lives.

Do I do this perfectly? No. But I am slowly surrendering my desires to His. It is fruitless and painful to fight and rebel against the creator of heaven and Earth. And why would we want to disobey Him? He has our best interests in mind—always.

Today, let us commit to the Lord our thoughts, words and actions. The menu is up to Him. All we must do is follow His recipe for our lives.

PRAYER

O Father, I need You! I commit this day to You and Your perfect plan. Let me follow You; let my desires be Yours as I make choices today. I thank You that You love me enough not to season my poor plans with Your blessings. May my actions and words today, Lord, be pleasing to You and allow others to see Your light and power. Amen!

Journal: Do you still find yourself bumping up against the wall of your own will? In what ways are you still rebelling and fighting God's plan for your life?

—Carol Van Atta

FEBRUARY 12

Becoming a Love Channel

A new command I give you: Love one another. As I have loved you, so you must love one another. By this all men will know that you are my disciples, if you love one another.

JOHN 13:34-35

All through the Bible, God commands us to love one another. In Mark 12:31, Jesus says that the second greatest commandment, after loving God, is to love my neighbor as myself.

I've heard people say, "I love my job; it's the people I can't stand." Our work is a known quantity, but people are different all the time.

All people are created by God and are loved by Him. This is why it is imperative that we, as Christians, learn how to love everybody we meet each day. By loving unconditionally, I open doors to future ministry in the lives of others.

I am always amazed by how people respond to love. When I encounter a grumpy salesperson and sincerely talk to that person in love, his or her demeanor suddenly changes. The world is truly dying because of lack of love.

When God places a person in my life who is impossible for me to love, I have learned to treat this as a divine opportunity for God to do His best work. If I will only ask God to love that person through me, He begins first to change the way I think and feel about the person. Eventually, I develop a true love for the person. I heard a wise old woman once say, "If you walked a mile in his shoes, you might not make as good a showin' as he has."

Whatever your question today, love is the answer.

PRAYER

Lord Jesus, show love through me to everyone I meet today.

Journal: Give that impossible person to God and ask Him to love that person through you.

—Carole Lewis

FEBRUARY 13

THE NEED FOR LOVE

A new command I give you: Love one another. As I have loved you, so you must love one another. By this all men will know that you are my disciples, if you love one another.

JOHN 13:34-35

What an exciting thing to be loved! God wants us to love and to be loved. And isn't it great to feel God's love? That's what He wants us to share with others.

I was in the waiting room at the hospital with one of our deacons who was awaiting the completion of his wife's surgery. Such conversations, when waiting, can go in any direction and, most of the time, in many directions. As we talked about the many opportunities at church, he said he was amazed how people in First Place keep coming back!

Our church offers many discipleship programs, but First Place is one which people continue to attend. They go through a three-month session and then participate in a different First Place class the next session. The only conclusion I can come to is that people keep coming back because in First Place they know they are loved.

Typically, someone enrolls in First Place thinking only of the need for weight loss. But God uses His people to meet the need for His love. During First Place, people experience the love God intended us to give each other, "warts and all!" as my husband says. We need to value each other in spite of the "warts and all" and feel God's love through each other.

PRAYER

Dear Lord, I ask You to fill my heart with Your love and remove my focus on self. Let me bring Your love to each person who crosses my path today that they may see Jesus in me. I am so thankful for the many friends You have placed in my life to love me as You love me, Lord, warts and all.

Journal: Share love with someone you have not seen in over a year by writing today's verse and a brief personal note in a note card. Mail it today.

—Karen Rhodus

FEBRUARY 14

LOVE IS THE *ONLY* CURE

A new command I give you: Love one another. As I have loved you, so you must love one another. By this all men will know that you are my disciples, if you love one another.

JOHN 13:34-35

Loving others seems easy enough to a Christian. But sometimes *showing* that love is difficult. When we are hurt by the actions or words of another, we don't want to love the person. But God tells us we must. When we harbor resentment, we end up grieving the Holy Spirit.

Since the events of September 11, 2001, our love has been tested. While loving those who lost their lives or gave their lives in rescue attempts is easy, loving those who caused the actions became impossible for so many.

Have you unconsciously wondered about someone who looked "different" or talked with an accent? It isn't intentional, but our subconscious minds wonder. We ask the question again and again: *Why did this happen?*

Answers don't come easily. What we know is that God is sovereign and He still loves His children. And He still commands us to love others. I have learned from experience how harmful it is to harbor resentment and anger against someone who hurts me.

When we love in the face of adversity, we show the world that our love for God is real.

In the past nine years, First Place has taught me so much about love. God's love surrounds us as we minister to each other in our groups. God's love keeps us going when we face setbacks and feel discouraged.

God's love will always see us through—even when terrible things happen.

PRAYER

Dear Lord, help me to love as You have loved me. Lead me to those who need to know about Your love.

Journal: Make a list of the people you see every day or very often. Think of ways to show your love and appreciation for them. Plan to carry out at least one demonstration of love every day for a week.

—Martha Rogers

FEBRUARY 15

YOUR BEST FACE FORWARD

A new command I give you: Love one another. As I have loved you, so you must love one another. By this all men will know that you are my disciples, if you love one another.

JOHN 13:34-35

Soft lights on the Christmas tree, the laughter of children, the aroma of food being prepared—all these things were in stark contrast to the face of the middle-aged man who sulked around this holiday gathering. His face showed the bitterness he felt toward some of the guests.

I thought, *If his face froze that way, how would someone out in the street describe it? Unhappy? Angry? Troubled? Mean? Would anyone say, "This man must be a Christian"?*

No way.

Love brings a softness. It brings a glow and a gentle youthfulness that defies age or difficult circumstances. A lack of love brings coldness and harsh lines to the face and dulls the eyes. It makes the person seem older and is as hard to hide as is love. Even in a crowd it shows and brings a chill in the air.

Does your face show whose disciple you are?

PRAYER

Forgive me, Lord, when Your love doesn't show through me.

Journal: What does your face show? Ask God and be prepared to make any necessary changes He shows you.

—Betha Jean Cunningham

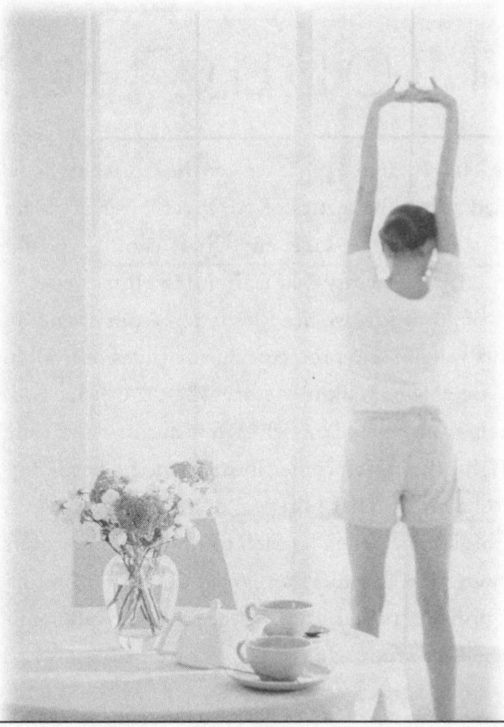

Everyday Victory for Everyday People

SECTION TWO

INTRODUCTION

God's intention for us, His children, is that we live the Christian life victoriously. Many believers haven't learned about the tactics of our great adversary, Satan. His work is to undermine us at every turn. And so, sadly enough, it is quite possible for us to know Christ and never experience the victory that is found in Him.

During the good times of life, we need Jesus to be our friend and guide. We also need Him as our mighty warrior and protector during times of trials, trouble, heartache and grief. Most of us are able to walk in victory when times are good, but during the worst times we need help from beyond ourselves. It is during these tough times, when we have no strength to fight, that Jesus comes in to fight the battle for us the way a big brother would fight someone who has hurt us.

The readings in this section focus on each of the 10 memory verses from the First Place Bible study *Everyday Victory for Everyday People.* The writers in this section acknowledge that they are just ordinary people learning the secret of walking in victory. Working through the First Place Bible study while reading the devotionals and memorizing the verses can help you live in victory too.

One of the powerful memory verses in this section is 2 Corinthians 10:4: "The weapons we fight with are not the weapons of the world. On the contrary, they have divine power to demolish strongholds."

God's weapons are spiritual, not physical. Learning how to let God fight our daily battles with the enemy will transform us from weak-kneed Christians to men and women who walk victoriously through each day.

My prayer for each of you, as you read this section, is that you grow strong and courageous. I pray that your fear level shrinks and your faith level grows to new heights. There truly is everyday victory for everyday people like you and me.

—Carole Lewis

FEBRUARY 16

NOTHING TOO DIFFICULT

Now what I am commanding you today is not too difficult for you or beyond your reach.

DEUTERONOMY 30:11

God's amazing promise in Deuteronomy 30:11 holds great comfort for me. When I meditate on it, it yields great riches in my everyday life.

Physically, when I just don't want to eat right or exercise, I take comfort in the fact that God will help me do the right thing if I will only ask Him for help. Some mornings I show up for exercise grumbling and complaining, but God always sends someone or something to encourage me and make my exercise time sweet. Over time I've learned that a large part of success in anything is simply to show up.

Some days I am mentally lazy. If I pray and ask God for help, He comes through and helps me to prioritize my tasks, so they don't seem insurmountable. Just getting a couple of unpleasant tasks done early seems to spur me on mentally.

Spiritually, this verse gives me the support I need to make the right choice. When I wake every morning, I know I can take time to meet with God for my quiet time, or I can live the day in the flesh. Since I want the best, I will often ask God to wake me even before the alarm goes off—and He does!

God offers me a tremendous amount of comfort in the emotional area of my life. He assures me that He hasn't sent anything into my life that is too difficult for Him to handle. Even though I am dealing with some huge issues that could wreak havoc in my emotional life, God keeps me on course.

With Him, nothing is too difficult.

PRAYER

Lord, help me realize today that anything I face is not too tough for You to handle.

Journal: Is there something that you believe God is commanding you to do? Share your reluctance, fears or rebellion with Him and ask for His help.

—Carole Lewis

FEBRUARY 17

Losing More Than Weight

Now what I am commanding you today is not too difficult for you or beyond your reach.

DEUTERONOMY 30:11

First Place gave me inspiration and courage to lose weight—and also to do far more in my life than I'd hoped or dreamed.

You see, I was a stay-at-home mother for 20 years. After my children were grown, I felt God calling me to attend college. After so many years away from school, I was scared. I wasn't sure if I could do it.

When I opened my Bible study and I read the very first memory verse—Deuteronomy 30:11—my fears quietly left me. Somehow in my heart I knew that God *was* commanding me to go to college. I knew that with His help it would not be too difficult or beyond my reach.

As it happened, I enrolled in college on the very same day that I had graduated from high school 25 years before! Only God could have set those dates in place to make the beginning of college so special for me. And for all its challenges, college was a rich experience for me because He made it so.

First Place helped me lose more than weight. It helped me lose fears about myself. It helped me to realize that God will not call us to do something that is too difficult. God knows each one of us, and He knows what we can do.

All we have to do is trust Him.

PRAYER

Father, Your name is so wonderful to me. Help me follow Your commandments for me. Help me to know that nothing is too difficult or beyond my reach when You are leading the way. Thank You for believing in me.

Journal: Is God asking you to do something today? If you're feeling that it is too difficult or beyond your reach, tell Him about it and place it in His hands.

—Tina D. Smith

FEBRUARY 18

STRONG WILL OR STRONG WON'T?

Now what I am commanding you today is not too difficult for you or beyond your reach.

DEUTERONOMY 30:11

"Reach." This is an action word—as in "reach for a cookie," which is one choice we can certainly make; or a better choice, "reach for the ceiling," which we do while exercising.

God first spoke to Moses, who then delivered His commands to the Israelites. The will to obey precedes carrying out His greatest commandments, which come down to two actions: to love and obey God. Not difficult—right?

If *only* it were that easy!

Personally, I battle weight control daily. But before First Place I considered it a losing battle. I now realize the battle is not mine but God's. And His greatest battle with me is not controlling my weight but commanding my obedience. Oswald Chambers said, "The battle is fought in the domain of the will."[1]

So the questions is always, What am I willing to be, to give or to do for Him? To obey I must make adjustments. First, I determine what it will cost me to obey—passing on a cookie, eating healthy vegetables and drinking water, measuring food, making a call, exercising, filling out a Commitment Record. Of course, the cost to me is nothing compared to the price Jesus paid for my salvation. Still, obeying God is always a battle fought within the will.

I once read that the difference between perseverance and obstinacy is this: Perseverance is strong "will"; obstinacy is strong "won't."

Reaching involves exercising the will. Do I reach for perseverance or obstinacy? Whenever we grasp for cheesecake or chocolate, we must remember to extend our reach beyond our grasp.

PRAYER

Lord, I'm ashamed that I often count the cost to follow You before I obey.
Guide me when I reach for inappropriate things. May I worship You today as
I reach out to You in prayer and strive to obey Your commands.

Journal: What adjustments can you make today to obey, thus allowing God more control in your life?

—Judy Marshall

FEBRUARY 19

As Hope Grows Stronger

Now what I am commanding you today is not too difficult for you or beyond your reach.

DEUTERONOMY 30:11

I put off joining First Place for many years because I felt the Bible study, the exercise and the other commitments would be too difficult for me to maintain. I hadn't had a lot of success in maintaining healthy disciplines in my life.

After talking with Carole Lewis and picking up her spirit of encouragement, I felt a flicker of hope. I promised to at least give it a try.

In the first session I attended, the first memory verse was this one from Deuteronomy. As I studied it and let it soak in, this verse became my motto for my endeavors to keep the commitments. The hope grew stronger.

It was not easy or natural for me to make the changes I needed to make. I had to pray that the Lord would help me to even like eating healthy foods—and I really had to pray that He would take away the desire for the unhealthy foods I craved. But at each step, I felt His help and support.

As the sessions progressed, I ate more of the healthy foods and less of the sugars and fats I had eaten before. The exercise I dreaded became a time of pleasure as I walked or rode my bicycle around the neighborhood. The fresh air and exercise gave me more energy, and I began to enjoy every aspect of the program.

At the end of the first session, *18 pounds* had disappeared. Within the next four months I reached my goal of losing *40 pounds*.

Victory is possible for everyday people—every day.

PRAYER

Dear Lord, may I always remember that what You command me to do is not too difficult for me or beyond my reach.

Journal: Make a list of both short-term and long-term goals. Pray over them and ask God to help you fulfill each one.

—Martha Rogers

FEBRUARY 20

WITHIN REACH

Now what I am commanding you today is not too difficult for you or beyond your reach.

DEUTERONOMY 30:11

I've never known weight loss to *not* be difficult. Then I encountered First Place.

I had spent a lifetime trying every new diet program available to achieve control of my weight. I failed over and over again. The only reason I considered trying once more was the fact that I was so miserable with myself the way I was.

Now, here I was in a Bible study, with God's Word telling me that the very thing I thought to be impossible was *not* too difficult. The only real difficulty was believing it!

First, I had to accept the idea that God was commanding me to eat right and take care of my body. Second, I had to accept that God really cared about how I treated my body and what I ate. Then, I learned that this was not even my own body! God had sacrificed His Son for me, and the Holy Spirit lived within me. I had not fully comprehended how deeply God cared for me.

Finally it sank in. His Word assured me that taking care of myself was not too difficult, nor was it beyond my reach. I could do this. God believed in me. God! The maker of heaven and Earth! The Master Artist! The great I Am! He believed in me. He was telling me that I could do this. He was on my team. He was cheering for me. He was providing me with all that I needed to achieve victory. With God on my side, how could I fail?

My part was, and continues to be, accepting His Word as true—every day.

PRAYER

Lord, forgive me when I don't obey Your commands. Forgive me for not believing that You believe in me. Thank You for cheering me toward victory!

Journal: Is there anything in your life that seems too difficult for you? What action would allow you to take a leap of faith and let God show you that He can give you victory in this area?

—Roberta Wasserman

FEBRUARY 21

Making the Right Promises

It is better not to vow than to make a vow and not fulfill it.

ECCLESIASTES 5:5

One of my greatest strengths is also one of my greatest weaknesses.

You see, I'm deeply moved when I see people hurting, and I want to help them. But sometimes I make commitments I am unable to keep.

Awhile back, I heard from a friend about a woman who was in a terrible family situation. The woman lived in my city, but her home was at least 75 miles from mine. I got her telephone number and said that I would make contact. Of course, I wasn't thinking that it was Christmas week or that I was reeling from a death in my own family or that I didn't have anyone to stay with my mom, whose care is my responsibility, while I visited this lady.

The promised phone call and visit never happened.

I can tell you this: When we make promises we can't keep, the enemy uses our own words to defeat us. Now I've learned that before I make a promise when I'm overloaded and unavailable, I need to present the problem to God and ask if there is someone else He could send. There will be times when that person is me, but there are also times when He will provide in another way.

And I am learning how to ask God to help me make only those promises He wants me to keep—those which He will give me the time and resources to meet.

PRAYER

Lord, help me to carefully consider the cost before making a promise I can't keep.

Journal: Is there something you have promised to do that you could do today? Ask God to help you do it.

—Carole Lewis

Is There Anything Greater?

It is better not to vow than to make a vow and not fulfill it.

ECCLESIASTES 5:5

This is one of the most important verses the Lord has used to minister to my heart, mind and body. As I meditated on it, I knew He was challenging me to make a vow to Him concerning my physical body. He had already helped me to see that taking care of "His temple" was a vitally important goal. Now I had to commit to it!

Making a vow to the Lord helps me to stay focused on what is important—my fellowship with Him and eating healthy foods. Making a vow reminds me that He has vowed to give me comfort, courage and strength. It keeps me thinking about His love and grace every day. A vow to the Lord helps me stay faithful to my commitments.

I've been moving forward to control my weight for four years now. Ecclesiastes 5:5 gives me encouragement to keep on going when I become weary with myself. Through this verse, the Holy Spirit gently and lovingly reminds me of the vow I've made to God and provides inner power to continue on the good path the Lord has planned for me.

To enjoy life to the fullest and to be in fellowship with my heavenly Father—is there anything greater? Praise His name today!

PRAYER

Heavenly Father, thank You for Your precious word to me. In Ecclesiastes 5:5, I am told it is better not to vow than to make a vow and not fulfill it. Please continue to help me keep my vow unto You, Lord.

Journal: What vows have you made to God in your First Place program? Which ones have been hard to keep, and why?

—Luane T. Clemmer

FEBRUARY 23

DOING WHAT WE SAY

It is better not to vow than to make a vow and not fulfill it.

ECCLESIASTES 5:5

After morning worship several years ago, a friend and I were telling each other our joys and needs. She asked me to pray for her child, who was ill. I assured her that I would. After visiting with other church family members, my husband and I shared the prayer need together as we drove home.

When I've been faithful to keep a vow, my spirit is at peace.

More recently, however, I arrived home on another busy Sunday, aware that I could not remember all the requests for prayer. I also realized that at the end of any given week there were specific requests that I had completely forgotten. God's voice inside me seemed to say, "Don't say you will pray for them if you are not going to do it!"

After that, I asked God to show me how to improve my behavior. He began to teach me how to be a better listener, how to pray even as I listen and how important it is to pray with people at the time they ask for support. I activate the First Place discipline of writing the prayer request in my journal. When I am unable to make the commitment to pray, I see that the individual's need is brought to one of the prayer teams in our church.

Sometimes I still forget. God knows my imperfections. But His perfect faithfulness shines through when I take practical steps to perform those commitments He has called me to keep.

PRAYER

Lord, You know how easy it is for me to say I'll do something and then to forget it. Help me to be more deliberate about my commitments. Give me the ability by Your strength and grace to keep trying and never give up.

Journal: What commitments has God called you to fulfill today? Where do you think you are succeeding? Failing?

—Nan Olmstead

FEBRUARY 24

IN THE PINK WITH OUR PROMISES

It is better not to vow than to make a vow and not fulfill it.

ECCLESIASTES 5:5

When we were children, if my friends and I said something and really meant it, we signaled our honesty by crossing our heart. Or we'd say "Scout's honor." Or we'd "pinky swear." (Of course, having your fingers crossed behind your back could cancel any of these signs of truthfulness!)

The promises we make as adults tend to carry more weight than playtime pledges made by children. Yet there are moments when in our haste to pacify a person or situation, a vow leaves our lips before we even realize what we're committing to and what it will cost us. If we're not responsible for what we say, the result can be disappointment and wounded relationships.

When we fail to fulfill our vows, we must face the unpleasant consequences. First, we must realize sin is inherent in any broken vow. In essence, we have lied. Even if the vow was seemingly small or unimportant, we must seek forgiveness from God and the person to whom the promise was made. Left unchecked, we may fall into a pattern of covering up one lie with another.

Second, a broken vow destroys trust. Trust takes time, sincerity and healing to rebuild.

Next time, before a vow leaves your lips, stop. Make sure your fingers aren't crossed behind your back. If they are, remember, silence is golden.

PRAYER

Dear God, thank You for always keeping Your promises to us. Help me to follow Your example, so the words of my mouth will be pleasing to You.

Journal: Do you need to mend any broken promises? If so, what is your plan for reconciliation?

—Tarena Sullivan

FEBRUARY 25

A CLASH OF LIONS

Be self-controlled and alert. Your enemy the devil prowls around like a roaring lion looking for someone to devour.

1 PETER 5:8

Once, after reading this powerful verse, I did some research on lions. What I found surprised and delighted me.

I learned, for instance, that the oldest lion—usually the one without any teeth—has the loudest roar. When the lion pride is on a hunt, the oldest lion will lay on one side of the clearing while the young lions congregate on the other side. When the prey enters the clearing, the old lion roars his loudest roar and the prey immediately runs the other way—into the clutches of the young lions.

After learning these lion facts, I changed the way I look at the enemy. Yes, he is a powerful foe, but I also think of him as old and toothless. The verse doesn't say that the devil *is* a lion but that he prowls around *like* a lion. He likes to roar loudly, hoping to paralyze God's children with fear so that we might run right into the very traps we're trying to resist.

Are you afraid that you will never lose the weight? Or that you will never get a better job? Or that your marriage is doomed to failure? Or that your rebellious child will never come back to God?

If so, think about who really has the power in your situation. Jesus, the Lion of Judah, is able to accomplish anything on your behalf today—if you will only ask Him.

PRAYER

Dear Lord, help me to face my fears today and be self-controlled and alert. Help me to lay all my fears at Your feet so that You are able to work freely on my behalf.

Journal: List every one of your fears today and give them to Jesus. Do this every day until the fear begins to leave. Write out Ephesians 6:11: "Put on the full armor of God so that you can take your stand against the devil's schemes."

—Carole Lewis

FEBRUARY 26

LEARNING THE ABCs

Be self-controlled and alert. Your enemy the devil prowls around like a roaring lion looking for someone to devour.

1 PETER 5:8

Rules! Rules! Rules! Like the laws of God that Moses handed down to the Israelites, rules seem to dominate our day-to-day life.

When there's an overabundance of things to remember, I like to arrange the information in bite-sized pieces. Then life becomes manageable, and I'm more likely to remember what I need to do.

For example, when it comes to keeping my head straight about physical health needs, I've devised an ABC system that may help you to stay alert and focused too:

- **A**im for fitness. Exercise at least three times each week. (I walk whenever I can, use stairs, park far away from stores and lift groceries twice when unloading the car.)
- **B**uild a healthy base. Choose sensibly when planning meals and control portions.
- **C**ommon sense. Pray, try to be self-controlled and alert, and put Christ first in all things.

Using this simple memory tool, I am often able to stay focused on God's healthy plan for me, even when I hear the roar of temptation.

PRAYER

Lord, I am grateful that You sent Jesus to free me from the Law that I could never uphold. How much easier life is, Lord, when I allow You to control me—as simple as ABC. Thank You for keeping me alert to my enemy's schemes and standing guard over me. Help my self-control become God-controlled today.

Journal: What laws, or rules, are dragging you down, and how can you break them up into bite-sized pieces to make them more manageable?

—Judy Marshall

FEBRUARY 27

DECLAWING THE FOOD LION

Be self-controlled and alert. Your enemy the devil prowls around like a roaring lion looking for someone to devour.

1 PETER 5:8

At a recent First Place meeting, a woman said she had just realized there truly is a "food lion"! She was making a pun, of course, of the name of the big grocery-store chain where many of us shopped, and we all laughed.

But in fact there is a "food lion" prowling around who tries to steer us away from our food plan. He is the one who seems to tempt us with the birthday party celebration the very same week we start our new food plan. He is the one who litters our paths with obstacles that make it more difficult to follow the meals planned that day. His goal is to get us to pick up and eat anything that will keep us from true victory.

Our invisible enemy has many ways of doing this. That's why we need to practice self-control through the power of the Holy Spirit. We need to be aware that an enemy exists.

And each time we decline his temptations, we grow stronger and more able to resist the next ones.

PRAYER

Lord, please help me to be self-controlled and alert in my food choices. I know there is a roaring lion tempting me to change my goals and rob me of my victory, but You have defeated him.

Journal: Do you have some upcoming special events that may tempt you to go off your food plan? Ask God to strengthen you, and then list specific ways you can resist temptation.

—Roberta Wasserman

FEBRUARY 28

P.E.R.S.E.V.E.R.E.

Be self-controlled and alert. Your enemy the devil prowls around like a roaring lion looking for someone to devour.

1 PETER 5:8

I'm amazed how often I forget that I'm a target. When I get up in the morning, quickly pray to God and then rush the kids off to school and head for work, I forget that close on my heels is a vicious lion. Later, when it's obvious that my adversary has bitten me, I remember my Father's words: Be aware and ready—always.

The following simple plan works for me, and I believe it will work for you too. The acrostic is PERSEVERE.

Pray without ceasing (morning, noon, night *and* in between!).

Enlist others in the fight. The lion does not like it when two or more gather.

Rejoice in the Lord. Praise and worship of God disturb the lion!

Submit to God's control each day, allowing Him to lead.

Encourage others on this journey to be wary and prepared.

Victory—remember Christ has already secured victory through the cross! Remind the lion that he's defeated.

Enlarge your arsenal of weapons. Keep God's armor on as protection against teeth and claws!

Repent—don't let unconfessed sin leave an opening for the enemy to sink his teeth in.

Eat according to God's bountiful and healthy plan. Take in both His Word and His food choices, allowing Him to make you strong and resilient spiritually and physically.

PRAYER

O Lord, deliver me from the evil one. Please protect and guide me. You alone, Lord, have the power to defeat the devil, and You are my shield and fortress.

Journal: What wounds has the enemy inflicted on you? What bandages are you applying? What will you do to avoid being wounded again?

—Carol Van Atta

GOD HAS GREAT TACTICS!

The weapons we fight with are not the weapons of the world. On the contrary, they have divine power to demolish strongholds.

2 CORINTHIANS 10:4

The Bible says that Satan wants to rob, kill and destroy—these are his tactics. So it is very important that we learn how to focus on God's tactics—which are to give us good gifts that give us life and build us up.

After the tragic death of my daughter, Shari, I have been able to see God's tactics at work in our family.

The morning after Shari's death, my granddaughter Cara received her acceptance letter to Texas A&M University. This in itself was a great gift to us all, because we knew it was the desire of her heart to study there. And there was more.

Cara decided to put her name into the pot for a roommate because she felt that people she didn't know would be more accepting if she was sometimes distant or withdrawn because of her mother's death. Well, wouldn't you just know what God would do in this situation? He gave Cara a Christian roommate and two Christian suite mates! One of the suite mates had also tragically lost her mother just a few days after she turned 18, during her senior year of high school. God used His divine tactics in Cara's life to show her how much He loves her, even in the midst of loss.

As Christians we belong to God. Yes, the weapons of this world are terrible. It is comforting, though, to know that we are not the ones doing the fighting. What is true for Cara—and for me—is also true for you. God has every situation all worked out for us, and He worked it out before the foundation of the world.

PRAYER

Dear Lord, today I want to experience Your divine power in my life. Show me Your power that I may testify to the lost world around me.

Journal: Write in your journal about the war you are engaged in today. Ask the Lord to use His divine power on your behalf. Be sure to thank Him in advance for His help.

—Carole Lewis

MARCH 2

His Word Is Our Weapon

The weapons we fight with are not the weapons of the world.
On the contrary, they have divine power to demolish strongholds.

2 CORINTHIANS 10:4

The Word of God is a powerful spiritual weapon, though we may not think about using His Word in this way. But when God talks about His armor (see Eph. 6:10-18), the Word of God is the only offensive weapon mentioned. All other parts of the armor are used for defense.

This verse from 2 Corinthians tells us to be on guard against strongholds—those situations or struggles that began as mere thoughts but have become so consuming they are now holding us hostage. These include unforgiveness, bitterness, anger and a negative view of ourselves.

In the Gospel of John, Jesus says the truth will set us free (see 8:32). The place we will find truth is in God's Word. If we use anything else to battle strongholds, we are using a weapon of the world—we are trying to win in our way and in our power.

The only way to demolish strongholds is to become intimate with God's Word. The First Place commitments to Scripture reading and memorization will help you greatly. Then when Satan comes to attack with lies through your thoughts, you have God's Word—His truth—to replace those thoughts before they begin to gain power over you.

God promises that His Word has divine power, or His authority, to demolish strongholds. Let's start tearing them down!

PRAYER

Dear Lord, thank You for providing me with the truth in Your Word.
Help me to discipline myself to read and memorize Your Word daily.

Journal: List the lies Satan has used in your life to create a stronghold. Write a prayer asking God to take your thoughts captive.

—Tarena Sullivan

MARCH 3

WEAPONS OF MASS HOPE AND HEALING

The weapons we fight with are not the weapons of the world.
On the contrary, they have divine power to demolish strongholds.

2 CORINTHIANS 10:4

Even as a Christian, I came to the program still resisting the Bible's term for compulsive eating—"gluttony." But for too long I had attempted to battle my weight problem with the meager and ineffective weapons of this world. As each one failed, my depression increased. Some of these methods hovered on the edge of the extreme. I was unable to find freedom, and these worldly strategies became tiresome. When I admitted that my struggle was a spiritual struggle, I finally began to win the fight.

It is so easy to forget that although we live in the world, we do not wage war as the world does. The false weapons of the world are as worthless as the false gods we are attempting to slay.

What I found in First Place was not another diet but what I think of as a wonderful and usable arsenal of weapons of mass healing and hope. By committing myself to the group, to daily Bible study, to balanced eating and to regular physical exercise, I found that in Him all things *are* possible!

As the old strongholds in my life crumble, God is replacing them with His grace, strength and hope. The divine weapons God has provided allow us to defeat the enemy and claim the land He has promised for us.

Since God has given us the power—all that's left is for us to use it.

PRAYER

Dear heavenly Father, we commit to putting on the entire arsenal today—
the belt of truth, the breastplate of righteousness, shoes shod in the gospel of peace,
the helmet of salvation, the shield of faith and the sword of the Spirit.
If You are for us, who can be against us!

Journal: What ineffective weapons of this world are you using to fight a spiritual battle? Consider writing your own prayer incorporating the pieces of God's full armor as described in Ephesians 6:10-18. Commit to praying it daily. Journal what happens.

—Carol Van Atta

THE MASTER COMMANDER

The weapons we fight with are not the weapons of the world.
On the contrary, they have divine power to demolish strongholds.

2 CORINTHIANS 10:4

On September 11, 2001, my family and I sat at the breakfast table in horror. How helpless we felt, watching the newscasters narrate the intentional crashing of two planes into the World Trade Center. Thousands of lives were destroyed. War began. Biological warfare followed. Fear, anger, uncertainty and loss were evident everywhere.

In the days that followed, the media showed us many different expressions of horror and grief. Commentators also explained the nature of terrorism and the strategies this country would use to fight it. Fighter planes, counter-terror measures and the best modern weapons were described.

Some leaders called the country to prayer and patience for the long road ahead. Others talked angrily about "attacking," "wasting" or "nuking" the enemy! The emotional responses of children and adults were addressed. Medications and methods of coping were offered as remedies.

At our breakfast table today, we continue to grapple with such tragedy, grateful that we can view it from the mind-set of faith. Because we know God—the Master Military Commander—our weapons are not of this world. They have divine power to demolish spiritual stongholds.

We must never forget that we are victorious only when our enemies are placed in God's hands.

PRAYER

Lord, we are learning how precious is the gift of each new day.
Give us patience, strength and courage to stand for the truth against
any enemy we encounter—with the right weapons.

Journal: How have you seen God's divine power demolish strongholds in your life?

—Nan Olmsted

THE UNSEARCHABLE THINGS

Call to me and I will answer you and tell you great and unsearchable things you do not know.

JEREMIAH 33:3

I have realized since the death of my daughter that God is the only One who can do the work that needs to be done in the life of each of my family members. This was always true, but many times in the past I have thought that *I* knew the solutions to everyone's problems.

Maybe we're all like this—so ready to believe we always know the right thing to do. Then comes a moment when we have no words, no wisdom, no strength in ourselves.

When the doctor came into the hospital waiting room to tell us that Shari was gone, there was stunned silence for what seemed like an eternity. My heart went cold and empty. All I knew to do was to pray. I don't remember a word I said, but I know the Holy Spirit began to pray for all of us as I cried out to God.

In the days and weeks that followed, all I could do was step aside and watch God work. My whole family has been amazed at the "unsearchable" things He has done for each one of us.

One Sunday night, Shari's husband, Jeff, had been talking for about an hour to their 15-year-old daughter, Christen, about her fears. After they finished talking, Christen picked up the remote control and started looking for something they could watch on TV. She came to a channel where Joel Osteen, a local pastor, was preaching. They watched for 30 minutes while Joel went over every single thing Jeff had talked about with Christen.

It is comforting to know that God is interested in the smallest and largest details of our lives, and it is comforting to know that only He can—and does—orchestrate events and people to meet our deepest needs.

PRAYER

Father, today I am calling out to You. I desperately desire to know those great and unsearchable things You have for me.

Journal: Write about your greatest need and ask God to do His supernatural work within you.

—Carole Lewis

MARCH 6

KNOWN BY NAME

Call to me and I will answer you and tell you great and unsearchable things you do not know.

JEREMIAH 33:3

It was clear that Sheri felt her prayer concern was a deep, personal need. But we couldn't help but be amused when she asked us to pray that God would awaken her early the next morning, so she could get to her exercise class before work.

Sheri was a First Place leader. Along with four other leaders, Sheri and I had been involved in this great program for several years. As leaders, we have prayed, cried, laughed, shared and struggled our way through facilitating our groups. All along the journey, God has showed us that the simplest truths are the most important ones. By studying and memorizing Scripture together, we are called consistently by God's Spirit to know how deeply He loves us and how much He cares about the tiniest details of our lives. While we laughed with her that morning, we all wrote the request in our notebooks, assuring her we would pray.

The following week, Sheri came in laughing and excited. She shared that the very morning she wanted us to pray, she had set the radio alarm to awaken her with music from an "Oldies but Goodies" station. When the alarm first sounded, she hit the snooze button. When it sounded again, the words of an old song rang out: "Sher-er-er-er-er-er-ery Ba-ay-by!"

Sheri's husband, Doug, rolled over and said, "Well, I think that's for you!" She made it to exercise class on time. Our sharing time was filled with praise to God for not only knowing us by name but also for hearing us when we call and answering in personal and life-changing ways.

PRAYER

Father, it is difficult for us to believe that You are here to help us on a daily basis to do the disciplines that are so difficult at times. We praise You for the joy of calling to You, our perfectly consistent Lord, and for the simple truth that You hear us when we call.

Journal: Write about the great and wonderful things God has said to you this week—things just for your ears.

—Nan Olmsted

MARCH 7

GREAT AND WONDERFUL THINGS

Call to me and I will answer you and tell you great and unsearchable things you do not know.

JEREMIAH 33:3

God always has a way of teaching us something new, even from Scripture we think we know so well.

One Sunday my husband and I attended church in another state with our son and his family. They were celebrating a month of missions emphasis as many churches do in the month of November. Scripture verses on beautiful posters were hanging all over the church on the walls and doors. Just before we entered the main sanctuary, I noticed that one of the posters was emblazoned with Jeremiah 33:3. *How was it connected to missions?* I wondered.

After a few minutes of meditating I realized the connection: When we call on His name and seek His face, He will show us where He wants us to be. He will also give us direction to reach the place. Then I saw the whole picture. Answering the call to missions comes as a result of calling on God and having Him give a vision of what can be done in the place where He wants a person to serve.

God can do the same for us. He will show us great and wonderful things through His Word and through His plans for our lives.

PRAYER

Lord, show me today where You want me to serve You. May I see the vision of the great and unsearchable things You have for me to learn.

Journal: Write a prayer using Jeremiah 33:3; in your prayer, call on Him to reveal where He wants you to serve Him.

—Martha Rogers

MARCH 8

THE PHONE'S FOR YOU

Call to me and I will answer you and tell you great and unsearchable things you do not know.

JEREMIAH 33:3

Inventions are wonderful displays of God's creative genius. I love them—well, *most* of them. My least favorite is my answering machine—especially when it's beeping obnoxiously when I'm trying to take a well-deserved "Calgon, take me away" moment.

The answering machine has taught me something though. It's made me realize I have an internal answering machine of sorts, and I engage it at certain times when I don't want to be bothered. That is to say, I've learned how to tune people out. Unfortunately, I sometimes tune out God too.

Sometimes, for instance, when I'm tempted by poor food choices, I turn on my answering machine. When the Holy Spirit tries to get through to me and tell me to pass up some calorie-laden horror, He sometimes hears this message: "Sorry, I'm not available at the moment."

Fortunately, God loves me enough to always keep an open line to His heart. He's faithful to answer my call anytime, for anything. Where would I be and how would I feel if He used an answering machine, had call waiting or put me on hold? He has caller ID and determines my need, even before I place my call to Him, and I expect His direct line to be open 24 hours a day.

Shouldn't I always be ready and willing to answer His call too? He has great and unsearchable things He can hardly wait to tell me.

PRAYER

Lord, thank You that I can call to You anytime and immediately
You're ready to listen and help. Help me to listen for Your first call.
Give me Your strength to answer and obey.

Journal: Is there a specific time you tend to put God on hold or turn the volume down? What are some of the great and unsearchable things God has told you lately?

—Judy Marshall

MARCH 9

FREE TO THE CORE

Call to me and I will answer you and tell you great and unsearchable things you do not know.

JEREMIAH 33:3

For the first time in my life I was opening the Bible every day to read and study God's Word. Each new Scripture in the First Place Bible study was like a treasure, a jewel to behold.

The mere fact that the God who had created the heavens and the whole Earth would speak to me simply amazed me. I mean, who was *I*? Just one in a jillion people struggling with weight issues. Just an ordinary person with a desire to lose excess weight. My alleged ordinariness and insignificance had trapped me into believing nothing great could happen for me.

Jeremiah 33:3 set me free. Yes, God was telling me that if I called to Him, He would answer me. He would not just answer me, but He would also tell me great and unsearchable things I did not know. Of course, I wanted to know more and was honored that this magnificent God would share things with me.

Getting hold of this new reality freed me at my very core. I had doubted my worth so deeply, because the world esteems thin people. The First Place program helped me to rebuild my self-esteem through the truth that since God created me, He has a very special plan for my life.

Today, I know that I am not *just ordinary*. Like you, I am extraordinary enough that Jesus Christ died on the cross for me. Personally, God has taught me great and unsearchable things I did not know—including who I really am in His eyes.

PRAYER

Lord, thank You for setting me free. Thank You for being available to hear my prayers. Thank You for speaking back to me.

Journal: Tell God your understanding of how He views you. Describe how because of these truths your life is different from the way it was in the past.

—Roberta Wasserman

MARCH 10

LOUDER THAN WORDS

We make it our goal to please him, whether we are at home in the body or away from it.

2 CORINTHIANS 5:9

During her 39 years on this earth, my daughter learned a valuable lesson: Shari knew that if she would just spend time with God early in the morning, He would bless her day with goodness.

Beth Moore is a great teacher and friend who spoke at Shari's memorial service. The night before the service, as family and friends gathered at the church, Beth said that she had talked to the teacher of one of Shari's daugthers, Amanda, who is 13. The teacher told Beth a story about Amanda, who frequently was late for things. Since Amanda is such a good student, the teacher was reluctant to talk about the problem.

One morning, after Amanda was late again, the teacher said, "Amanda, I am puzzled as to why you're late so much of the time." Amanda replied, "It's my mom. She just can't get through with her Bible study so that we can leave on time."

After Shari's memorial service a friend came up to me and said, "I don't want to die before I have made some changes in my life. My kids need to see me reading my Bible, instead of those romance novels."

Make it your goal to please God today. You will never be sorry. What you do speaks so much louder than what you say.

PRAYER

Lord, I want to please You today with everything I do and everything I say. Help me to make pleasing You my greatest priority.

Journal: List some areas of your life that are not pleasing to God right now. Give God permission to make the necessary changes in your life so that it will be pleasing to Him.

—Carole Lewis

MARCH 11

WHOSE LIST ARE YOU FOLLOWING?

We make it our goal to please him, whether we are at home in the body or away from it.

2 CORINTHIANS 5:9

I love to make lists. I write down all the things that need to be done, block time slots on a sheet of paper and plan my day. That paper then contains my goals for the day.

Sometimes I meet my goals and sometimes I don't. Sometimes I grow frustrated if things interfere with my goals. At those times, I need to remember that perhaps God preempted my goals and placed His goals into my day– things He wanted me to do and people to whom He wanted me to relate.

Again and again I have to ask myself, *What is more important—His goals or mine?*

God's goals are more important. This is why we need to pray for His leading as we make our lists. We need to be in tune with Him as we set our goals for any given day so that we can hear His leading. Then throughout the day we need to be flexible enough to allow interruptions and changes to take place, according to His will.

PRAYER

Lord, show me Your plans for my life. Help me to be in tune with
You as I use each moment of the days You give me.

Journal: List how many of your goals are the same as God's goals. How might your life be different if you sought His direction while planning the next hour, day, week, month and year?

—Helen McCormack

MARCH 12

MAKING THE MAIN THING

We make it our goal to please him, whether we are at home in the body or away from it.

2 CORINTHIANS 5:9

What is your aim in life?

In First Place, are you aiming to please God or are you aiming to lose weight? I can guarantee that you will succeed at pleasing God if you just try. It pleases our Father when we aim to please Him. So we hit the mark just by trying.

The decision to go all out and give God first place in your life does take a bit more, though. It takes real commitment and effort. It requires you to make the same decision over and over again, sometimes on a moment-by-moment basis.

I am discovering that the major component of the victorious life is focus. Just what are you focused on? Are you allowing yourself to be fragmented into 1,000 different directions or are you focused on the main thing—your relationship with God?

Are you spending too much of your time on the couch watching soap operas? Of course not! But do you drop everything to watch a specific show? Do you make time for Bible study or is it left to chance, depending on how the rest of your day is going?

As with anything worth doing, you must plan your work and then work your plan. Just because one day you decide to make God first in your life, doesn't mean you always will. Over and over again every day you must make the same decision to keep Him in first place.

PRAYER

Dear Father, help me to focus my aim on You.

Journal: A life unplanned and unchecked is prone to return to failure-ridden patterns. What three things could you do today to keep your focus on God?

—June-Marie Avery

MARCH 13

STAYING ON COURSE

We make it our goal to please him, whether we are at home in the body or away from it.

2 CORINTHIANS 5:9

The big holidays have passed and this verse is haunting me. It is my goal to please my Lord—but as I look back on the last few weeks, I realize I have pleased my enemy, the devil, more than I've pleased God.

In terms of weight, I hate to admit that the "roaring lion" certainly has more to devour (see 1 Pet. 5:8). Not only do I feel guilty and less mentally alert—but we won't even discuss how snug my clothes are fitting!

I have asked God to forgive me for overloading my plate with unhealthy choices and amounts. Now I have to forgive myself and do what needs to be done to get back on-track.

Here's what I know: It is far easier to stay on the program during a First Place session than out here on my own. But that should not be the excuse. God has given me the training to stay on the program when away from my group. Once again, though, I've blown it. So this week I will not only face my group—but even worse, I'll also face the scales.

Even so, my God is faithful; and when I'm away from First Place, I will strive to be more faithful to Him, so I can serve Him better.

PRAYER

Abba Father, forgive me for not taking care of myself. When I don't take care of myself, I cannot do my best for You. Pleasing You is my goal.

Journal: Are you on track with your weight-loss program? If not, ask God to help you and then list several ways you could begin again today.

—Betha Jean Cunningham

ARE YOU BITTER OR BETTER?

However, I consider my life worth nothing to me, if only I may finish the race and complete the task the Lord Jesus has given me—the task of testifying to the gospel of God's grace.

ACTS 20:24

Years ago, I began asking God to make me into a godly woman. I didn't have a clue that my prayer would be difficult to answer without my sharing in the same kind of suffering Jesus endured.

Four years ago, my husband was diagnosed with stage-four prostate cancer. God is the only reason Johnny is alive today, and God has given us the most wonderful four years together.

Two years ago, my 89-year-old mother came to live with us full time. My mom, Frances, has always been my hero. I have counted it a joy to be able to take care of her now that she is unable to care for herself.

And I have already spoken of my daughter, Shari, who was killed by a drunk driver in November 2001. This event is so fresh that I haven't had time to look back and see God's hand. The one thing I know is that He will bring good from this awful tragedy. I know this because God and I have a history, and that history says He loves me.

Do I believe that God caused these events to answer my prayer? Certainly not. I do believe, however, that the promise of Romans 8:28 is absolutely true: "And we know that in all things God works for the good of those who love Him, who have been called according to his purpose."

God wants to use every event, whether good or bad, to conform us to the image of His Son, Jesus. I have heard that painful circumstances can make you bitter or better. I want to be better when I reach the end of my personal race.

PRAYER

Lord, I thank You that You are a loving God who wants good for those You have called, those of us who belong to You. Praise Your holy name!

Journal: If you are right now facing some seemingly hopeless situations that are keeping you from running your race, think about God's faithfulness to you and then write about your circumstances from that perspective.

—Carole Lewis

LACE UP YOUR SHOES!

However, I consider my life worth nothing to me, if only I may finish the race and complete the task the Lord Jesus has given me—the task of testifying to the gospel of God's grace.

ACTS 20:24

There are times when I can throw a great one-woman pity party! I often ask God why He puts up with me.

But God knows how to redirect my attention to keep it off myself. Invariably God will place people in my path who need a shoulder to cry on. As I listen, I shoot up an "arrow prayer" to God, seeking the help I need in handling things His way. When they have said all they can say, I quietly assure them they are not alone—others have had similar problems. I try to assure them that God's grace and love is available to all who call on His name and believe on His only begotten Son, Jesus.

Maybe this does more to help me out of my pity party than it does to help the other person. I don't know. What I do know is that I can then put on my jogging shoes and get on with my race. Perhaps this is one of the reasons God puts up with me and even brings people across my path—He knows I love to tell others about His grace, His love and what He has done for me.

On the other hand—maybe He is using others to show me how blessed I am!

PRAYER

Thank You, God, for giving me the opportunity to share You with others.
Thank You for being my Abba—my Father.

Journal: Describe the last time you told someone in pain about the healing love and compassion of the Lord.

—Betha Jean Cunningham

MARCH 16

WILLING TO LIVE FOR HIM

However, I consider my life worth nothing to me, if only I may finish the race and complete the task the Lord Jesus has given me—the task of testifying to the gospel of God's grace.

ACTS 20:24

I can't remember when I was not a Christian. I can't remember when I didn't know that Jesus died to save me from my sins and that He has a place prepared just for me.

Despite this great beginning, it was the First Place program and meetings that have helped me find a new purpose for my life. I now realize that I *must* live for Jesus. My direction is clear and my mission is focused. I strive each day to put Christ first.

Colossians 3:23-24 says: "Whatever you do, work at it with all your heart, as working for the Lord, not for men. . . . It is the Lord Christ you are serving." First Place has made me realize that my life is nothing unless I do all for Jesus. The program has opened so many doors for talking about Him. If we are called by Him to serve, it matters not whether it is to teach, preach, sing, visit a shut-in or be a First Place leader or member. We are to do the task God has placed before us and do our job heartily for the Lord.

God has placed a special calling on my life to serve Him and witness for Him through the First Place program. How thankful I am that I have been able to do just that. I have learned that I only need to be willing to live for Him and to seek His will and He will do the rest.

PRAYER

Lord, thank You for the opportunity to live for You. Help me realize that my body is Your holy temple. May I never fail to tell those who are lost about Your love.

Journal: How could you live your life today so that someone can see that you're living for Jesus?

—Carolyn W. Owen

NO CHANCE ENCOUNTERS

However, I consider my life worth nothing to me, if only I may finish the race and complete the task the Lord Jesus has given me—the task of testifying to the gospel of God's grace.

ACTS 20:24

Several years ago, a group of ladies and I traveled from our small town in Alabama to the Atlanta area for a First Place workshop. After the first session, we realized the workshop was about how to start a First Place group. We already had a successful program in our church, so we decided to wait—until after lunch, of course—just to see what we *could* learn.

During lunch, I had the opportunity to meet Kay Smith, the associate national director for First Place, and we immediately began discussing food. You see, I am a chef by trade, so food is my business.

Not long after, members of our group suggested that I come up with a First Place menu to offer the people in our area. It wasn't long before the restaurant where we met became a favorite destination for First Place members from surrounding counties. After a few months, several other churches began offering First Place, with hundreds of people participating in the program.

As First Place continued to grow in the area, a local grocery store, with the help of employees participating in the program, even set up a First Place section in the store. Another company sponsored a cooking show that featured First Place-style recipes. This led to the cookbook *Healthy Home Cooking.* A few months later, I was asked to join First Place as their food consultant and to assist with the preparation of foods at conferences.

All of this from a "chance encounter"? I think not! Our heavenly Father gives us special gifts and He wants us to use them for His glory.

PRAYER

Heavenly Father, help me find where You want me to be.
Give me a ministry that will testify to Your grace and love.

Journal: Do people see Jesus' purposes in the work that you do? Share how the grace of Jesus has fulfilled your life.

—Scott Wilson

MARCH 18

THE QUALITY OF OUR RACING STRIDE

However, I consider my life worth nothing to me, if only I may finish the race and complete the task the Lord Jesus has given me—the task of testifying to the gospel of God's grace.

ACTS 20:24

It was a crisp Monday morning when I attended the memorial service of a high school classmate.

I have attended many funerals and memorial services that had an evangelistic tone—but this was the first where the plan of salvation and the sinner's prayer were printed and given out together with the information about the deceased. Talk about finishing the race in style!

Oddly enough, my friend had only been a Christian for five months! He found Christ as his Savior while planning his wife's funeral! God used his wife's death as a way to lead him to Christ.

There is no way to know how many people may have learned about God's love and sacrifice because of the deaths of my friend and his wife. But they both completed their tasks and went home to receive their prize from the Lord.

My friend, as I said, had only been a Christian a short time. From his death I have realized that it isn't how long we are in the race that counts but how we run the race while we are in it.

PRAYER

Father, may I finish my race leaving no doubt about Your love and grace for Your people.

Journal: Ask God how He would like you to finish your race and then write down what He tells you.

—Betha Jean Cunningham

March 19

His Power, His Might

"Not by might nor by power, but by my Spirit," says the LORD Almighty.

Zechariah 4:6

After my daughter's death, her husband was faced with the awesome task of finishing the job of raising their three girls—ages 19, 15 and 13.

In the days after the funeral, there were so many things to do, one of which was moving back into Houston, so they would be closer to all of the family. Jeff's employers were gracious and gave him time off during the holidays to work out a plan; yet a couple days before he had to go back to work, he was still overwhelmed with all there was left to do.

That Sunday night, as Johnny and I were driving home from the airport, I called Jeff to see how he and the girls were doing. I could tell by his voice that he needed some clear direction.

After we got home, I cried out to God to give Jeff the direction he so desperately needed.

Jeff called me the next night to tell me the owner of his company had called that day. He told Jeff that his situation was much like being on a plane. The flight attendant instructs you that if there is a loss of cabin pressure, put the oxygen mask on yourself first before you put a mask on each of your children. He told Jeff, "You must survive if your girls are to survive." He told Jeff that he wanted him to start working some every day, even if it was only for a half day at first.

There is no doubt in our minds that the Holy Spirit prompted Jeff's boss to deliver these powerful words at such a critical time. Jeff had no power or might, but God's Spirit did what needed to be done.

Prayer

Lord, You know the areas of my life in which I have no strength or power to straighten things out. Take charge and intervene on my behalf today.

Journal: List problems that you have no power to fix. Ask the Holy Spirit to supernaturally intervene in each of these areas.

—Carole Lewis

MARCH 20

A PRESCRIPTION FOR VICTORY

"Not by might nor by power, but by my Spirit," says the LORD Almighty.

ZECHARIAH 4:6

All during my "dieting career," I had relied upon my own strength and/or the power of diet foods, fads or pills. I followed the diet du jour and popular fads like a groupie. I experienced the thrills of sudden weight loss and then fell into despair when the weight, accompanied by extra pounds, returned at the end of the diet.

Over and over again it was the same thing: My expectations of each of these methods were always high, and their (and my) failure was certain.

Memorizing Zechariah 4:6 made me aware that my success did not depend on my strength or how much willpower I possessed. God never intended for me to enter a battle under my own strength. I needed only to have faith in God and be obedient to His teaching.

Today I know my victory does not require a prescription for diet pills. The victory belongs to God, and the path I must follow is obedience. As I allow God's Holy Spirit to teach and guide me, I will reach my goal.

My strength is limited and my willpower is often subject to my emotional state. But God's Spirit is able to endure and lead me to victory!

PRAYER

Father, thank You for providing the necessary strength and power through Your Holy Spirit. Help me always to call upon and be obedient to You.

Journal: How has dependence upon your own strength affected your health? Ask God to fight the battle for you.

—June Chapko

MARCH 21

POPPING THE PITY-PARTY BALLOON

"Not by might nor by power, but by my Spirit," says the LORD Almighty.

ZECHARIAH 4:6

I just hate to be alone sometimes—especially when I throw one of my pity parties. Such parties always begin just when I run out of steam and willpower. By party time I've made a long list of multiplied gripes. Each one is so full of hot air that I could fill up balloons and decorate! And with this negative sing-song litany, I've run my friends off. So it's me—alone again.

Ever been to one of these parties? I've got just the remedy. It's found in Zechariah 4:6: "'Not by might nor by power, but by my Spirit,' says the LORD Almighty." This verse has reminded me so many times that I'm never really alone. Saying it aloud can turn the most pitiful pity party into a real celebration for two—the Holy Spirit and me.

Even when we are not faithful to ourselves, God is always faithful. He is ever present to help when we're not strong, to hold us when we're lonely, to heal us when we're hurting, to hug us when we're happy and to high-five us when we obey Him.

And because one of His great promises is that He will never leave us, I can assure you that He will always show up for your pity party and turn it into a real celebration.

PRAYER

Lord, thank You for Your promise to be with me by Your Spirit at all times.
Thank You for faithfully being ready to help, hold, heal, hug and high-five,
even before I realize I need You.

Journal: Describe the last time God came through for you, whether to help, hold, heal, hug or high-five.

—Judy Marshall

MARCH 22

God Knows You Can

"Not by might nor by power, but by my Spirit," says the LORD Almighty.

ZECHARIAH 4:6

This Scripture provided the key to victory for me in the area of my weight. My whole life I had tried to follow food plans—only to fail over and over again. I would set out with the very best intentions. In the beginning I would have success, but over time my willpower ran out.

Then I learned that I could count on His willpower when mine failed. God has the power through the Holy Spirit to lead me into victory in all areas of my life. My role was to learn to follow His will, not my own. My will would have been to eat everything I wanted, anytime I wanted, as much as I wanted and still remain thin!

As I slowly followed the First Place program, my life began to be transformed in many areas, including physically. I did gain victory over my weight through the power of Jesus Christ.

I know you can too.

PRAYER

Lord, thank You that I do not need to depend on myself to achieve victory. Thank You for providing all that I need to be free of issues regarding weight.

Journal: What methods have you tried to achieve victory in regard to your weight? How have you felt after you failed to reach your goals? Ask the Holy Spirit to help you follow His will.

—Roberta Wasserman

MARCH 23

SEEDS OF FUTURE WORTH

"Not by might nor by power, but by my Spirit," says the LORD Almighty.

ZECHARIAH 4:6

Several years ago I was blessed by a Bible teacher—a friend who had been recently widowed. Her face was radiant, her eyes sparkled, and her smile lit any room. When asked if she ever thought of remarrying, she would say with conviction, "God is my husband; He promises that in Isaiah 54:5." She knew from experience that her needs would be met by the Lord Almighty.

I remembered those words almost 25 years later when my husband passed away. I thank God for a precious friend whose words would remind me—"'Not by might nor by power, but by my Spirit,' says the LORD Almighty" (Zech. 4:6). And He has been my husband, as well!

When we tell someone how God has helped us, we never know what impact we might have on others, even in years to come.

PRAYER

I thank You, Father, for beautiful friends whose words impact our lives.
I thank You for carrying me through the rough times by Your Spirit.

Journal: List some ways you could be a friend to others and tell them your experiences with God. If you are hesitant, ask Him to empower you by His Spirit.

—Betha Jean Cunningham

MARCH 24

HE LOVES YOU SO MUCH

Therefore, there is now no condemnation for those who are in Christ Jesus.

ROMANS 8:1

It is Saturday morning as I prepare to write this devotional entry. The phone rings, and it's the wife of a family member who has had many problems over the years. Her husband has turned around 180 degrees and is now on track again. His wife just called to tell me they had been praying for us every day, and we had a wonderful chat about the Lord.

After I hung up the phone, my 89-year-old mom told me that she woke up the other night worrying about this family member because she didn't think we were doing anything for him. I told her, with an edge to my voice, that he was doing fine—he is happy, working every day and going to church every Sunday.

As I walked back to my desk, I realized that my snappishness with my mother came from the fact that I felt condemnation and guilt that I hadn't done enough to help this member of my own family. I asked God to forgive me and then went back to tell Mom—more cheerfully—all that is going on in his life and that I talk with his wife often. She smiled and was immediately at peace.

And now I know what it is I need to write about: The enemy wants to continually condemn us for what we have or haven't done. For those of us in Christ Jesus, there is never condemnation, only unconditional love and acceptance.

Just for today, allow God to show you how much He loves you. You'll be glad you did.

PRAYER

Dear Lord, I know that when I feel condemnation, it is not from You. Help me to realize that as Your child, I am covered in Your love and grace.

Journal: List areas of your life in which you suffer guilt and condemnation. Ask God to help you give each of those areas to Him—for good—so that you can be free.

—Carole Lewis

MARCH 25

No Condemnation Is a Great Thing!

Therefore, there is now no condemnation for those who are in Christ Jesus.

ROMANS 8:1

Having spent a lifetime trying to achieve victory in regard to my weight, I had developed a very condemning spirit. It seemed that the harder I tried to lose weight, the more weight I gained.

The root of my problem, I learned, was a deeply held belief that I was a failure, and I felt tremendous guilt over past failures. *Why couldn't I lose weight?* I would start off with the best intentions. I would compare myself to others who had done better than myself. No matter how hard I tried, though, I would eventually fall off my diet. That's when the guilt and condemnation would overwhelm me.

To comfort myself, I would throw away my good intentions and binge on foods I had denied myself. My thoughts told me it was no use—there was no point in trying anymore. I was defeated once again.

When I became part of First Place and read today's Scripture, I was filled with hope. I was set free from the negative belief that I was a failure. After all, if Jesus Christ lived within me, then victory was mine.

It took time, but I learned that if I began to feel any condemnation from not being perfect, those thoughts were not from the Lord. He always gave me grace to press on toward my goal. A condemning spirit was just an obstacle that needed to be overcome by the power of Jesus Christ in me.

PRAYER

Lord, thank You for setting me free from guilt and condemnation. Thank You that Jesus Christ resides in me and that I can be victorious.

Journal: What negative thoughts overwhelm you at times? Write a prayer of faith, asking the Holy Spirit to release you from this burden.

—Roberta Wasserman

MARCH 26

WHAT'S EATING YOU?

Therefore, there is now no condemnation for those who are in Christ Jesus.

ROMANS 8:1

Sometimes what we're eating is not as bad as what's eating us.

We eat to bring comfort or to numb our feelings. We despair over past mistakes or hurtful memories. These unpleasant feelings can eat us alive.

But there's good news today! Jesus paid our debt, and God has thrown away the record of our sin. We allow the enemy to cause us to despair over God-forgiven sins of the past. God has forgiven us, so we have no reason to hang on to feelings of condemnation.

The bedrock truth is this: *God loves us.*

No matter where we go or how we respond to God, He loves us deeply. He longs for our fellowship, our praise and our worship. He constantly pursues us, seeking to draw us into a loving relationship.

And here is another bedrock truth: *God is faithful.*

God has shown this to me over and over again in the past few years. Now whenever I see the word "faithful" in the Bible, I lift up my heart to God in thanksgiving.

When the enemy comes to blame, claim or shame, we need to lift up Christ and claim the blood that was lovingly shed for our sins. We are new creations because of Jesus and His work on the cross. Hang on to that love. Accept that forgiveness.

PRAYER

Father, Your Word says we are new creatures in Christ. The old things are no more, and the new things have come. Help me to wrap my mind around these truths.

Journal: What hurt or shame from past sin are you still holding? Think about your newness in Christ and write a love letter to Him, releasing your hold on the past.

—Becky Sirt

MARCH 27

How to Walk Free Within

Therefore, there is now no condemnation for those who are in Christ Jesus.

ROMANS 8:1

What do you do with guilt? How do you experience God's love and forgiveness?

I recently discovered the answers to those questions at the First Place Fitness Week in Roundtop, Texas. On Friday night, the speaker instructed over 100 women to be silent—we could not talk to each other from 9 P.M. on Friday until 9 A.M. on Saturday. She called this a social fast. What an incredible, life-changing experience this was for many of us attending the retreat.

It was in the silence of that night, in a small rose garden, that I talked alone and aloud to God for the first time. When I heard my sins in my own words, my heart broke and tears of godly sorrow streamed down my face. As I walked from the garden, I felt free and full of God's love and forgiveness. My life had been changed.

What do you do with guilt? Confess it with godly sorrow.

How do you experience God's love and forgiveness? Accept it with all your heart.

If you want to live and walk free within, you can.

PRAYER

Lord, thank You for Your call to silent communion with You. Thank You for the gardens of new life and possibility in Spirit that always open when we come to You. Thank You for Your love that results in forgiveness and freedom.

Journal: After you spend time in prayer, enter the "rose garden" of your journal and confess whatever the Holy Spirit has brought to mind.

—Kathy Runion

MARCH 28

A GREAT REWARD

Those who know your name will trust in you, for you, LORD, have never forsaken those who seek you.

PSALM 9:10

As I write devotionals on the memory verses for *Everyday Victory for Everyday People,* I am amazed that only weeks have passed since Shari's death.

Our Christian friends from First Place and our church have bombarded the throne of God with prayers on my family's behalf. We have received hundreds of cards, phone calls and e-mails. Every single day I talk to someone who says, "I pray for you constantly that God will strengthen you and your family as you grieve this loss."

The Lord hears and answers the prayers of His children. When you intercede for someone who isn't able to pray for their own needs because of something they are going through, you are telling God that you trust Him to intervene in the circumstance with His strength and power. Every word of God is true and powerful, and prayer is the medium we use to tap into His power.

In First Place, we have learned that each day spent without prayer is a day we choose to live in the flesh. You've heard the biblical saying, The spirit is willing, but the flesh is weak (see Matt. 26:41). Begin today to discipline yourself by setting aside a definite time each day for prayer, Bible reading and Bible study. If these activities are not part of your life, commit yourself anew to seeking Him in deeper ways.

Then when trials come your way, I can assure you that God *will* reward you greatly.

PRAYER

Lord, I want to become a mighty prayer warrior. I ask Your precious Holy Spirit to impress my heart with the needs of those I love so that I may lift them up to You in prayer.

Journal: List the names of people you personally know who need God's strength today. Ask Him to strengthen them and let them know in some small way today that He is with them.

—Carole Lewis

MARCH 29

FAITHFUL IN ALL THINGS

Those who know your name will trust in you, for you, LORD, have never forsaken those who seek you.

PSALM 9:10

Business, family, financial and personal crises—plus the illness and death of my husband—have taught me that God will not forsake me! Sometimes I haven't walked with God, but that's because He has picked me up in His arms and carried me.

At 66, I'm still learning to depend on God for every need in my life. Recently the washing machine gave up. It had literally been held together with baling wire! As I unplugged it, I told God that He had promised to be my husband and that the washer was now His problem. I live on a widow's income (Social Security!) and did not have money in the budget to replace this appliance.

The next morning, to my amazement, a man from church called to tell me he understood that I needed a washing machine and that he had one in his pickup truck ready to deliver if I wanted it. God had used another couple to furnish it, and I'm grateful to God and to them!

Not long ago I had made the decision to drop out of First Place for the upcoming session because I could not afford the new materials. Before I could call my leader, she called me. She told me I had a scholarship! God used His people to handle my needs.

I can't wait to see what God is going to do about my transportation problem!

PRAYER

Abba Father, thank You for Your faithfulness. Thank You for never forsaking me.

Journal: Do you need the Lord's provision in a specific area today? Write to Him about your concern and ask Him to carry you. (Don't forgot to record His response—no matter when it comes!)

—Betha Jean Cunningham

MARCH 30

HIS KISS OF COMFORT

Those who know your name will trust in you, for you, LORD, have never forsaken those who seek you.

PSALM 9:10

I had read stories of martyrs, and I couldn't imagine raising my arms in praise and proclaiming "Jesus is Lord" as I was being burned at the stake! I wasn't sure if, on that fateful day at Columbine High School in Colorado, I would have said "Yes, I believe in God." And while neither of these scenarios seemed likely to me, I did have a situation that I was afraid could shake my faith.

The sunshine of my life is my precious granddaughter, Madeline, who has been in and out of the hospital her whole life. I wondered, *What if something terrible happens to Madeline? Would I really trust God even then, or would I turn away from Him in bitterness and blame?*

As I memorized Psalm 9:10 for First Place, God showed me something new. In the past I had always focused on God's promise never to forsake me—but this time I realized it also meant I could trust in Him, no matter what happened to me! I had to make a decision: I decided then and there to claim His promise that I would trust in Him, and I'm so very glad I did.

Just a few weeks ago, my sweet Madeline gave up her fight and went home to the Lord. Although I grieve, I can testify that His promise is true. I trusted Him as I kissed Madeline good-bye, and I've trusted Him every day since.

And I trust that I'll kiss her hello again someday!

PRAYER

Lord, thank You for Your many precious promises—especially for Your promise that our faith will hold strong in times of trouble.

Journal: What secret fears do you harbor? Write them down, lift them to God and claim His promise that you *will* trust in Him, no matter what problems you face.

—Kathy Hickey

MARCH 31

THE FINGERPRINTS OF GOD

Those who know your name will trust in you, for you, LORD, have never forsaken those who seek you.

PSALM 9:10

Several years ago, my life seemed to be turning into a bad soap opera as I experienced a triple-whammy of difficulties. First, I was diagnosed with cancer. Shortly thereafter, my best friend, Annette, moved out of state. And then a tornado flattened my new house! My life was literally turned upside down, giving me the perfect opportunity to explore the promise found in Psalm 9:10!

I discovered that the promise Jesus made—"I will never leave you or forsake you"—carries the same message when read forward or backward! (Okay, so it's a little awkward when you say it backward, but it does work!) I wonder if Jesus said it that way for the times in our lives that are so mixed up that we don't know if we're coming or going!

Now, years down the road, my bout with cancer is just a vague and bad memory. Annette is still my best friend—thanks to a covenant promise and the technology of e-mail! And the house stands again!

Sometimes I pull my old journals out from under the bed, blow off the dust bunnies, read my account of those years and marvel again as I see the fingerprints of God on every page.

PRAYER

Lord, thank You for Your promise never to leave us or forsake us! We trust You to walk by our side as we go through every difficult moment of our lives.

Journal: What difficulties have you and God walked through together? Write them down and record your praises for the lessons He taught you during those hard times.

—Kathy Hickey

APRIL 1

SOURCE OF ALL CREATION

Those who know your name will trust in you, for you, LORD, have never forsaken those who seek you.

PSALM 9:10

If you want to know God better, then study His *name*. The various Hebrew names of God provide a very rich study.

One of my favorite verses is Psalm 63:1: "O God, you are my God." From the Hebrew this verse is translated "O Holy Three-in-One, Thou art my Only One." When we grasp the love and desperation of the heart from which these words flowed, the rest of the psalm has a deeper and richer meaning.

Jehovah is a Hebrew word that speaks of God's being, His essence. "Jehovah" tells us God is, was and always will be. Lamentations 3:21-32 tells us about eight characteristics of Jehovah. These verses show us that when we remember these eight characteristics, we can have hope. Jehovah is merciful, compassionate, faithful, good, our deliverer, just and righteous, long-suffering and kind.

If we can see God as having these characteristics, it is easier to trust Him.

Another word for God, *Elohim*, means "the source of all creation." This means He created us and planned the details of our existence. In support of this truth, Jesus told us that God knows our needs before we ask Him (see Matt. 6:8). God could easily have met all our needs without our saying even one prayer. But He wants us to *know* Him. He wants us to believe that He wants to provide for our needs. He wants us to have faith that He will keep His promises.

PRAYER

O Holy Three-in-One, Thou art my Only One. Your Word tells us in Psalm 139:7-10 that no matter where we go, You are with us and aware of our every circumstance. Thank You for Your faithfulness and for the many names You bear. Your name is mighty and worthy of our praise.

Journal: Write a love note to God and tell Him what He means to you today.

—Becky Sirt

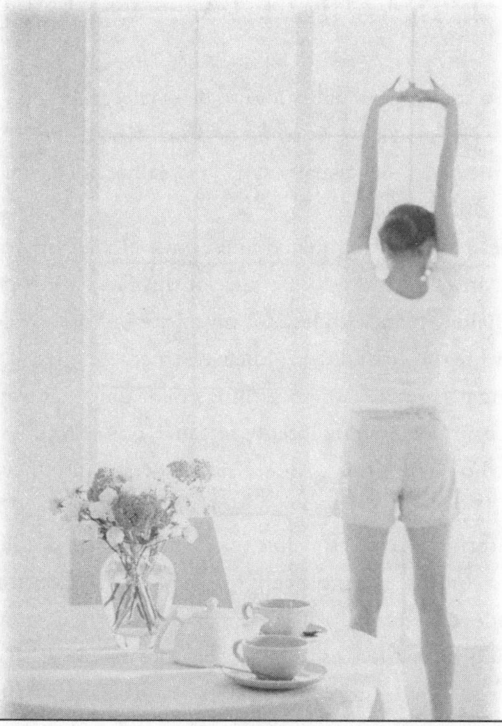

Life Under Control

SECTION THREE

Introduction

Those of us born with a strong personality love to be in charge. When I lead a First Place class, I can always spot the people with strong personalities. If they've had a bad week, when they get up on the scale, they usually say, "I'm really out of control." I spot them because I am one of them.

People like me desire to control our families, our weight, our circumstances—and just about every other area of life as well! Because of this facet of my personality, I lived the Christian life for 30 long years with Jesus as my Savior but not my Lord. Until I relinquished control of my life to Christ, I never knew real victory.

If we have a strong personality, we want things to be done our way. I am still learning that when I'm in control, He isn't. Florence Littauer, one of my mentors in the faith, says that those of us who possess this strong, choleric personality "have a problem with the sovereignty of God."[1]

Here's what I'm learning: God is not able to do the work He would like to do in our lives until He has total control. The Bible verses used in this section teach all of us what it means to live life under Christ's control. We learn how Christians should talk. We learn how we are to think and what it means to be "crucified with Christ" (Gal. 2:20). And we learn how to be content—even during times of stress. And we learn that our tongues can be weapons the enemy uses, unless they are under Christ's control.

I believe that God wants complete control of you and me so that our lives will overflow with the hope that is found only in Him.

My prayer for you comes from the second verse used in this section, Romans 15:13: "May the God of hope fill you with all joy and peace as you trust in him, so that you may overflow with hope by the power of the Holy Spirit."

—Carole Lewis

JOY THAT BLOSSOMS

Restore to me the joy of your salvation and grant me a willing spirit, to sustain me.

PSALM 51:12

In October 1997, my husband, Johnny, was diagnosed with prostate cancer, which had metastasized to his bones. Before this news, I had always thought of myself as a strong person who could find something positive in every situation. As we left the hospital after receiving the bad news, I began to cry like I had never cried before. Johnny hadn't eaten a bite all day because of all the tests, so he was very hungry. We decided to stop at a little restaurant on the way home, so he could eat. I cried all the way to the restaurant, all the way through dinner and for the next three days.

On the third day, I looked at Johnny and said how sorry I was that I couldn't be strong for him when he needed me so badly to be strong. He looked at me and said, "How do you think I would feel right now if you weren't sad?" My countenance immediately lifted; we had a good laugh about that statement, and God began to fill me again with His hope and joy.

It has been four years since those first dark days of his diagnosis, and I have come to see the manifold blessings God has bestowed on the two of us, even though Johnny still has cancer. I've heard it said that happiness happens, but joy blossoms in the storm. Through this time, Johnny and I have both learned to experience joy, even when we aren't happy about some particular circumstance of the journey we are taking.

PRAYER

Dear Lord, You are the source of my joy. Grant me a willing spirit today for whatever lies ahead.

Journal: Write down one problem that is causing you to experience a lack of joy. Ask God to give you back your joy and to grant you a willing spirit to sustain you in the days ahead.

—Carole Lewis

SUSTAINING JOY

Restore to me the joy of your salvation and grant me a willing spirit, to sustain me.

PSALM 51:12

When you hear the word "salvation," what comes to mind?

Many people think of going to heaven. True, through His saving grace, Jesus can rescue us from a miserable eternity. But is there more? If we accept His salvation only to get that "ticket to heaven," why would we need Him to lead healthy lives here?

How many times have you enthusiastically started a diet, only to quit after a period of time? You retreat to the old ways of living, indulging in whatever you'd been denying yourself; and before long, the pounds are back—maybe with a few more added. You feel physically miserable, and the ache in your heart is still there. You wonder, *How will I have the strength to get back on track, if I ever do?*

Thankfully, Jesus can give us this strength. He not only provides eternal life but also an abundant earthly life, and the strength to continue in it. In Psalm 51, David laments his many sins. He earnestly prays, knowing that God can restore his former joy. He also knows that the Lord can give him the desire to be obedient as well as the strength to sustain that obedience.

Isn't that what we all want in First Place—and in life? Don't we all want enthusiasm, an obedient heart and endurance? All of these things are possible through Jesus. He yearns to save us from spiritual torment after death as well as in our present struggles. All we have to do is accept His hand. He is waiting, ready to give you the healthy life you dream of.

PRAYER

Lord, please bring back the joy, dedication and power that I need to live the abundant life You want for me. Thank You for Your sustaining love.

Journal: Write a prayer of praise to God for the grace He offers each of us.

—Laura Hartness

APRIL 4

A Home Full of Joy

Restore to me the joy of your salvation and grant me a willing spirit, to sustain me.

PSALM 51:12

When my husband and I moved into our home 14 years ago, I took great joy in keeping house. It was spacious, bright and cozy. I had an abundance of room for everything, and I made trips to the department store to fill any empty spaces. Believe it or not, I enjoyed cleaning, vacuuming, rearranging furniture and hanging pictures.

However, I recently discovered that my joy in taking care of my home had diminished and many times was outright drudgery. My energy was depleted just thinking about cleaning closets. I needed more space!

During my quiet time recently, I shared with God my dissatisfaction about my home. In a short time, this verse from Psalm 51 came to me. I believe God was using my situation with my physical home to point out a problem in my spiritual life—in the home of my heart. God reminded me how joyful and excited I had been when I first invited Jesus into the home of my heart 27 years ago. I took great care to keep it bright and in good shape. I even went out of my way to find opportunities to share Christ with others. Lately though, I had been complaining to God about how busy I had become, and I had even made excuses like, "I'm too tired."

That was when I realized I needed to be restored, revived and sustained. Only God can do that. He will pour His strength and energy into you, as you memorize His Word and spend time with Him in prayer. He can give you the joy you once felt, even when you're tired or busy. Then you can return to caring for your home—both the inner one and the outer one—joyfully doing all that you need to do.

PRAYER

Dear God, I want always to experience the joy of my salvation—no matter how many years pass by. Grant me a willing spirit to get me through life's challenges.

Journal: Write a prayer asking God to restore His joy to every area of your life.

—June Chapko

APRIL 5

JOY IN THE DESERT

Restore to me the joy of your salvation and grant me a willing spirit, to sustain me.

PSALM 51:12

After years of experiencing a wonderful, personal relationship with Jesus Christ, I understood for the first time what David was saying in this verse.

I experienced spiritual breakthrough after joining a First Place group in Mountain Home, Arkansas, in 1994. I learned through the nine commitments how to have a special time with God. Praying regularly did not come easily; I really had to commit to it. But God was so faithful to honor my effort that I soon grew to treasure this time. I felt true fellowship with God in my daily quiet times.

Then came a time when everything went dry. I sensed almost a silence from Him. Days and weeks went by, and as I prayed and read His Word, I felt no connection to Him. I thought this season would pass, but it did not.

I began to plead with God to show me what I was allowing to block my fellowship with Him. After praying Psalm 51:12 for days and weeks, God began to show me areas of sin that I was allowing to get in the way. After confessing and repenting of these sins, He answered my heart's cry. He filled me with the joy of His salvation and granted me a willing spirit.

PRAYER

Lord, I pray that I will always know the joy of Your salvation
and enjoy true fellowship with You.

Journal: Describe a time in your life when the faithfulness of God lifted you out of a spiritual desert.

—Jill Jamieson

APRIL 6

Joy Restored

Restore to me the joy of your salvation and grant me a willing spirit, to sustain me.

PSALM 51:12

My younger brother was recently killed in a terrible accident. The paralyzing grief gave way to a growing sadness. Many things deep inside me were affected, even though I often did not understand my feelings or reactions at the time. My inner turmoil impacted how I treated others, and even more, it directly impacted how I treated myself.

We may try to smother the discomfort with different kinds of temporary relief: overactivity, alcohol, inappropriate relationships or the misuse of food. But overindulgence is often a symptom of an accumulation of unresolved painful experiences. If we are dominated by long periods of painful emotions such as grief, guilt, anger or shame, and we fail to deal with these troubling emotions, troubling results are sure to follow. We attempt to quench the fire of past and present pain with quick fixes, but these only add fuel to our dysfunction.

Instead, we need to turn to God and allow His grace to revive and renew us. Having joy restored involves honestly facing the source of pain and loss and then walking through restoration with a commitment to make right those things that can be righted and adjusting to what can't be changed!

Pain can make us bitter or better. When we rest in God, joy comes to us—not because all places are full of joy, but because God, who *is* joy, can come to be with us in all places.

PRAYER

Father, may I be Your instrument to bring joy to joyless places. Use my pain for another's gain. Make me an instrument of Your peace and joy.

Journal: What situations are you allowing to block God's joy in your life? Ask God to take away the joy blockers from your life and give you courage to conquer them. Find at least one opportunity today to bring joy to a joyless situation.

—Dr. Bill Heston

APRIL 7

NOT BY COINCIDENCE

May the God of hope fill you with all joy and peace as you trust in him, so that you may overflow with hope by the power of the Holy Spirit.

ROMANS 15:13

Right after my husband, Johnny, was diagnosed with prostate cancer, we received a video and a subscription to a newsletter called *Cancer Communication*. The video featured a doctor speaking about prostate cancer. I was still in a state of shock then, and I have no idea which of our First Place members sent these items to us.

As we were seeking the right treatment, we researched everything available about the disease. At our First Place Fitness Week, just before Johnny's diagnosis, I met a wonderful couple who lived in Bakersfield, California. The husband was diagnosed with the same disease just a few months after we met. Not coincidentally, he was seeing the same doctor in California that I had been reading about in the newsletter sent by the First Place member.

The man's wife began to e-mail me, urging that we come for a consultation with their doctor—an oncologist who specializes in prostate cancer and whose patients come from all over the world for treatment.

Johnny had finished his 13 months of hormone therapy, and we were at a crossroads. So we decided to go to California to get a second opinion. We ended up choosing this doctor as our primary physician. Today, we are under the care of an oncologist in Houston, but he follows the instructions of our doctor in California.

God specializes in difficult assignments; He is truly the God of hope. He orchestrated all of these "random" events in order to give us hope and fill us with joy and peace.

PRAYER

O Lord, may I trust You with every perplexing circumstance in my life today. Fill me with joy and peace as I trust in You so that I will overflow with hope by the power of Your Holy Spirit.

Journal: Confess to God areas in which you have lost your joy and peace and ask Him to fill you with hope again.

—Carole Lewis

APRIL 8

The Way to Freedom

May the God of hope fill you with all joy and peace as you trust in him, so that you may overflow with hope by the power of the Holy Spirit.

ROMANS 15:13

Do you ever wish you could be free to forget the Nine Commitments and indulge in whatever your heart desires? When I became pregnant in 1999, I granted myself this wish for nine months—and it cost me dearly.

During my pregnancy, I went far beyond the normal weight gain and put on 90 pounds. By God's grace I gave birth to a healthy boy; however, I was damaged physically, emotionally and spiritually. Doing my own thing had not brought me the fulfillment I had been looking for.

A year ago I returned to First Place. With God's help, I have shed 70 pounds and learned some valuable lessons. There have been times when I've thought that the nine commitments were keeping me from things I really wanted. This simply is a false belief. I realized that I had used junk food to replace God in my life. Overindulgence brought bondage and emptiness, instead of true happiness.

Only in doing God's will do I find the freedom to live in true peace and fullness. God's rules aren't there to keep us from life but to save us from physical and spiritual death. C.S. Lewis wrote, "We are far too easily pleased."[2] By that, I think he meant that we think we can be completely satisfied by what the world offers—but we're wrong.

God has so much more in store for us than we would naturally strive for. All we have to do is trust Him and follow His direction.

PRAYER

Lord, only You can fill me with true joy and peace. Be in my life every moment this day so that I can know the hope that only You can give.

Journal: Make a list of the eternal blessings God has poured into your life. Thank Him for each one individually.

—Laura Hartness

APRIL 9

LETTING HIS POWER REIGN

May the God of hope fill you with all joy and peace as you trust in him, so that you may overflow with hope by the power of the Holy Spirit.

ROMANS 15:13

Overflowing hope is a treasure I do not take lightly. Having survived breast cancer twice, I consider each new day a gift from God. Having lost a lot of weight and gained my life back, I count every minute as precious.

I began First Place in June 2000, weighing over 300 pounds. I had a very low self-esteem and feared dying of a heart attack more than cancer. I was desperate! I had drudged through every possible diet I could afford, and First Place was my last-ditch attempt. I knew that I was being disobedient to God in my eating habits and choices.

Memorizing Romans 15:13 was like a spring of fresh water to my soul. I needed the hope, joy and peace that God gives to His children. I decided that this time I would allow God's power to reign in me. One year later, I am still pressing on—but 60 pounds lighter! God has blessed me with the privilege of leading a First Place group Bible study, which challenges me to encourage others to live balanced lives.

We all need hope; we all need the power of the Holy Spirit. Reading Romans 15:13 makes me realize that by God's power I can abound in hope and I can minister, not only to people in the First Place program, but also to others who are experiencing various trials in their lives.

PRAYER

Thank You, Jesus, for the joy and peace that overflows with hope when I trust in You and only You.

Journal: What do you hope for today? Journal your thoughts as a prayer to your Father.

—Jeannie Gramly

APRIL 10

POWERED BY HOPE

May the God of hope fill you with all joy and peace as you trust in him, so that you may overflow with hope by the power of the Holy Spirit.

ROMANS 15:13

Many times during my life I have been unhealthy, miserable and hopeless. When I asked myself why, I could only come up with one reason: I was trusting in my own strength to get me out of whatever condition I found myself; I was not trusting in God to deliver me.

There is no joy or peace when I trust in myself. Ultimately, I will fail if I am relying on my own strength. But with Christ as my source of strength, I am free to be at peace and experience true joy. I am confident that God will come through, no matter what my circumstance.

When we trust in ourselves, we have no hope; but when we trust in the God of hope, we can experience His joy and peace, overflowing with hope in all areas of our lives. Spiritually, my hope of salvation comes through Jesus, who says, "I am the way and the truth and the life" (John 14:6). Emotionally, my hope of experiencing peace comes through the Holy Spirit who provides the fruit of "love, joy, peace, patience, kindness, goodness, faithfulness, gentleness and self-control" (Gal. 5:22)—all wonderful Spirit-controlled emotions! Mentally, I can have the hope of wisdom and insight through the Word of God, which is truth—the only truth! Physically, I can have hope because God created my body to honor Him, and He provides me with everything I need to live (see 2 Pet.1:3).

PRAYER

Lord, teach me to trust in You so that I can experience Your peace and overflowing joy.

Journal: Describe how God's hope is touching each area of your life: spiritual, emotional, mental and physical.

—Nancy Taylor

APRIL 11

Overflowing Hope

May the God of hope fill you with all joy and peace as you trust in him, so that you may overflow with hope by the power of the Holy Spirit.

ROMANS 15:13

Hope. Those who study human behavior tell us that we cannot live without it.

Who needs a professional to analyze that one? Hopelessness is no fun. Hopelessness doesn't feel good. Hopelessness is cousin to helplessness and brother to worthlessness; and, frankly, worthlessness is how I feel about life when hope is drained from me.

I think I know why Paul prayed for the believers in Rome to have hope—because without hope, life stinks.

Okay, so that's a given. But suppose I'm feeling hopeless about a situation, a relationship, my work, my future—my weight? Where can I, how can I, hope? Here is Paul's insight: Hope comes from God. And God has so much of it to offer that He's giving it away free!

God can freely give out hope because it is His to give. And what's more, God is not stingy in His giving. Paul says that your hope will *overflow*. Sometimes I would be satisfied with even a trickle of hope—but an overflow? Now that's worth seeking!

God's hope comes packaged with joy and peace. All we need to do is trust Him. If yesterday was a hopeless day, don't be discouraged. Pray to the God who can make your day overflow with hope.

PRAYER

Lord, replenish my supply of hope from Your boundless reservoir.
Let Your flow become my overflow.

Journal: Write a prayer asking the God of all hope to begin a new flow from His reservoir to your heart.

—Rob Heath

THINKING ON THE TRUTH

Finally, brothers, whatever is true, whatever is noble, whatever is right, whatever is pure, whatever is lovely, whatever is admirable— if anything is excellent or praiseworthy—think about such things.

PHILIPPIANS 4:8

Shortly after my husband, Johnny, was diagnosed with cancer, he told me the worst times for him occurred while he was driving. Alone in the car, he would worry about the future and how long he might live.

One day as he was driving along, he said to God, "If I only knew how long I have to live." A mile or two of highway went by. And then he said it was as if God put a billboard in front of him with only two words on it: "Nobody does."

From that day, Johnny says, he's had a different perspective on his disease. Truly, none of us know if we will be here tomorrow. Our thought-life can get us into so much trouble when God isn't given permission to control it.

Our daughter, Shari, told Johnny shortly after his diagnosis that she had been battling depressing thoughts about his cancer when God reminded her that everyone's future is uncertain and that she could be gone before he was. As you know now, this ironically proved to be true.

Satan is a great manipulator, and he uses fear to fill our souls with deep unrest. Take control of your thoughts today. When feelings of hopelessness, worthlessness or despair come into your thoughts, chase them away with the truth of your situation—which you will find through prayer and God's Word.

PRAYER

Dear Father, help me to think about You and the truth of my situation today. Fill my mind with thoughts that are true, noble, right, pure, lovely, admirable, excellent and praiseworthy.

Journal: Write down all the thoughts you entertain that are the opposite of Philippians 4:8. Ask God to replace these thoughts with the truth of this verse.

—Carole Lewis

APRIL 13

LIVER AND ONIONS?

Finally, brothers, whatever is true, whatever is noble, whatever is right, whatever is pure, whatever is lovely, whatever is admirable— if anything is excellent or praiseworthy—think about such things.

PHILIPPIANS 4:8

Getting life under control has been a struggle for me—because I'm addicted to chocolate! I eat the stuff when I'm happy, sad, sick or need comfort. You get the picture!

First Place taught me that chocolate is not always a healthy choice. I desperately wanted to be true to the program and noble for my Lord. I wanted to be a pure and lovely person—without chocolate on my hands and face. I wanted folks to admire my disciplined life.

At first I thought I'd found the perfect verse to help me out—Philippians 4:8. Armed with this truth, I would head down the chocolate aisle reciting the verse under my breath. But what was that scent I was smelling?

I found that just reciting a verse does not always work. Chocolate is "excellent" in my eyes! Through time in prayer, I finally discovered the secret to conquering that aisle: I took the food I disliked the most—liver and onions—and repeated it under my breath as I walked down the candy aisle.

Much to my horror I do not always repeat these words quietly enough. Often someone will stop me and ask, "Why are you saying, 'Liver and onions'?"

All I can say is that this can be a great way to open up a conversation that leads to witnessing for our Lord!

PRAYER

Lord, fine-tune my desires so that I want only those things that honor You.

Journal: Make a list of the healthy foods that you really enjoy. Thank God for giving you food that nourishes and sustains your health.

—Betha Jean Cunningham

APRIL 14

REPEAT AFTER ME

Finally, brothers, whatever is true, whatever is noble, whatever is right, whatever is pure, whatever is lovely, whatever is admirable— if anything is excellent or praiseworthy—think about such things.

PHILIPPIANS 4:8

There are times in my life when people say things that really hurt me. I'm sure you have experienced this too. We can say, "Sticks and stones may break my bones, but words will never hurt me"; but the truth is that hurtful words can cut us to the core.

When I'm badly hurt, I become angry—I do not feel I deserve to be treated so unkindly. But I can't dwell in that hurtful place, so I confess my anger to God and get on with life by repeating Philippians 4:8. God's wants me to dwell on better words: His! I need to think about the things that are true, noble, right, pure, lovely, admirable and praiseworthy.

When I obey God's direction to "think about such things," I find that I have not only forgiven the person who hurt me but I'm also praising God for the good things He has done for me.

I thank God for the truth that He gives us in Philippians 4:8. I thank God I have Him to walk with me through this journey of life. His Word is something I can really depend upon.

PRAYER

Thank You, Abba, for Your words that show me Your love.
Discipline me to become more like You.

Journal: Has someone hurt you with unkind or unfair words? Forgive that person by faith and ask God to show you how to respond to the person with compassion and wisdom.

—Betha Jean Cunningham

APRIL 15

NOT "WHATEVER!"

Finally, brothers, whatever is true, whatever is noble, whatever is right, whatever is pure, whatever is lovely, whatever is admirable— if anything is excellent or praiseworthy—think about such things.

PHILIPPIANS 4:8

I have an acquaintance who almost always says "Whatever!" in a haphazard way. In this way she effectively shuts down conversations she's reluctant or unwilling to continue. Not long ago I became frustrated trying unsuccessfully to pursue the topic we were discussing.

I later took my frustration to God and asked for His wisdom. That week Philippians 4:8 appeared as my memory verse. God poured His love on me and answered my prayer. I used the attributes in this verse to make a list of my friend's best qualities, one for each day of the week. Then I used each one as a basis for a prayer for God's ongoing work in her life.

As time went on, I watched for an opportunity to engage her in conversation. And it came! As we discussed a difficult work project, she tried to end our conversation with a disdainful "Whatever!"

Before my usual frustration could surface, I quickly responded, "I have been wanting to tell you how *admirable* I think you are."

She stopped short. "What?"

I repeated my statement. Then I went on to explain that I thought it was admirable of her to complete her project early and then help a coworker finish hers. Instead of gruffly walking away, she said, "Thank you for noticing."

It seemed to me she stood a little taller and returned to her desk.

I thank God that He showed me how to help another human being feel good about herself. In Christ, I stand a little taller too.

PRAYER

Lord, help me always to respond to others in ways that are noble, right, pure, lovely, admirable, excellent or praiseworthy.

Journal: Write down the name of someone who you know needs uplifting. Ask God to show His love to that person through you.

—June Chapko

APRIL 16

FEEDING YOUR MIND

Finally, brothers, whatever is true, whatever is noble, whatever is right, whatever is pure, whatever is lovely, whatever is admirable— if anything is excellent or praiseworthy—think about such things.

PHILIPPIANS 4:8

What a difference a subtle shift in attitude makes! This truth was recently brought home to me while I was leading a First Place group for men in our church.

About 12 of us had gathered at noontime, and one man said he was motivated to lose weight because he was attending his high school reunion in a month. He wanted to lose weight to impress his old cronies. It was obvious he was only interested in losing pounds—not in reaching for the goal of a balanced Christian life.

The attitude this man had was reflected in other areas of his life. Seldom did he arrive on time or complete his Bible studies. After the weigh-in, he complained loudly about the program. "This thing does not work!" he challenged with great authority.

The other group members generally sat in silence and let him ramble. He would complain, "I've eaten exactly like you said, and I haven't lost a pound."

He obviously didn't like my response when I told him, "That isn't physically possible. If you exercise and follow the program's food plan and eat right portions, you *will* lose weight. Your body has no choice. It isn't what you write down on the Commitment Record that matters: It's what you put in your mouth that adds up."

Similarly, what you feed your mind will determine what you think. Are you negative, critical or obsessed with sleazy thoughts? Paul gives a remedy for this: Feed your mind things that are true, noble, right, pure, lovely, admirable, excellent and praiseworthy.

PRAYER

Dear Father, I desire to be a person who has a mind that thinks on higher things. Give me wisdom and discipline to feed my mind the nourishment it needs.

Journal: Select one of the "mind foods" listed in Philippines 4:8 that needs to be added to your "life list." Write a plan for including new sources of positive thinking.

—Bill Heston

APRIL 17

AN ETERNAL PERSPECTIVE

I have been crucified with Christ and I no longer live, but Christ lives in me. The life I live in the body, I live by faith in the Son of God, who loved me and gave himself for me.

GALATIANS 2:20

What does it mean to be crucified with Christ? I visited recently with a precious friend, who is 34 years old and who has had stage-four breast cancer since she was 28. We talked about her and her husband's battle with this disease and how Christ is sufficient at every bend and turn of the journey.

I believe that to be crucified with Christ means four things:

1. Our physical life must cease to be our primary concern.
2. We realize that we live and breathe by the life of Christ which is now in us.
3. The life we live in the body is just a spot on the continuum from creation until the time when Jesus returns for His Bride.
4. Only what we do in the way of Kingdom work will last after we are gone.

To be crucified with Christ means that we die to our wants and wishes. We rest in the knowledge that God wants good for us and that He will take care of us and protect us when we let Him control our life.

Most of us spend a lot of time telling God what we want and what He needs to do for us. Today, try asking God what He wants and what He needs from you.

Then sit quietly until you hear Him speak to your heart.

PRAYER

Lord, I don't fully understand what it means to be crucified with Christ. Teach me this important truth.

Journal: Make a list of the worries of this life that consume you. Ask God to crucify your flesh and help you see the bigger picture of His plan for you.

—Carole Lewis

APRIL 18

LIVING SACRIFICE

I have been crucified with Christ and I no longer live, but Christ lives in me. The life I live in the body, I live by faith in the Son of God, who loved me and gave himself for me.

GALATIANS 2:20

The word "crucifixion" brings to mind the picture of a cruel death on a cross. According to *The Holman Bible Dictionary*, "The cross on which Christ was crucified became the means by which Jesus became the atoning sacrifice for our sins. It also became a symbol for the sacrifice of self in discipleship and death of self to the world."[3]

Have I been crucified with Christ? Do I sacrifice my own desires and amibitions? Am I dead to the world's pull?

The apostle Paul urges us to offer our bodies "as living sacrifices" (Rom. 12:1). This means presenting ourselves as living sacrifices, worshiping Him and making our lives an appropriate offering.

Many times I am a very reluctant sacrifice. My hands are not open in obedience but are clenched in fists of refusal. Often my eyes are not open to see Him but are squeezed tight in the pain of letting go. My face does not mirror the peace of joyful submission but reflects a grimace of disgust. Too often I am not found kneeling humbly before Him but am squirming to break free.

If I am to be a living sacrifice, holy and pleasing to Him, I know I must adopt the attitudes of a servant—and freely offer my body, mind and spirit in acts of worship to Him.

I long to be His fragrant offering.

PRAYER

Lord, as I come before You today with myself as my offering, please humble me and allow me to worship with a pure heart. May everything I think, say, do and eat today be a rich sacrifice, holy and pleasing to You, worthy of my Christ.

Journal: List areas of your life that you must let go of in order to become a pleasing sacrifice. How will you let go of them?

—Judy Marshall

APRIL 19

DIE TO LIVE

I have been crucified with Christ and I no longer live, but Christ lives in me. The life I live in the body, I live by faith in the Son of God, who loved me and gave himself for me.

GALATIANS 2:20

Put me to death.
Tear off my tough, crusted shell of sin—
It runs deep.
Flush hatred and bitterness from my mind—
Its roots hold me fast.
Carve jealousy and dissention from my heart—
It is becoming part of me.
Purge sinful actions from my body—
They cover me like a heavy chain.
Stay my wandering feet—
They stray so easily.
Put me to death!

Live in me.
Surround me with a soft covering—
It must be pliable.
Saturate my mind with love and peace.
May I overflow with all that is You.
Fill my empty heart with the knowledge of You.
Keep me in Your Word.
Guide me to loving actions.
May I serve obediently and completely.
Speed my feet on the narrow path.
Hold me fast and true.
Live in me!

PRAYER

Lord, thank You for giving Yourself for me. May I always yield to Your work in my life so that You can live through me.

Journal: Are you allowing God to perform surgery on your body, mind and heart? What does He need to remove so that you are an empty vessel He can fill?

—Helen McCormack

APRIL 20

CHANGE MY "I" SIGHT

I have been crucified with Christ and I no longer live, but Christ lives in me. The life I live in the body, I live by faith in the Son of God, who loved me and gave himself for me.

GALATIANS 2:20

As an overweight person, one of my biggest problems was that I had bad "I" problems. Here's what I mean.

"I" couldn't understand why I had a weight problem.

"I" didn't think it was fair that my friend Teri could eat anything she wanted and be so skinny.

"I" couldn't figure out why I couldn't lose weight.

"I" didn't think I should have to exercise to lose weight.

"I" just knew I was going to grow old and fat.

"I" didn't think it was fair that I was tired all the time.

"I" couldn't stay on a diet because "I" didn't like fruits and vegetables.

"I" couldn't eat breakfast because food makes me sick when I first get up out of bed.

"I, I, I"—yes, I had some really bad "I" problems.

Then I learned that our enemy the devil loves to keep our "I"s out of focus. He delights in keeping our vision turned toward our problems. Before I came to First Place, I was just about fed up with my "I"s. I was ready to turn my eyes on Jesus.

That is what I have learned to do. And now "I" no longer live, but Christ lives in me. Where I used to seek to be thin, I now seek the kingdom of God and His righteousness. Once my "I"s became Kingdom eyes, the thing I was seeking the most—weight loss—was added to me (or should I say deleted from me!).

I was seeking to be thin, and I have lost weight in First Place. But more important, Jesus changed my "I" sight.

PRAYER

Thank You, Jesus, for my new Kingdom eyes.

Journal: List the "I"s that keep you from focusing on living a balanced life in Christ. For each one, list a thought from God's Word that shows you His perpective.

—Beverly Henson

APRIL 21

THE SECRET OF CONTENTMENT

I have learned the secret of being content in any and every situation, whether well fed or hungry, whether living in plenty or in want. I can do everything through him who gives me strength.

PHILIPPIANS 4:12-13

Those of us living in America have a hard time fathoming physical hunger or real want of any kind. Americans are probably the best-fed and most overfed people in the world.

We can, however, identify with everyone else in the human race in regard to the struggle for daily contentment. I have had many people share with me how, after reaching their weight goal in First Place, they still struggle with being content. When they started the program, they thought that they would finally be content when they lost weight. Instead, they have discovered that they have only traded the compulsive behavior of overeating for some other compulsion such as shopping.

True contentment is found only in Jesus Christ. He is the One who heals all our diseases and delivers us from our compulsions.

May we learn the secret of being content in any and every situation, whether overweight or thin, whether living in a mansion or in an apartment. We can truly do anything and everything through Him who gives us strength.

PRAYER

Dear Lord, teach me the secret of being content where I am right now.

Journal: Make a list of the areas in which you lack contentment. Ask God to give you His contentment and the strength to overcome your compulsions.

—Carole Lewis

APRIL 22

Confident and Content

I have learned the secret of being content in any and every situation, whether well fed or hungry, whether living in plenty or in want. I can do everything through him who gives me strength.

PHILIPPIANS 4:12-13

To be content is a choice. It is a state I must choose by an act of my will.

To be content is to accept whatever circumstance God places before me, knowing that He has the outcome figured out. Whether it is a time of waiting, struggle, grief, uncertainty or blessing, God desires for me to cling to Him.

Choosing to be content can be a powerful witness for Christ, since our world does not foster that condition in us. Discontentment and the hunger for more material things are hallmarks of our culture and its values. But God calls us to live a life with different priorities.

Through First Place, I have learned that the struggles others face can put my own life into proper perspective. One widowed woman who was facing cancer surgery and treatment stands out in my memory. She was the greatest testimony to contentment that I've ever met. She walked in confidence with her Lord. Everything about her radiated the light of Christ. Her spirit of faith gave much honor and glory to God.

To be content, we must have confidence in the One who made us. When we realize that He made us and cares for us, we can face anything.

PRAYER

Lord, help me to be content with whatever situation You provide for me.
You are able to give me the strength and ability to accomplish anything.

Journal: List several times when God provided for you in the midst of difficult situations. Thank Him for His faithfulness.

—Pattie Perry

APRIL 23

BLESSINGS IN A HARD SITUATION

I have learned the secret of being content in any and every situation, whether well fed or hungry, whether living in plenty or in want. I can do everything through him who gives me strength.

PHILIPPIANS 4:12-13

As the cancer progressed in my husband, Ray, I watched his faith in God grow. His walk with God became noticeably more intimate.

Ray told everyone that he was in a win-win situation. If God allowed him more time to live, it was a miracle and he was the winner. And if God took him home to heaven, he was an even bigger winner. One of the nurses who cared for him during his last few days commented later that Ray had a living faith and a dying faith.

During his illness, Ray used every opportunity to share with others his faith in God. One of those people was a single woman who had moved away from her church and rejected her Christian upbringing. Ray explained to her that she would not be truly satisfied until she got her life straight with God and was active in a church—and this was only hours before he went to be with the Lord!

Ray's attitude and actions have made it easier for me to get through the lonely days and nights. Do I miss Ray? You had better believe I do. And when I need to, I let the tears flow.

And at the same time, the way that Ray passed from this life builds my faith. Knowing he was facing death, Ray was a stronger witness than ever for his Lord.

PRAYER

Lord, please help me to be content in every situation. Give me the wisdom and power to face any trials or obstacles I may face today.

Journal: Give examples of times in your life when you were able to be a witness for God, even in the midst of difficult circumstances.

—Betha Jean Cunningham

APRIL 24

Decidedly Content

I have learned the secret of being content in any and every situation, whether well fed or hungry, whether living in plenty or in want. I can do everything through him who gives me strength.

PHILIPPIANS 4:12-13

When I accepted the challenge to become a First Place leader, I knew very little about the program. As a nurse I knew about nutrition and food exchange lists, but I was still 50 pounds overweight. I assumed that leading adults through a Bible study and weight-loss program couldn't be that difficult!

So I thought.

As the day of my first class approached, I found myself overwhelmed by the magnitude of my undertaking. Thoughts of fear crept in. I was certainly not a biblical scholar—I wasn't even comfortable praying out loud!

The one thing I did have on my side was God. I prayed for His strength and guidance and watched with amazement as God worked through me to teach, support and uplift the members of my class.

Then I was faced with another challenge: my 90-year-old father was hospitalized with heart failure. I had to be the strong one for my mother. I was the nurse who asked the questions and then explained the answers to my mother. I was my father's advocate in making life-sustaining decisions. I had always dreaded the day that this would happen. I knew I wasn't really strong and I feared I would crumble under the pressure.

But God had a different plan for me. He gave me His strength. He gave me the peace I needed to make difficult decisions. Because of Him, I had no fear, no guilt. I was content with my decisions.

What a comfort God is!

PRAYER

Lord, no matter what challenge lies ahead for me, I know that I can face everything with Your help. Thank You for teaching me the secret of contentment in all I do: faith in You.

Journal: What overwhelming challenge lies ahead of you right now? List the ways in which God has promised in His Word to help you through this challenge.

—Marie Muller

"I CAN" CONFIDENCE

I have learned the secret of being content in any and every situation, whether well fed or hungry, whether living in plenty or in want. I can do everything through him who gives me strength.

PHILIPPIANS 4:12-13

I didn't want to go through a Bible study to help me lose weight.

I thought if I did that I would have to admit several things: I was fat, I wasn't living up to the standards God had laid out for me, and I wasn't being the kind of witness for His kingdom that I should be.

To make things worse, after my mother died in 1995 from stomach cancer, my weight escalated over a period of three years to a whopping 220 pounds! I knew I had to do something about it—or die.

I finally got up enough courage to join First Place. In the first session, Philippians 4:13 was quoted to me: "I can do all things through [Christ] who gives me strength."

At home I wrote the verse on a card and put it on the refrigerator door. Every time I was tempted to go to the fridge, I'd read that verse.

Then one day those words became real to me: I realized I *can* do all things through Christ! He gives me the strength to say no to the food that has always controlled my life. I realize now that to give Christ first place in my life means that He will help me to be the kind of witness He wants me to be.

I have lost 80 pounds—but only through the grace of God. That's what I have to tell everyone who asks me, "How did you do it?"

To God be the glory!

PRAYER

Lord Jesus, thank You for reminding me that I can do everything—but only through You! Lord, help me do this, not for my glory, but to glorify You.

Journal: What is it that you want to do? List several goals you would like to achieve and explain tell how each of them will glorify God.

—Shelley Wilburn

APRIL 26

INVITED TO JOIN

Do not think of yourself more highly than you ought, but rather think of yourself with sober judgment, in accordance with the measure of faith God has given you.

ROMANS 12:3

I've heard it said a lot: Pride comes before the fall. To put it in today's vernacular, we set ourselves up to fall when we start to believe our own press.

The people I know who are accomplishing the most for the cause of Christ are those people who have a clear sense that their success has nothing to do with their talents or abilities. Instead, they know, as author Henry Blackaby put it, success has everything to do with "watching to see where God is working and joining Him."[4]

We can never take credit for the great things that happen in or through us, because we know that God is the One doing the work. Rather, we can be grateful that He is allowing us the privilege of coming along for the ride.

When God invited me to join Him in the work He was already doing with First Place, I had a choice. I could stay where I was in my comfortable job, or I could join Him for the most joyous ride I could have ever imagined. God could have chosen someone else if I had turned down His invitation, and His work in First Place would have still gotten done. But I am so grateful He gave the opportunity to me!

PRAYER

Lord, help me remember that You are God and are able to accomplish anything with or without my help. Thank You for allowing me to work with You as You work.

Journal: What opportunities is God giving you to join Him in His work? Thank Him for working through you to get the job done.

—Carole Lewis

APRIL 27

EQUAL-OPPORTUNITY KINDNESS

Do not think of yourself more highly than you ought, but rather think of yourself with sober judgment, in accordance with the measure of faith God has given you.

ROMANS 12:3

Have you ever met someone who was truly humble? You automatically feel so at ease around that person and know that you can be yourself without fear of being criticized.

A few years ago I lived in East Texas and had a neighbor who wore a boot-camp style haircut and drove an old pick-up truck. He was the nicest guy you could ever hope to meet. He couldn't do enough for me—or for anyone else for that matter. He ran the Young Life group in our small town, and all the kids (including my own) loved him. He could always find a smile and normally would have you laughing in a few minutes. If I hadn't lived next door to him, I probably would have never known that he owned an enormous Purex bleach company.

My neighbor lived in a 10,000-square-foot home with a huge indoor pool. His house was nestled on a huge tract that included a large lake that we would ski and fish on. Though in the world's eyes he "had it all," he never once gave the impression that he was better than anyone else. He was just an ordinary man with a generous and kind heart. I know that was because of his relationship with Jesus.

My neighbor was a servant and always treated everyone with respect and dignity. His humility was and is a witness to me of the attitude I must make my own every day.

PRAYER

Lord, help me to always treat others with love, respect and dignity.

Journal: Describe a time when someone touched your life with unexpected kindness.

—Rick Crawford

APRIL 28

SOBER JUDGMENT, GOOD ADVICE

Do not think of yourself more highly than you ought, but rather think of yourself with sober judgment, in accordance with the measure of faith God has given you.

ROMANS 12:3

How often do we avoid pointing out areas of concern we feel for friends and loved ones because we fear hurting their feelings or, worse, we fear having them lash out in anger and end up having *our* feelings hurt.

A few years ago, my daily exercise routine was interrupted by a broken wrist. Days turned to weeks and weeks turned to months, and I looked forward to the day the cast would come off, so I could get back to exercising. Then a friend who was unaware of my dilemma inquired, "How's your exercise program coming along?"

In response, I told her of my travails. Gently, but firmly, she wondered if, just perhaps, there were some exercises I could do without using my wrist!

She was bold enough to point out the obvious, and I was thankful for her answering God's call to challenge me to get back on track. Indeed, there were several exercises I could do; it was out of pure laziness that I'd not pursued them. This dear friend was confident enough to risk hurting my feelings in order to bring a greater good—God's good—to my attention.

I want to be available to God, as my friend was, when He needs me to have the courage to nudge others back onto the path of obedience and health.

PRAYER

Lord, forgive me for making excuses for my disobedience. Use Your saints to point Your way to me when I'm lost; and open my ears, eyes and heart to listen and obey.

Journal: Whom do you know who needs a word of admonishment and encouragement? Pray for that person now, and ask God to give you an opportunity to talk with this person this week.

—Bruce Barbour

APRIL 29

SINGIN' A DIFFERENT TUNE

Do not think of yourself more highly than you ought, but rather think of yourself with sober judgment, in accordance with the measure of faith God has given you.

ROMANS 12:3

For several years, I played keyboard in the band of a well-known Christian artist. One weekend we were on a plane going to Los Angeles to perform a concert for a youth conference. I was sitting across the aisle from the guitarist. I was showing him a piece of choral music that I had written and which had recently been published. As a joke, he mentioned to the stewardess that I was a "famous composer" and showed her the music with my name on it. She was quite impressed and asked me for my autograph. Later when she was giving out the refreshments, she gave me twice as much as she did to anyone else. Soon another flight attendant asked for an autograph. By this time, I was feeling pretty good about myself.

On the ride back from L.A., it was a different story. We had a different flight crew. After we had been seated, the flight attendant came to tell me that I had to get off the plane because they had assigned the seat to someone else. They moved me to the last seat on the plane—right in between two big bikers. I felt like a human sardine. Later when the flight attendant opened a soft drink, it sprayed all over me. Without an apology, she just handed me a napkin and went on. And she hadn't brought me any peanuts!

At this point, I could clearly see what the Lord was trying to teach me. I couldn't help but laugh at the whole situation and realize that the pathway of humility is always the best road to take. Anything special about me is a gift of God. Even our faith is a gift straight from His hand.

PRAYER

Lord, help me to think soberly of myself and to walk humbly with You.

Journal: In what areas are you thinking of yourself too highly? To whom can you show more honor? In what ways can you place others above yourself?

—Jeff Nelson

APRIL 30

"PRIDE BUMPS"

Do not think of yourself more highly than you ought, but rather think of yourself with sober judgment, in accordance with the measure of faith God has given you.

ROMANS 12:3

My salvation occurred within the workings of the First Place ministry. What I thought was a rededication, God later revealed as a true conversion. This time I had a broken repentant heart when I said the sinner's prayer—an attitude I'd never had before.

Since that time I have asked for a passion for the Lord and His Word. I watch as He daily answers my prayers and gives me the desire to follow Him. And yet, in working out my salvation in fear and trembling, I have experienced some major, spiritual "pride bumps" cluttering the way.

I recently felt God asking me to step down from a ministry that He had used me to put into place. At first I resisted, but then I sensed my spiritual greediness, confessed my sin and obeyed the Lord.

Whenever we get too full of ourselves, we need to consider the examples God has set forth in the Scriptures. When Jesus rode on a donkey into Jerusalem on what we now call Palm Sunday, the people celebrated His coming by waving palm leaves and shouting words of praise as He rode by. They were praising Jesus—not the donkey He rode. This reminds me that He can use anything to accomplish His plans—even a donkey. Yet He chose to use me. Why? I don't know.

I have prayed, "Lord, let me see myself." This is one prayer I would like to revoke, but He won't let me. He continues to show me a broken vessel, which He lovingly keeps on the potter's wheel and gracefully remolds, one stroke at a time.

PRAYER

Lord, show me my spiritual pride and give me the grace I need to surrender everything to You.

Journal: List achievements in your life that you have allowed to become idols of spiritual pride. One by one, surrender them to God and reaffirm your dependence on Him.

—Denise Peters

M A Y 1

DOING THE WORD

If anyone considers himself religious and yet does not keep a tight rein on his tongue, he deceives himself and his religion is worthless.

J A M E S 1 : 2 6

I awakened very early on Thanksgiving morning, 2001. The bedside clock said 4:00 A.M. We had a big family dinner planned at our home at noon, and there was a lot to do to get things ready. I rolled over thinking, *I don't really need to get up this early*. Yet a gentle nudge got me on my feet and into our living room to meet with my Lord.

In that predawn hour, the Lord directed me to the book of James. I read it and reread it, meditating on the words James had written so long ago. Among other things, the Lord seemed to be telling me to be aware of how I use my words—an admonition I would need sooner than I expected.

Later that day when we got the news at the hospital that Shari was with Jesus, I immediately remembered how tenderly God had summoned me that morning to spend time with Him. I believe that God, knowing what lay ahead, was already sorrowing for us all and wanted to spend some personal time with me.

I was also aware of what I had read that morning. I had asked God to use me in a powerful way to bring glory to Him, especially by the spoken and written word.

Why don't you get your Bible right now and read the first chapter of James? Verse 27 tells us what God considers to be pure religion—and it isn't what we say but what we do.

P R A Y E R

Dear Lord, I ask You to keep a tight rein on my tongue today. Use me and let me bless and not curse people with my words.

Journal: Ask God to reveal how something you have said has wounded another person—it could be someone in your immediate family. As He shows you, ask His forgiveness and then, before the day is over, ask the person you wounded to forgive you.

—Carole Lewis

Revealing Words

If anyone considers himself religious and yet does not keep a tight rein on his tongue, he deceives himself and his religion is worthless.

JAMES 1:26

The tongue is a highly developed organ used for taste and speech. But that doesn't begin to describe the power of the tongue. Words can be sweet, bitter or anywhere in between, depending on their use. We have all been in situations in which words have had the warmth and peace of a fireside recliner or have pierced us through like stinging swords. Given the choice, would you choose the company of a soft-spoken person or one freely dispensing a tongue-lashing? I'd take the soft-spoken one any day!

From a biblical perspective, the meaning of "tongue" is much different. The Bible says that the tongue actually reveals what is in our hearts (see Matt. 15:18). Words are the expression of our true nature. What we choose to say reflects who we are inside and can bring a blessing or a curse to those around us. Like the bit in a horse's mouth or the rudder of a ship, the tongue can control the direction of a person's life. How we choose to use our tongue, which has potential for both good and bad, can either honor our Lord or grieve Him, can either praise God or cause separation from Him.

The tongue can also refer to unique language of a people or nation. If we are truly God's children, shouldn't we learn to speak His language fluently, so others will know we're related to Him?

PRAYER

Lord, thank You that I can daily read Your Word and become more fluent in Your language. May others know I belong to You because of the words they hear from my mouth.

Journal: When have you recently misused words? To whom were they directed? How can you rectify them?

—Judy Marshall

KEEPING A TIGHT REIN

If anyone considers himself religious and yet does not keep a tight rein on his tongue, he deceives himself and his religion is worthless.

JAMES 1:26

These are harsh words to most of us! We are all guilty of gossiping and saying things that we later regret. Let us take to heart what James says about our tongues. Christians cannot go around speaking badly of others—if we do, our religion is worthless.

When we don't let God control our tongues, they can become weapons by which we slander, criticize and hurt others. Let's turn this potential weapon into a tool that builds others up and glorifies our dear Lord.

Before making a derogatory comment about someone or something, think about this Bible verse and remember what the Lord says about keeping a "tight rein" on our tongues.

PRAYER

Father, we know we disappoint You when we use our tongue to hurt others. Help us to think before we say anything hurtful.

Journal: Have you gossiped about someone, even under the guise of a "prayer request"? Write a note asking forgiveness from anyone you have hurt in this way.

—Joe Ann Winkler

MAY 4

Do You Speak His Love?

If anyone considers himself religious and yet does not keep a tight rein on his tongue, he deceives himself and his religion is worthless.

JAMES 1:26

My tongue has been a problem since the days of my childhood when I said whatever popped into my head, sometimes to the extreme embarrassment of my mother.

As I contemplate this verse, I remember so many apologies I had to give because my mouth and brain were not in sync. This verse has helped me to really think about what I say to or about others.

When we hurt others with words spoken in anger or defense, we are letting our human nature be in control. When we submit our lives to the Holy Spirit, letting Him be in control, our words are kinder and more understanding.

Words have the power to heal or hurt, to soothe or agitate, to convey hate or love. Words may build up relationships or tear them down. Like wildfire, words spoken in anger or in haste can spread quickly, destroying everything in their path. On the other hand, words spoken in love can spread a mantle of kindness over a relationship.

Do your words spread the peace and love of God's Word? With our words, we have the opportunity to share God's love with countless lost, hurting souls. We find these people everywhere—on the street corner, at the office, at school, on vacation and even in our churches.

Let us strive to make *all* our words acceptable in His sight (see Ps. 19:14). With the Holy Spirit in control, our words have the potential to make a tremendous difference for good in the lives of others.

PRAYER

Heavenly Father, guide my thoughts and words today to be focused on You and Your great love and lead me to share Your love with others.

Journal: Describe a time when God used you to speak His Word to someone else. What happened as a result?

—Martha Rogers

MAY 5

One Kind Deed

If anyone would come after me, he must deny himself and take up his cross daily and follow me.

LUKE 9:23

One of my greatest helpers in First Place was a lady who had never been in the program. Her name was Mary Elizabeth Headland, and she was my mom's best friend. Mary Elizabeth was one of those rare people who understand the true significance of this all-important verse.

Mary Elizabeth was a wonderful chef, and she helped cook at most of our Fitness Weeks. Her needs always came after those of the people around her. She went home to be with the Lord in February 2001, and I can truly say that our world is poorer because she is gone. But her legacy didn't end with her death.

Her daughter, Sue, carried on this selfless service when my daughter, Shari, was killed. Upon hearing our devastating news, Sue called me right away. "I'm coming," she said, and that was all. She and another dear friend, Mary, came to help me and stayed until after the funeral.

These women truly personified this verse by taking on all the servant jobs that were so needed at the time. For three full days they shopped, cooked, served and cleaned up—again and again. Our house was full of family and friends and God sent these servants to care for our every need.

To me, denying self means that we do what needs to be done when it needs to be done, instead of doing what we might want to do when we feel like doing it. I once saw a plaque that read: "One kind deed is worth many kind thoughts." The kindness we show in times of crisis will be remembered forever because that is when Jesus is loving others through our deeds.

PRAYER

Dear Lord, teach me what denying self really means. Help me be Your voice, hands and feet in my world today.

Journal: Ask God to show you someone today who needs your touch and His love. Tomorrow, write in your journal about what happened today.

—Carole Lewis

MAY 6

A Simple Question

If anyone would come after me, he must deny himself and take up his cross daily and follow me.

LUKE 9:23

Jesus is speaking to me today as I read this verse. He wants me to listen carefully—and then He wants me to make a choice.

Here's the simple question He's asking: Do you want to follow Me?

It's crunch time. No waffling here. Do I really want to follow Jesus, rather than chasing after my hopes and dreams?

Assuming I'm ready to make the choice to follow Jesus today, what's the first thing I need to do? Jesus' words to His disciples are also intended for my ears and my heart: I need to trust Him and His Word. Will I let my heart be ruled by fear or the peace of God? Will I take control or turn everything over to Him?

His beckoning hands are open. His ways are perfect. He is watching my struggle and, if I go with Him, He will give me peace.

But the choice is mine.

Will I choose to take up His cross and be His follower today?

Will you?

PRAYER

Open my eyes today, Lord, and lead me. Show me the way to go and strengthen me in my mind, body and spirit to be a Christ follower.

Journal: What are three things you can do this week that will equip you to be a better Christ follower? Who do you need to pray for rather than praying for protection for yourself?

—Bruce Barbour

MAY 7

BEARING THE CROSS, EVEN IN WEAKNESS

If anyone would come after me, he must deny himself and take up his cross daily and follow me.

LUKE 9:23

Today I sit in Loveland, Ohio, with a broken heart, weeping with so many others who weep. Today, November 26, 2001, Shari Lewis Symank, Carole Lewis's daughter, will be laid to rest.

I write this as a witness to the way God has glorified Himself through Carole Lewis. Carole is one of my spiritual warfare heroines. Keeping my eyes fixed on Jesus, I cannot help but recognize the threat Carole and the ministry of First Place have been to the kingdom of darkness in the battle over souls.

Carole is a woman who continues to take up her cross daily, even through life's adversities. Her family has been struck numerous times with unthinkable tragedy, yet she continues to fight the good fight, pick up her cross and deny herself. Carole and the First Place family are a part of the Body of believers that is forging forward to follow Him!

Thank you, Carole, for being a spiritual warrior who continues to show me how to seek first the kingdom of God.

PRAYER

Lord, cause me to recognize those that need intercession and encouragement. Use me to lift and strengthen a tired heart.

Journal: List ways that you are picking up your cross daily and following Jesus.

—Denise Peters

MAY 8

THE FREEDOM OF SELF-DENIAL

If anyone would come after me, he must deny himself and take up his cross daily and follow me.

LUKE 9:23

My dad was a great businessman. He taught me that the more "I" words that I use in a business letter, the less effective the letter is in communicating my thoughts and requests. He's sent back to me my letters with each "I" circled—it was like getting back a test in school, because my total would be circled at the top.

This made me crazy, until I saw that my focus was all wrong: I was seeing things only in my own way, and that made me unable to see any other perspective. My intentions may have been right, but until I put the recipient's desires before my own, I would not be able to really make any progress.

Jesus knew this all too well. He knew that He had to follow the Father at all times—and He calls each of us to do the same. Self-denial is not natural to us, but it is the first step to true freedom in the Christian life. By laying down my own desires and dreams, I am free to truly follow Jesus—the only true source of light in my life.

Do my thoughts and prayers have too many "I" words? Who, or what, am I putting between Jesus and me today?

PRAYER

Jesus, I give up the right to my own desires and ask You to forgive me for running ahead of You. Slow me down today, Lord, and take my hand.

Journal: Tell how you first came to Christ. How did He draw you? What was your response? Then recommit your life to following Him with all your heart.

—Bruce Barbour

MAY 9

TUESDAY BLESSINGS

Let us consider how we may spur one another on toward love and good deeds. Let us not give up meeting together, as some are in the habit of doing, but let us encourage one another—and all the more as you see the Day approaching.

HEBREWS 10:24-25

I normally lead the First Place leader's class at church. When the new materials came out in September 2001, I decided to lead a member's class as well so that I could see if the materials worked as we had envisioned they would, or if changes were needed. This class proved to be full of the sweetest women—and I also had the joy of having my daughter, Shari, and my niece, Julie, in my group!

One week, a lady who is handicapped and uses leg braces to walk shared how hard it had become for her to attend class. She had moved in with her mother and had to get a taxi to bring her about 35 miles to class. When Shari heard that it cost $75 dollars in taxi fare, she immediately told the lady that she would pick her up each Tuesday.

During the sessions, they became great friends and spent each Tuesday together.

First Place is such a wonderful place to practice this verse. We have the opportunity to show love by praying for our class members. We can also show love by learning to encourage our fellow class members with a note, e-mail or telephone call.

Do you know someone who could use your encouragement today?

PRAYER

Father, help me to learn how to spur others on to love and good deeds by loving them and doing good deeds for them myself.

Journal: Make a list of the needs of people who are close to you. Ask God to show you how you might meet a need this week.

—Carole Lewis

May 10

Encouraged to Continue

Let us consider how we may spur one another on toward love and good deeds. Let us not give up meeting together, as some are in the habit of doing, but let us encourage one another—and all the more as you see the Day approaching.

Hebrews 10:24-25

Being the only First Place leader in my church placed a great responsibility on me. I felt called by God to lead my members on a continuing basis—but to be honest, I became discouraged as some either dropped out or were habitually absent from meetings.

I questioned my ability to lead and to teach, and I prayed that God would raise up another leader. In my humanness, I asked God, "Are you sure I am the one to do this?"

His answer came in this memory verse, "Let us not give up meeting together, . . . but let us encourage one another." God revealed to me in this verse that it is never up to me to decide whether I am to stop leading my group. I am to be obedient in doing what He has called me to do. All He expects of me is that I meet with others and encourage them. It is God's responsibility to deal with members concerning their obedience.

Now as I lead my First Place class, I no longer feel personally responsible for absent members. I encourage those who are present and try to spur members to love one another and do what God calls them to do.

I still pray that God will raise up additional leaders, but until that happens, I will continue being an encourager to those whom He sends my way.

Prayer

Lord, I confess my fleshly bent to succumb to discouragement. I am thankful You are always there to spur me on, encourage me and uplift me.

Journal: Have you considered ways to spur someone toward love and good deeds? Write down a plan of action and follow through with it!

—June Chapko

MAY 11

JOINING TOGETHER IN WORSHIP

Let us consider how we may spur one another on toward love and good deeds. Let us not give up meeting together, as some are in the habit of doing, but let us encourage one another—and all the more as you see the Day approaching.

HEBREWS 10:24-25

As a preschool worker, I learned a simple song to sing to the children—a song my husband and I would adapt from time to time, changing the words to fit the occasion. When we drove with our grandchildren to church, we sang the song using these words: "I like to go to church, to hear Jesus loves me."

Now that I'm living alone and away from my grandchildren, I still sing as I drive to church. I know that I can worship God anywhere, but there is something special about meeting with other Christians—praising God and hearing His Word together. As I drive alone I sing: "I like to go to church, to sing Jesus loves me." (In my case, this amounts to making a joyful noise, with the emphasis on *noise!*)

When I'm in a worship service, I love to look around at the smiles that come as favorite hymns are sung. Sometimes I even notice tears of joy. In these special moments, I feel like our voices are joining the saints from all of history, singing before the Lord of the ages who received our voices as a sweet sound in His ears! On my way home I think of the great reunion we will experience one day, when all the children of God gather around His throne to adore Him. And I sing, "I like to go to church, to see my happy friends."

Going to church opens the door to God—and to eternity.

PRAYER

Thank You, God, for the opportunity to worship in Your house with other believers.

Journal: Choose a psalm and sing it to your own melody as an offering of worship to the Lord. Write down ways in which worshiping with other believers encourages you. Share your thoughts with someone this week.

—Betha Jean Cunningham

Encouragement from Many Sources

Let us consider how we may spur one another on toward love and good deeds. Let us not give up meeting together, as some are in the habit of doing, but let us encourage one another—and all the more as you see the Day approaching.

HEBREWS 10:24-25

I am *not* a morning person. And yet for weeks I got up and drove to a 6:15 A.M. First Place class. The motivating factor was the prayer support I was getting from the group while my husband and I were separated because of work situations. When it came time for me to drive to where Ray was working, I could feel the prayers going with me. How I needed that support!

Later when my husband was diagnosed with a rare terminal cancer and had to return home for surgery and treatment, the folks in my group and in my church not only prayed for us but also came to visit. The women in my class prayed and sent notes on a regular basis, and we received encouragement and gifts from the small church we attended.

We were back home only a short time when it became necessary to put Ray in the hospital. The presence of God, family, friends, visits, cards (some from prayer groups across the country) made it easier to accept what was happening.

I can tell you that receiving encouragement is a blessing from God!

PRAYER

Heavenly Father, thank You for caring people who give encouragement when the going gets rough. Thank You for Your constant presence in every situation.

Journal: Have you contacted someone whom God has put on your heart? Have you been an encouragement to people just as you have been encouraged by God and others?

—Betha Jean Cunningham

MAY 13

What Do You Really Desire?

Let us consider how we may spur one another on toward love and good deeds. Let us not give up meeting together, as some are in the habit of doing, but let us encourage one another—and all the more as you see the Day approaching.

HEBREWS 10:24-25

It's been proven in many weight-loss programs: Attendance is a key to success. This Scripture speaks of the same principle and explains why it is true.

You see, we need each other as we try to make changes in our lives. We need each other for support and encouragement. Being together reminds us of our goal. It is easy to isolate yourself when you struggle with being overweight, because you sometimes don't feel good about yourself—on the outside or the inside. So you want to hide in embarrassment and shame. Then to comfort yourself from the negative emotions that are surfacing, you turn to food. Not many of us have been known to binge in front of a crowd. Typically this behavior is done in isolation. We use food to numb the pain inside, but this only perpetuates our physical struggle.

What you really desire, though, is the love and fellowship of others—isn't it? We are relational beings. And we need connections with other people—for support, encouragement and laughter.

Not one of us can do without help on our journey.

Are you trying to go it alone?

PRAYER

Lord, forgive me for all the times I have isolated myself and turned to food for comfort. Thank You for providing me with others to help me along the way.

Journal: Have you reached out to others for support as you strive toward your weight-loss goals? Can you encourage someone else who is trying to achieve victory?

—Roberta Wasserman

MAY 14

PEACE THROUGH AND THROUGH

May God himself, the God of peace, sanctify you through and through. May your whole spirit, soul and body be kept blameless at the coming of our Lord Jesus Christ.

1 THESSALONIANS 5:23

The first letter to the Thessalonians is one of the sweetest epistles ever written to the churches. It is obvious that Paul, Silas and Timothy loved these people very much and were extremely proud of them. And this verse is one of my absolute favorite memory verses. I often use it to close letters and notes to my dearest friends.

What I love about this verse is that you can pray it for your friends and loved ones, knowing that God wants to answer your prayer. It begins by telling us that God is the God of peace. We hear so much about peace today, yet there is no peace. War is taking place all over the world.

Today, meditate on the fact that God is the God of peace and ask Him to fill you with His serenity. After that, ask Him to sanctify, or purify, you through and through.

The next part of the verse talks about the need to live a balanced life—a truth that is at the very core of the First Place program. Paul prays that our whole spirit, soul and body will be kept blameless until our Lord Jesus Christ comes again. What a beautiful prayer for us to pray for ourselves and for those around us.

We can never go wrong by praying God's Word back to Him.

PRAYER

Lord, fill me with peace and help me to understand that You have set me apart—spirit, soul and body—to serve You.

Journal: What does it mean that God "sanctifies" you? Describe ways in which you see His peaceful work of sanctification in your life.

—Carole Lewis

MAY 15

What He Wants for Me

May God himself, the God of peace, sanctify you through and through. May your whole spirit, soul and body be kept blameless at the coming of our Lord Jesus Christ.

1 THESSALONIANS 5:23

The very first thing First Place did for me was to give me back my hope. I'd lost hope that I could do God's will. I'd even lost hope in my ability to serve God.

The truth is that I was saying no to many opportunities to serve in my church because I felt that my extra weight and my general physical condition prohibited my serving. I wanted to be a counselor at youth camp, but I knew that I could not physically handle the required walking. I wanted to sing in the choir, but my extra weight caused such an extreme sweating problem that I felt I would be detrimental to the group.

But in my hopelessness, God took over and began to sanctify me. I realize now that sanctification is not my idea of what I want for me but God's idea of what He wants to do for me.

I am now in a state of mind and spirit where I allowed Him to sanctify me—that is, to set me aside for His purposes—whatever the cost.

Make this commitment to God today: I want to be used by you. You will be amazed at what He does in and through you.

PRAYER

Father, today I submit to Your will. I pray that You will continue to change me into a person You can use whenever, however and wherever You please.

Journal: Are you doing your part to help attain the physical goals you would like to accomplish in First Place? If not, what do you need to do to make things right?

—Kay Smith

MAY 16

NOTHING MISSING, NOTHING BROKEN

May God himself, the God of peace, sanctify you through and through. May your whole spirit, soul and body be kept blameless at the coming of our Lord Jesus Christ.

1 THESSALONIANS 5:23

In this blessing, Paul shows us that we are not responsible for our righteousness or for the preservation of any part of our being. The God of peace has assumed these responsibilities.

This reference to peace is powerful. The Hebrew word for peace is *shalom.* "Shalom" doesn't just mean the absence of conflict; it also conveys the idea of complete wholeness. Someone once described God's shalom peace as "nothing missing, nothing broken." When you plug that thought into this Scripture, you arrive at the awesome understanding of God's willingness to set us apart and preserve us until we are totally whole again.

This Scripture falls at the end of a list of very specific instructions that Paul gave to the Thessalonians. God always leads us to a life of balance. On the one side, we need to do all that we can do; on the other, we must absolutely rely on Him to take care of us.

PRAYER

Father, I thank You for Your peace and for Your preservation. Show me the balance between what I can do and what I need to leave to You.

Journal: What areas have you been trying to handle yourself that you should be leaving to God?

—June-Marie Avery

MAY 17

Ask the One Who Knows

May God himself, the God of peace, sanctify you through and through. May your whole spirit, soul and body be kept blameless at the coming of our Lord Jesus Christ.

1 THESSALONIANS 5:23

When I joined the First Place program last September, I weighed 182 pounds. My size-16 jeans were so tight that I could hardly get them on, and my self-esteem was at an all-time low. I was depressed and thought, *If I could only lose weight, I'd feel better about myself.*

Through the program and God's Word, I have learned that He doesn't want me to be ashamed of myself. I have learned that God is proud of me just the way I am. The more I read His Word, the better I feel. And to my surprise and delight, I have begun to lose weight.

To date, I have lost 27 pounds. I have learned so much about food groups and food portions. And best of all, I have let Jesus take control of my life and my eating habits. I came closer to God through the Scriptures that we read and memorized each week.

Seeking to do the will of the Father has blessed me more than I originally realized. Jesus has become my strength, my courage and my will to succeed. I have needed to know God more than I needed to lose weight. My life has been empty without Him as I sought answers but failed to ask the One who knows all things.

Now I know whom to turn to when I need a friend to help me. I turn to Jesus, my best friend, my redeemer, my salvation.

PRAYER

Father, I pray that Your comfort, strength and mercy will inspire people to believe that all things are possible through You and that You are our refuge in times of need, as well as times of rejoicing.

Journal: Do you feel shame today because you think God is not proud of you? Turn that feeling over to God, praising Him that you are not loved and accepted because of your performance but because of His Son, Jesus.

—Karen Duffy

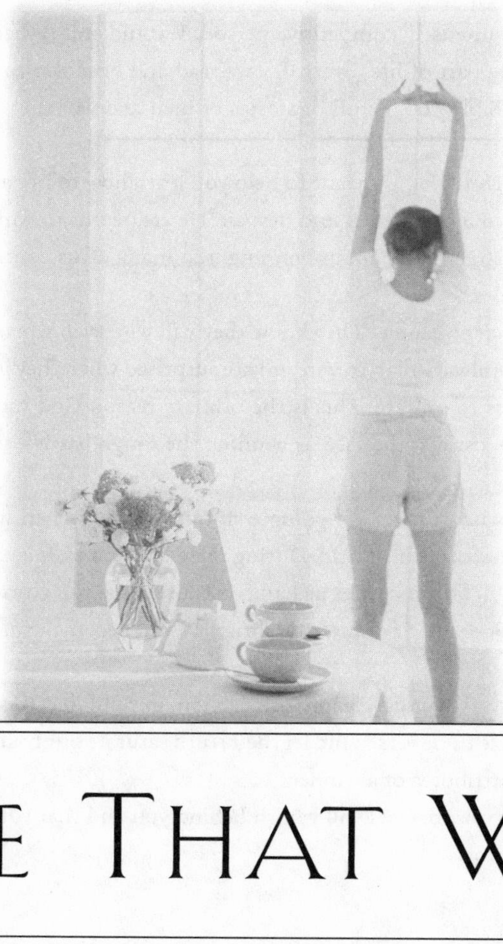

LIFE THAT WINS

SECTION FOUR

Introduction

Although I am not an intensely competitive person, I would still rather win than lose. Winning and losing are part of life. Every day we read and hear stories of great victory and great defeat. The Bible, too, is full of stories of men and women who won or who lost—or did both.

This section, *Life That Wins,* is meant to help you learn how to live as a winner. God never intended for us to live in defeat and despair. He created us to win. Until we learn what the Bible wants to teach us about winning, too many of us continue to lose too many of our daily battles.

Winners are confident people. They know they will win, even when their prospects are bleak. True winners always plan to win and are surprised when they lose. Winners are people the world wants to imitate. This is the primary reason God wants us to live as winners. He wants the lost world to see us winning the tough battles, so they will want what we have.

Winning is easy when things are going well but difficult when we're confronted with the trials and troubles of this world. During these dark times, it is essential to know that we don't have to fight the battles at hand, because Jesus has already won the war. Thanks to our great God and Savior, Jesus Christ, we can become winners every day of our lives.

The 10 Scripture verses undergirding this section, in combination, teach us how to win. When we memorize these verses and let their truth saturate our hearts, our lives take on the attitudes and attributes of a winner.

My prayer is that your defeats will vanish behind you and that your life ahead will be characterized by victory.

—Carole Lewis

MAY 18

GIVE IT UP!

But God demonstrates his own love for us in this: While we were still sinners, Christ died for us.

ROMANS 5:8

At our First Place conferences and Fitness Weeks, one of our most popular seminars is the one presented by our chef, Scott Wilson. People just love to see someone demonstrate how to prepare a recipe; and they like even better the prospect of getting to taste the finished product.

The apostle Paul gives us a mental picture when he tells us that "God demonstrates." Paul is saying that in a very specific way, God chose to show us the extent of His love for us: "While we were still sinners, Christ died for us."

We have all heard stories of someone who has heroically given his or her life for a friend—even for a stranger. But how often do we hear of someone giving his or her life for a sworn enemy? Sin is the sworn enemy of God. The Bible says that God cannot even look at sin, yet God sent Jesus to give His life to demonstrate that He loves us even though we are sinners.

If there is known sin you are still hanging on to today, I implore you to demonstrate your love for God by giving Him permission to take it from you. Too often we stay stuck in guilt and shame, asking God over and over to forgive us but making no movement toward becoming free. Admit to God that you know you can't give up this particular sin by yourself. Ask Him to come to your assistance and work in you and deliver you. Later there will be time to ask Him to forgive you for hanging on to the sin for so long.

Christ came that we might experience freedom. Our sin keeps us in bondage, which is the opposite of being free. We are free to triumph in Spirit!

PRAYER

Father, I know You want to set me free from this sin that I refuse to give up. Today I admit that I am powerless to give it up, but I give You permission to take it.

Journal: Write the one word that best describes the sin you're holding on to and write the word every day as you think about turning from it.

—Carole Lewis

MAY 19

KNOW YOUR WORTH

But God demonstrates his own love for us in this: While we were still sinners, Christ died for us.

ROMANS 5:8

I had spent a lifetime trying to be "good enough to be loved." The measure of my worth was based on my appearance and body size. I believed that if only I were thin, I would be lovable. This was such a lie.

In Romans 5:8, Paul speaks about God's unconditional love, which the ministry of First Place helped me to discover. Jesus Christ died for my sins, and that is the measure of my worth. I am already good enough—even with all my imperfections—based on the immeasurable price that was paid for me at Calvary. This same God who gave His life for me created me to have a relationship with Him.

Through journaling my prayers and reading God's Word each day, I finally connected with the God of the universe. Jesus Christ not only died for my sins, but He also helped me to achieve victory in the area of my weight. More and more of my time is spent on developing my relationship with God, rather than focusing on my weight problems.

When I lost weight, I gained far more than I could imagine. I gained a precious relationship with my Savior and Lord. That's the way God does things, it seems. He blesses us beyond measure.

PRAYER

Lord, thank You for dying on the cross for my sins. Thank You for showing me the true measure of my worth. Thank You for unconditional love.

Journal: Tell God the ways you have tried to earn acceptance, approval or love.

—Roberta Wasserman

MAY 20

BLESSED BEYOND MEASURE

But God demonstrates his own love for us in this: While we were still sinners, Christ died for us.

ROMANS 5:8

As I drove to work in the early dawn, the sun was painting the horizon with colors of pinks, blues and misty grays. It was a breathtaking canvas! I found myself praising and thanking the Lord for His beautiful creation.

From within I heard Him reply, "Be still and know that I am God."

As I quieted my soul before Him, oddly enough I began to notice American flags placed sporadically along the freeway—each flag waved gently in the morning breeze. I thought about the freedom our flag represents. (For example, we have the freedom to drive to work while listening to Christian music or to the preaching of the gospel.)

Near one flag was a church with a tall, stark cross outlined against the majestic sky. I was reminded of our spiritual freedom: "God demonstrated his own love for us in this: While we were still sinners, Christ died for us."

As I drove into the driveway at the church and saw the rows of flags in front of the building, I was so thankful that of all the places on Earth I could be living, I live in America—and I will live for eternity with my Lord and Savior, Jesus Christ.

PRAYER

Thank You, Lord, that the heavens declare Your glory. Thank You for Your still small voice that reminds us of Your love and the great sacrifice of Your Son.

Journal: List the daily freedoms you enjoy but often take for granted. Praise God for sending His Son to set the captives free.

—Pat Lewis

MAY 21

JUST AS YOU WERE

But God demonstrates his own love for us in this: While we were still sinners, Christ died for us.

ROMANS 5:8

When I was a child, my mother demonstrated food products in the local grocery store. Her job was to prepare and hand out samples of different products on sale that day. The hope, of course, was that by tasting the product, customers would actually make a purchase.

When I read Romans 5:8, I think about Mother's product demonstrations. God took great efforts to prepare His own Son to demonstrate His love for us. In our human body we only get to have a sample of His love. But because of this demonstration, we have tasted hope—the hope that comes from experiencing His love. This foretaste tells us that one day we will experience the fullness of His love when we slip from this world into eternity.

I am forever grateful to Jesus that while I was yet a sinner, He died to demonstrate God's love for me. I didn't have to lose weight first. I didn't have to get the victory over food first. I didn't have to have genuine love for exercise first. Guess what? Before any of those things, Jesus loved me and He loved you—just the way we are!

PRAYER

Thank You, Lord, for loving me just the way I am this day.

Journal: Yes, Jesus loves you! Tell Jesus that you receive His love and ask Him to step in and start the process of change that you so desire.

—Beverly Henson

MAY 22

UNFATHOMABLE LOVE

But God demonstrates his own love for us in this: While we were still sinners, Christ died for us.

ROMANS 5:8

The amazing promise in Romans 5:8 has been my life verse for many years. I began to love this verse back in 1984 when God was calling me into full-time Christian service. But to be completely honest, back then I was afraid of what He might do with my life if I gave Him complete control.

Growing up, I was very involved in the missions program of our church. I heard many missionaries speak; and I somehow picked up the warped idea that if I gave God control of every part of my life, He would probably send me to China or Africa where I would undoubtedly minister the gospel but also be miserable and lonely. This sounds silly now; but looking back, that warped view and my fears worked together to keep me in bondage.

When I discovered Romans 5:8, God started using it to build my faith. I began to believe that His plans for me are *always* good, even when the circumstances of my life are bad. God's assurance to me through this verse has literally carried me these last few years as we've dealt with my husband's, Johnny's, cancer. His assurance has been my constant companion as I have become the full-time caretaker of my aged mom, and has been my cloak of comfort as I have grieved the loss of my precious daughter Shari.

Today, I pray that you will memorize this verse and say it every day until it becomes part of who you are.

PRAYER

Father, help me to claim this verse for myself. May it become Your personal statement of love to me, Your child.

Journal: Write about something going on in your life right now that you find impossible to believe is God's plan for you. Ask God to show you how He wants to use your present circumstance for His glory.

—Carole Lewis

MAY 23

PRESENT AND FUTURE GRACE

"For I know the plans I have for you," declares the LORD, "plans to prosper you and not to harm you, plans to give you hope and a future."

JEREMIAH 29:11

I lost 70 pounds over the time of the first three sessions of First Place, and my relationship with God definitely improved. Then, in March 1998, during our fourth session, my world fell apart.

I had been having trouble with blurred vision in my right eye and loss of hearing in my left ear. My family doctor sent me to an ophthalmologist. He told me I had optic neuritis and ordered an MRI. I was feeling very confident that nothing would show up on the MRI.

When my family doctor got the results, however, he called me in right away and told me I had multiple sclerosis. I was immediately referred to a neurologist. I spent the next week in the hospital having intravenous treatment and more tests to determine if the MS was in my spine as well as my brain. Praise the Lord, it was not.

As it happened, I had my First Place materials with me in the hospital. These, along with the Bible and the support of other First Place members, got me through the initial shock of my diagnosis. My neurologist told me that one thing in my favor was that I had lost so much weight.

My left arm is now weak, but I continue to work four hours a day. Jeremiah 29:11 has really helped me, because I know that God has a plan for my life and that He has a hope and a future for me, despite the fact that I have MS.

PRAYER

Father, I praise You because, as Jeremiah 29:11 says, You do have a plan for me—a hope and a future. And what a blessing that is!

Journal: Write several reasons to be thankful today. What plans do you have for your life? Are they are in accordance with what God has planned for you?

—Vicki L. Harnly

MAY 24

In Jesus' Name

"For I know the plans I have for you," declares the LORD, "plans to prosper you and not to harm you, plans to give you hope and a future."

JEREMIAH 29:11

Letting God be God is probably one of the most difficult responses we have to learn as Christians. Our prayers can sometimes come out like marching orders for our Lord, as we present Him with a specific list of things He needs to do for us.

Then we're given a reminder that our lists don't always read the same as His. On October 31, 1990, my family saw our wants and needs, our prayer desires and especially our relationships with each other and with God change dramatically: I was diagnosed with pancreatic carcinoma and told I only had three months to live.

I suddenly had only 90 days to share a lifetime with my wife and two teenaged children. This was not the future my family and I had planned!

Peggy, my wife, began to pray—in fact, night after night she begged the Lord for my life. Every night after we had all gone to bed, she would go into another room and be facedown on the floor and cry out to God on my behalf.

During that time she sensed God giving her two responses: "For I know"—which meant that God was not surprised by my illness—and also "this is not a disease unto death"—which was great news!

Through this time we have learned what praying in Jesus' name is all about—praying only for that which is consistent with His perfect character and for that which will bring glory to Him. The hardest part is being willing to accept His answer, whatever it might be. And even though the jury is still out for me, He has changed my will.

PRAYER

Father, help me to know and accept Your will, not mine, for the glory of the Kingdom. Amen.

Journal: If you have a tendency to walk by sight, rather than by faith, how do you think you can find God's will in the face of adversity? What causes you to have greater faith?

—Rick Jones

MAY 25

THE GOD WHO HEALS

"For I know the plans I have for you," declares the LORD, "plans to prosper you and not to harm you, plans to give you hope and a future."

JEREMIAH 29:11

"When all else fails, read the directions." I was reminded of this by my 15-year-old daughter after my terminal cancer diagnosis on October 31, 1990.

Very quickly we claimed Jeremiah 29:11 as our family Scripture verse. What I learned from this short declaration changed everything. In Hebrew the word "declare" has an incredible translation and is derived from the word "oracle."[1] In a biblical sense, an oracle is a decree from God Himself, words spoken from the inner sanctuary of His Temple.

Wow! We sensed God's promise of welfare, and we were going to claim that for sure. And the Great Physician had revealed to my wife that my disease would not be fatal.

Our surgeon was not that optimistic, but he told us of a surgical procedure that could give me six months to a year more of life. With no other options available, we decided on the surgery.

On December 5, 1990, I underwent the procedure. The promise God had given to my wife had not yet been made manifest, but all heaven was about to break loose. After the surgery my body continued to heal, despite the doctors' warnings and misgivings.

Praise God, I have been cancer-free for 11 years.

What made the difference? Prayer and the power of our sovereign God—together with the fact that, for us as believers, the Lord controls the future.

PRAYER

Most powerful God, may I never be guilty of asking You to come bless what I am doing. May I, instead, always look to see where You are working and make myself available to be used of You in that place.

Journal: Describe how today would play out if your only desire was to bring honor and glory to God.

—Rick Jones

MAY 26

For God's Glory Alone

"For I know the plans I have for you," declares the LORD, "plans to prosper you and not to harm you, plans to give you hope and a future."

JEREMIAH 29:11

Unbelief is like a spiritual cancer that can spread and destroy the life of our spirit.

After my terminal cancer diagnosis, that process of raising a barrier against unbelief began as soon as I changed my focus from self to the grace supplier, God. Whether I lived or died, God was in control. Only He knew the plans for my future, so my family and I took our eyes off medical prognoses and set them firmly upon Him.

Actually, the barrier against unbelief began to rise right in the middle of my surgery on that December day in 1990 when the surgeon found that the cancer had spread. Turning to his assistants, he said, "Let's sew him back up. There's nothing we can do."

Later he told me that as he turned to walk away, he felt as if a hand had firmly gripped his shoulder and he heard a voice inside him say, "James, you can do the surgery. I gave you the talent. What would you want your doctor to do if this were you?" The voice was so strong that he turned around to see if someone was actually speaking. As he told me later, "I knew it had to be God."

After 12 hours of surgery, the surgical team had removed my entire pancreas, gall bladder, spleen, duodenum, 60 percent of my stomach and 60 percent of my intestines. According to the doctor, before they could close me up, the remaining pockets of cancer actually vanished.

God promised me a future and hope, and He delivered.

PRAYER

Most gracious and awesome God, I only want to be where You are, for I know You will provide comfort, love, encouragement, direction and everything else I need. Help me to raise high that barrier to my unbelief and reside always in Your glorious presence.

Journal: Are there areas of doubt and questionable belief that you and God need to address? When was the last time you asked, or had a craving, for the glory of the Lord?

—Rick Jones

MAY 27

MUSTARD-SEED FAITH

And without faith it is impossible to please God, because anyone who comes to him must believe that he exists and that he rewards those who earnestly seek him.

HEBREWS 11:6

As a First Place leader, I have talked with hundreds of women during the past 20 years. Most of them would be classified by the medical establishment as obese, and they have a real problem having faith in their situation. They have no problem believing that God *wants* to do something wonderful in my life or in the life of their friends; but they cannot personalize this verse and believe it to be true for themselves. They find it impossible to believe that God wants to reward them with a substantial weight loss if they will have faith. They also can't seem to believe that He wants to reward them in any other area of life.

Somewhere I have read that 80 percent of overweight men and women have experienced some sort of abuse in their lives. The abuse could be sexual, emotional, verbal or physical.

It is easy to understand why these people would find it difficult to express faith. If this devotional is speaking to you today, take heart. God knows where you are and He knows your faith is small. Praise His name.

The faith you need is not so much your faith in Him as *His faith in you.*

PRAYER

Lord, I ask You to show me today in some small way how much faith You have in me. Lead me to a Bible verse and bring someone into my life to teach me about this truth.

Journal: List all the areas of your life in which your faith is small. Ask God to begin the job of building your faith. Look up Scriptures on faith and start memorizing them.

—Carole Lewis

MAY 28

THINGS NOT SEEN

And without faith it is impossible to please God, because anyone who comes to him must believe that he exists and that he rewards those who earnestly seek him.

HEBREWS 11:6

Some time ago, I was helping First Place with the revision of their new program. The editorial work was nearly complete, but a publishing deal we had been working on had just fallen through. Panic and fear began to set in my heart as I looked for ways to get things back on track.

Then God brought Hebrews 11:6 to mind. Did I want to please Him? *Yes, I did.* Did I believe He is with us as we work diligently to seek His way? *Yes, I did.* Then there was only one thing to do. *I must have hope. I must believe in things not seen.*

As we pressed on, believing, we rested in the fact that God was fully capable of meeting our every need in His perfect timing. Not long afterward, and in plenty of time to get the updated program to market, God rewarded us with His perfect choice: a publisher excited about First Place who had been praying for just such a program for over a year!

Lesson learned . . . again.

PRAYER

Lord, when the day is dark, open my eyes to Your light and guide my steps away from fear to Your peace, comfort and confidence.

Journal: Turn over that one thing you are really nervous about to God and see what He will do.

—Bruce Barbour

MAY 29

Childlike Trust

And without faith it is impossible to please God, because anyone who comes to him must believe that he exists and that he rewards those who earnestly seek him.

HEBREWS 11:6

Here's how this verse reads in the *New Living Translation*: "So, you see, it is impossible to please God without faith. Anyone who wants to come to him must believe that there is a God and that he rewards those who sincerely seek him."

Why is it impossible to please God apart from faith? "Because anyone who wants to approach God," *The Message* says, "must believe both that he exists and that he cares enough to respond to those who seek him."

Why is it impossible to please God without faith? Because God loves us and wants to bless us; and if we don't believe, we won't reach out to receive His love. If we are only praying in hope and not in faith, we will quickly give up or pray, "If you're there and if you care, please do something about this."

How do we develop the kind of trusting faith that moves God to "reward" it? First, we have to get to know God through His Word and by fellowshipping with Him in prayer. Once we have read His Word, we will begin to see His promises to us. We then begin to believe these promises might actually apply to us. We are almost there! The faith of a child in his loving Father is within our grasp!

When we have the faith, we can know "both that he exists and that he cares enough to respond to those who seek him." We will have made the leap from praying in hope to praying in faith.

PRAYER

Father, I know You're there and I know You care! I know that You will take care of me!

Journal: Make a list of the areas of your life in which you have trouble believing God. Then search God's Word for promises that will replace the doubt with faith.

—June-Marie Avery

MAY 30

I SPY

And without faith it is impossible to please God, because anyone who comes to him must believe that he exists and that he rewards those who earnestly seek him.

HEBREWS 11:6

The world says, "Seeing is believing." The child of God says, "Believing is seeing Christ."

Tracy is a woman who needed Christ when I first met her. But I saw no interest on her part in a life of faith. Then, at my invitation, she came to a concert we had at church. At first, she seemed ready to leave. The music was loud and her baby was scared. But then some of us saw tears forming in her eyes. I was happy to keep the baby in back and let Tracy enjoy the music. Without the distraction of caring for her child, the Lord penetrated her heart with the message from the band. That evening she was brought into the family of God.

After pondering the entire incident, God showed me how important each step was in her coming to know Christ—from the prayers, music and child care to the absolute moving of the Holy Spirit.

Our job is just to be obedient and do only the part God asks us to do.

PRAYER

Father, increase my faith to understand that even the changing of diapers has a holy agenda. Let me see the call to obedience and seek You wholeheartedly.

Journal: Describe a time when you saw Christ in the smallest detail. When was the last time you splashed Living Water on someone?

—Denise Peters

MAY 31

MORE THAN ENOUGH

And without faith it is impossible to please God, because anyone who comes to him must believe that he exists and that he rewards those who earnestly seek him.

HEBREWS 11:6

Even as a little child, I never doubted that God existed. My parents taught me about the importance of faith. I still have a favorite piece of jewelry from my twelfth birthday—a pin containing a tiny mustard seed. Along with this gift came an explanation that emphasized Jesus' teaching that faith the size of a mustard seed is sufficient when we "plant it" by trusting in our great God.

In the past few years, I've faced trials that required me to exercise mountain-sized faith, and I thank God I was prepared. I didn't have to fake having faith or search for something I didn't understand. I was ready to rely wholeheartedly on the integrity of God's holy Word and to be confident that He would get me through this difficult time. After all, doesn't it take faith to believe God's promises to us? Doesn't His Word tell us that it is impossible to please God without faith?

I sincerely desire to please God, but many times I fall short. If I earnestly seek to know Him better, my rewards are numerous. I choose to believe that in my darkest hour God sends His light to illumine my way.

I call this faith—maybe it is small faith, but it is faith in a big God. For God, amazingly, this seems to be enough.

PRAYER

Thank You, Lord, for faith as small as a mustard seed that allows me to believe in a big God.

Journal: What trial are you facing that requires mountain-sized faith? Ask God for mustard-seed faith to believe He is big enough to handle it for you.

—Irene Bonner

JUNE 1

FRUIT OF THE VINE

The fruit of the Spirit is love, joy, peace, patience, kindness, goodness, faithfulness, gentleness and self-control.

GALATIANS 5:22-23

When I think of the fruit of the Spirit, I always see grapes. One reason is that the verse says "fruit" and not "fruits." While in California, I had the privilege of visiting a grape vineyard. I had read *Secrets of the Vine* by Bruce Wilkinson and wanted to see what grape growing was all about.

One thing I noticed immediately is that grapes grow in clusters. Some fruit, such as apples and oranges, grow alone. Not so with grapes. You never see one grape growing alone. So it is with the fruit of the Spirit. When a person's life exhibits the fruit of the Spirit, you usually see the entire cluster, not just one grape.

In First Place, the one fruit most of us single out and struggle with is the "grape" of self-control. We often wish this attribute had been left off when the fruit of the Spirit was listed.

It is my belief that God knows that without self-control it is quite impossible to be a balanced, healthy individual physically, emotionally, mentally or spiritually. Self-control is something you might need badly right now. You might even feel that there isn't one piece of fruit in your life right now, much less an entire cluster. Give God permission today to come in and rearrange your life so that it resembles a cluster of grapes, all the luscious fruit together in one place—your life.

PRAYER

Dear Lord, I want my life to resemble a beautiful, luscious cluster of grapes. Do whatever it takes to fill me with the fruit of the Spirit.

Journal: Tell God which fruit of the Spirit is entirely lacking in your life right now. He already knows what's missing but would like for you to tell Him and ask for His help.

—Carole Lewis

LIFE-GIVING WORDS

The fruit of the Spirit is love, joy, peace, patience, kindness, goodness, faithfulness, gentleness and self-control.

GALATIANS 5:22-23

On a recent Saturday morning, I was eating breakfast with my granddaughter, Tricia, who is five years old. She was unusually quiet. Suddenly she said, "Mimi, I need to tell you something." As I gave her my full attention, she said, "Mimi, you are the oldest person I know that is still alive."

Tricia was quite preoccupied with death at the time because of the recent death of her beloved Papa. Was she worried that I might also die, leaving her without either one of us?

Later, as I was committing to memory the verses from Galatians, Tricia's innocent remark came back to me. Her words were not spoken to cause harm, but I wondered how often we speak words that cause pain to someone because of a lack of the fruit of kindness in our lives. Although you can retract spoken words that are unkind or hurtful, it is much, much harder to undo the harm they have done.

I have a friend who told me recently that she remembered every unkind word ever been spoken to her, going all the way back to her school years. How many words do you remember that were spoken to you in kindness and how many that were unkind? Proverbs 18:21 says, "The tongue has the power of life and death, and those who love it will eat its fruit."

Ask the Lord to help you speak life to all those around you today so that your words will bear the fruit of kindness.

PRAYER

Lord, I pray that every word my mouth speaks will be acceptable to You and will build up and encourage, instead of hurt or cause harm.

Journal: Have you spoken unkind words to someone that could have hurt them or caused them harm? Ask God if He would have you go to them and ask forgiveness.

—Pat Lewis

JUNE 3

INSPECTING THE FRUIT

The fruit of the Spirit is love, joy, peace, patience, kindness, goodness, faithfulness, gentleness and self-control.

GALATIANS 5:22-23

When it comes to enjoying the fruit of the land, summer is the peak season for East Texas. No need for roosters to wake us up on Thursdays. In the cool of the morning, our farmers' market buzzes with excitement as area farmers unload their fresh produce under the shade trees.

Walking along in front of the tables, looking for the brightest fruits and vegetables, I'm reminded that God looks over our lives for the ripest fruit of His Spirit.

First stop, my favorite—tomatoes. Taking one in hand and turning it for inspection brings a smile to my lips, just like God smiles when I make that secret choice to love a difficult person in my life. Clutching a handful of peas or okra and wondering how much for a "mess," I realize it really takes a lot of kindness, goodness, faithfulness and gentleness to make a difference in my daily walk.

Last stop, melons—my most difficult purchase because I never know exactly how to select them. I'm told to press the stem end and smell, or squeeze a little or thump three times. It's rare for me to find a ripe one because mostly I just have to guess and grab. Patience and self-control are a little like melons; but whenever I ask God for either, He is always faithful to provide.

Joy and peace seem to rule when all of God's other bountiful fruits (and vegetables) come together to let His Spirit reach from us to those He brings to our gardens each day.

PRAYER

Lord, may the fruit of Your Spirit grow in the garden of my life today.
Help me to love others and give them room to fail and time to change,
just as You allow me the same luxury.

Journal: Who will enter your garden today needing the Holy Spirit's fruit? Ask the Spirit to show you what choices you can make to show love or self-control to those people.

—Judy Marshall

JUNE 4

A Smile on Your Workout

The fruit of the Spirit is love, joy, peace, patience, kindness, goodness, faithfulness, gentleness and self-control.

GALATIANS 5:22-23

As children of the living God, we should strive to show active evidence of the fruit of the Spirit in our lives every day and in every way. Now, here's a news flash: This also applies to our exercise routine.

As a recovering lazy person, I found that in the beginning, as I went out to walk each day, it was much easier to complain about how bad it hurt—how my back hurt, how my feet hurt and how much I hated to "have" to exercise. The more I complained, the worse it became to fit in my workout and the easier it was to make excuses not to do it at all.

Then I asked Jesus to change my heart toward my exercise. I began to have an excitement and anticipation for my workout every day, because I had a new walking partner. His name is Jesus. I walked with Him and talked with Him. He began to rub off on me. Before long, I liked exercise so much that I began to think of my walks as having a smile on them. I was filled with the Spirit, and the fruit was evident in my workout.

People would say to me, "You really enjoy walking, don't you?" The weight began to come off as I found a new love for moving.

So how about it? Is there a smile on your workout? Try it—you'll like it!

PRAYER

Father, give me a love and a joy for my exercise routine. I desire to be a walking example of the fruit of Your Spirit.

Journal: The older we get, the easier it is to do less moving and more complaining about having to do it. Ask the Lord to give you a new love for moving and let Him bring a smile to your face and to all you do.

—Beverly Henson

JUNE 5

STRENGTHENED BY JOY

Do not grieve, for the joy of the LORD is your strength.

NEHEMIAH 8:10

The last few years of my life have been filled with difficult circumstances. God has used this verse about the joy of the Lord so many times to give me abundant joy right in the middle of a situation in which I might want to grieve.

One day I was sharing with a friend about my mom, who, because of her diminished mental capacity, is unable to grieve with me the loss of my daughter Shari. Mom was the one who taught Shari to sew as a young girl. Mom loved Shari so much, and she doesn't even seem aware that Shari is no longer with us.

Yet even as these words of dismay came out of my mouth, I was immediately conscious that this, too, is a tremendous blessing. I suddenly felt joy that God had insulated my mom from this intense pain. Since she is almost 90 years of age and unable to leave her wheelchair, this knowledge would be a source of grief and pain that she could only absorb but not express. Mom had said when my sister, Glenda—my only sibling—died in 1994, "Children should bury their parents, not the other way around."

When we finally learn that God is good all the time, we begin to see the events in our lives as part of His plan to conform us to the image of His Son, Jesus. I wish I could say that I become more like Jesus when things are going great, but the truth is I seem to become complacent and wind up doing my own thing. I can rejoice in the fact that I grow more like Him when I share in His sufferings. It's not my joy but His that gives me strength.

PRAYER

Lord, You know the things I grieve. Strengthen me with Your joy today so that my life looks more and more like Your Son, Jesus.

Journal: Write about the area of your life in which you are grieving right now. Tell God what caused the grief and why you find yourself unable to let it go. Ask Him to take away your grief and fill you with His joy.

—Carole Lewis

JUNE 6

FATHER'S VOICE

Do not grieve, for the joy of the LORD is your strength.

NEHEMIAH 8:10

As a little girl, I grew up in a non-Christian home with an alcoholic father. My mother was a victim of domestic violence, and in those days shelters were not available. In this chaotic environment, I learned very early to turn to food for comfort. As a result, throughout my teens I struggled with food and weight problems and life-threatening eating disorders. I used food to suppress my feelings and pain.

When I came to the First Place program, I began my personal relationship with the Lord Jesus Christ. I learned to write out my prayers in a prayer journal every day. One particular day I was burdened for my estranged alcoholic father. I began to pour out my heart to God in my journal. I asked God to heal my father, and I pictured him totally recovered.

Two weeks later, my father died from the long-term effects of alcoholism. When I received the telephone call, my eyes landed on Nehemiah 8:10, the week's memory verse, which was written on a card stuck to my windowpane. In that moment, I experienced the joy of the Lord for the first time in my life.

In the difficult days that followed, at every moment I sensed Jesus near me. It was like I was on higher ground and could see everything through spiritual eyes. During my daily Bible devotions, Scriptures became illuminated and jumped off the page to me. My every need was met.

From then on I knew that I had the Father of the fatherless speaking to me. Our relationship deepened and I have met with Him first thing every single day for years now.

PRAYER

Lord, thank You for providing Your Holy Word to speak to me, so our relationship is not one-sided. Thank You for hearing my every prayer.

Journal: If you aren't already using a prayer journal, begin today to write and pour out your heart to God, instead of finding comfort in food and other things.

—Roberta Wasserman

JUNE 7

BURDEN LIFTED

Do not grieve, for the joy of the LORD is your strength.

NEHEMIAH 8:10

It has been said that joy is a state of mind, not a state of affairs. But consider some joy robbers that find a way of sneaking in our back doors to rob us blind!

One of today's most prevalent culprits is anxiety. "An anxious heart weighs a man down" (Prov. 12:25). I often find myself taking on the cares and struggles of others. I know it is the will of God that I care for people, but it is not His will that I allow these cares to become worrisome burdens.

Psalm 55:22 says "Cast your cares on the LORD and he will sustain you." The word "cast" means to heave—as one would throw a heavy sack of garbage into a can. In Psalm 68:19, God says He "daily bears our burdens" if we will just let Him.

Sometimes I spend more time worrying about something than praying about it. Worry causes me to lug my cares and anxieties around like sacks of garbage. When we worry, it's like trying to dance while carrying heavy baggage we need not carry.

It is possible to live in this world and not lose our joy, but we have to consistently give our worry burden to the One who can carry it lightly.

PRAYER

Lord, reveal to me those things that cause me to worry and fret, and help me cast those things upon Your strong and mighty shoulders!

Journal: Identify the worry you struggle with the most. Ask God to reveal the factors that make you prone to worry and record them in your journal.
Pray about what He has shown you.

—Vicki Heath

JUNE 8

JOY ROBBERS

Do not grieve, for the joy of the LORD is your strength.

NEHEMIAH 8:10

The writer of Hebrews admonishes us to "be content with what you have" (13:5). God blesses us with so much. Yet often we think it's not enough. Then we covet or resent the blessings of others, and our joy quickly goes down the drain.

I believe there are two major categories of "joy robbers" in our lives. The first is comparing and coveting. The second is busyness and overcommitment.

Nothing will rob you of your joy more quickly than discontentment and ungratefulness. When we focus on what others have—a larger home, better looks, better husband, better kids, stronger health—we are silently questioning God's goodness. Thankfulness is the secret to developing an attitude of gratitude. When we choose contentment over covetousness, our lives are enriched and we recognize the good gifts we receive from God.

A close second to the joy robber of discontentment is busyness. Americans seem to be the busiest people in the world. If we're not careful, the busyness of our lives distracts us from the blessings of God and dissipates our joy. As a mother of four and wife of a minister, I tend to "overbook my flight," as my husband describes it. When we overbook, we miss the opportunities to lie down in quiet green pastures where God can restore our souls (see Ps. 23).

Overcommitted people have a common vocabulary and often say, "If I don't do it, it won't get done." Psalm 127:1 says, "Unless the LORD builds the house, its builders labor in vain." We need to learn that saying no can be a holy thing.

PRAYER

Lord, help me today to say yes to the things that are needful and no to the things that distract me from You. I will listen to Your Holy Spirit to show me the difference. Help me also to remember Your goodness so that my soul may be joyful.

Journal: Write down those things you have been guilty of coveting; compare them to what has eternal value. Ask the Holy Spirit to give you more joy and reveal how you could become less busy.

—Vicki Heath

JUNE 9

SUSTAINING PRAYER

Do not grieve, for the joy of the LORD is your strength.

NEHEMIAH 8:10

As I was reading the context of this verse, I discovered that Nehemiah was a man strong in prayer. For the record: Nehemiah rebuilt the wall around Jerusalem in a record 51 days; the Bible says that Israel's enemies lost confidence because they recognized this was accomplished with the help of God. Because Nehemiah was strong in prayer, God's power was displayed to the enemy. Prayer is a powerful weapon in the mouths of God's servants.

My late husband was a prayer warrior. Bill loved to pray. Many nights after we had prayed together, I would fall asleep while he continued to pray. He prayed for our children and grandchildren, our extended families and friends, the sick and the hurting. He had a special prayer burden for the men of our church and community that they would become spiritual leaders of their homes. He also had a compassion for single moms and prayed much for them. It was not uncommon for our phone to ring during the night; I would awaken from a sound sleep to hear Bill praying fervently for someone in a crisis situation.

When Bill died, a woman told me of a dream she had. When the angels came for Bill, he was dressed in a uniform with many stripes on his sleeve. He truly was a man strong in prayer—a mighty warrior in God's kingdom.

As I have grieved his death over the last year, the memories of those prayers have comforted, strengthened and sustained me. The joy of the Lord is truly our strength when we are devoted in prayer to Him who is mighty in power.

PRAYER

Father, how I thank You that Your joy is my strength! Help me to experience that joy today and become strong in prayer that Your power would be seen in my life.

Journal: Focus on relying on God's strength today and ask the Lord to make you strong in prayer.

—Pat Lewis

JUNE 10

PEACE-FILLED PROTECTION

And the peace of God, which transcends all understanding, will guard your hearts and your minds in Christ Jesus.

PHILIPPIANS 4:7

We have a guard dog named Meathead. He belongs to the man next door, but he showed up shortly after we moved into our home, and he only leaves if his owner comes over to get him.

My husband, Johnny, made the mistake of feeding Meathead because he always looks hungry. Now he refuses to leave Johnny's side, and he won't even let visitors get out of their car unless Johnny tells him it's okay.

I know this is a weird way to illustrate what this verse means to me, but as I was thinking about it, I realized how much peace we have when we're home alone because of Meathead. When he is here, no one will be able to harm us.

God's peace, which defies our understanding, works much the same way. Because of Jesus and our accepting Him as Savior, our hearts and minds are guarded and filled with peace as we allow Him to take care of us. When I allow my mind to be filled with fear and start to think of all the "what ifs," I only need to call on my friend, Jesus, the guard of my life. He wants to fill me with His peace that truly transcends all understanding.

PRAYER

O Lord, help me today not to be afraid of the future and to realize that You are the guard of my mind and heart.

Journal: Confess to God areas in which you are lacking peace. Ask Him to guard your heart and mind today and to fill you with His peace.

—Carole Lewis

JUNE 11

BEYOND OUR OWN ABILITY

And the peace of God, which transcends all understanding, will guard your hearts and your minds in Christ Jesus.

PHILIPPIANS 4:7

God promises that we can have peace that passes understanding. We've often heard it said that God won't give us anything we can't handle. Many people think this means we will never have to face really hard trials.

It may surprise you to know that Paul suffered hardships in Asia that he said were *far beyond* his ability to endure! If you study 2 Corinthians 1, you'll see he "despaired even of life" (v. 8) and "felt the sentence of death" (v. 9). The word "sentence" in the Greek actually means "answer"[2]—Paul felt like the only answer was to go ahead and die, because he couldn't see any light at the end of the tunnel!

As I write this in late September 2001, there are thousands of people still trapped in the rubble of the World Trade Center. How can the families of those people stand that? They have nothing to put in a casket, nothing to touch, nothing to stand over and grieve. How do you deal with that? I think that's a situation far beyond the ability to endure.

But if you keep reading what Paul has written, he explains that there is a special surpassing kind of power, comfort and glory that God only gives in those truly terrible times that are beyond our ability to endure. So yes, there is a peace that passes understanding. No hardship, trial or tragedy is excluded from that promise.

PRAYER

Lord, I thank You for the promise that no matter what comes into my life, You will give peace that transcends understanding.

Journal: Think of things that you feel would be far beyond your ability to endure. Thank God that He has peace sufficient for even those hardships.

—Kathy Hickey

JUNE 12

COUNT YOUR MANY BLESSINGS

And the peace of God, which transcends all understanding, will guard your hearts and your minds in Christ Jesus.

PHILIPPIANS 4:7

The peace that passes understanding is a wonderful promise from God. But if we look more closely, it's a conditional promise. The previous verse says that God will give us this peace *if* we present our requests to Him by prayer and petition *with thanksgiving.*

I once read a story about a seven-year-old boy whose little brother had died unexpectedly. The night after his brother's funeral, the boy's mother was lying quietly beside him in bed. Out of the silence and darkness, the little boy said, "I feel sorry for us. But I almost feel more sorry for all those other people."

When she asked him what other people he was referring to, he said, "The people who never knew Tanner. Weren't we lucky to have Tanner with us for 20 months? Just think, there are lots of people who were never lucky enough to know him at all. We are really lucky people."

My granddaughter recently died—and how I need the attitude of this little boy! I can think of all the things I didn't get to do with her, or I can thank God for the 1,072 days I had with her. And if I want God's peace, I know exactly what to do, thanks to a great apostle and a wise seven-year-old boy!

PRAYER

Lord, so often I want Your peace, but I don't cultivate the condition You said I needed in order to experience peace. Give me a thankful heart today!

Journal: Make a list of things you are thankful for, and just see what a great attitude you have all day!

—Kathy Hickey

JUNE 13

INNER PEACE

And the peace of God, which transcends all understanding, will guard your hearts and your minds in Christ Jesus.

PHILIPPIANS 4:7

In a world overflowing with unrest, finding any source of peace is a treasure indeed. How much greater it is to find a peace that transcends all understanding!

World events disturb us and we long for deep peace. When something bad happens, we often begin sentences with the words "How could someone" or "Why would someone."

To me, the most interesting part of Philippians 4:7 is that God's peace is not just a feeling but a part of our intellect. Our hearts cry for peace as we struggle with everyday life. God's peace can fill that need. But our minds also need a sense of purpose and meaning in all that happens. When we keep asking why and there is no logical answer, we keep our spirits stirred up and restless.

God's peace can fill that inner need for rest. We don't need to look further for peace. We can find it by looking to God alone.

PRAYER

Lord, may I be fully satisfied with Your peace in all areas of my life. Help me to reach for You when I sense needs in my heart and mind.

Journal: What areas of your life need peace? What have you used to fill that void in the past? How can you fill it with God?

—Helen McCormack

JUNE 14

BEHIND THE SCENES

Let us not become weary in doing good, for at the proper time we will reap a harvest if we do not give up.

GALATIANS 6:9

When I read Galatians 6:9, I am immediately reminded of my friend and assistant, Pat. She is *the* most amazing person. She loves for me to clean off my desk, which just means more work for her. She never acts annoyed with all the myriad tasks she has to accomplish. When we had to downsize our staff from 25 to 5 people, Pat started wearing even more hats.

I have marveled to myself and to Pat that it's hard for me to understand how she never becomes weary. She doesn't even get the reward of accolades from being in the public eye, as I get all the attention for the work *she* has done. Pat has told me time after time that I don't need to worry, because God is allowing her to reap the full harvest of all He is doing in First Place by using her service to me to bless my life. She makes my life easier in thousands of ways, having gifts and strengths I don't possess.

A friend once told me she wonders if a lot of us will find out when we get to heaven that we don't have a big pile of rewards because we got them all here on Earth. She thinks it might be because we needed the praise of people more than God's. A quiet servant like Pat must delight the heart of God.

When you find yourself becoming weary, even though you are working hard and doing so much good, remember my friend, Pat, who allows God—and not the praise of people—to be her reward.

PRAYER

Dear Lord, I must confess that I love the praise of people when I work really hard. Teach me that You will reward me in ways the world knows nothing about.

Journal: Write about the areas in which you feel the least appreciated. Ask God to change the way you feel about needing the praise of people for what you do.

—Carole Lewis

JUNE 15

A LONG OBEDIENCE

Let us not become weary in doing good, for at the proper time we will reap a harvest if we do not give up.

GALATIANS 6:9

I have hit a dreaded weight-loss plateau. At first, I was quite frustrated. I called out to God and asked Him to please let me continue experiencing the weight loss. I was keeping my commitments, but I wasn't seeing the same results. Then I could feel myself starting to give up on making good choices. It started in little things like not recording everything on my Commitment Record. I wasn't trying to hide anything; I just wasn't taking the time to do it.

Before long, however, I was missing exercise time and not being faithful to writing in my prayer journal. As I continued to pray, I had to examine my motives. My behavior was characteristic of a fair-weather friend, and that was not acceptable.

The harvest principle reminds us not to become weary in doing good. I had allowed myself to focus only on weight loss as a fruit of the harvest. I was ignoring other benefits like lowered blood pressure, increased energy and the joy of obedience in keeping my commitments.

Now I am able to see the Lord working in my life to build perseverance.

PRAYER

Lord, when I take my eyes off You and Your plan for my life, I become weary. Help me to stay focused on doing good so that I may reap the harvest You have planned for me.

Journal: What can you do during this time of sowing and waiting for a bountiful harvest? Whom can you encourage along the way to do the same?

—Diana Robinson

JUNE 16

A NEW WAY OF LIVING

Let us not become weary in doing good, for at the proper time we will reap a harvest if we do not give up.

GALATIANS 6:9

Perseverance is the quality we most need if we are to achieve weight-loss victory. Diets are not successful, because they are a temporary fix to a long-term problem.

First Place promotes a new way of living and a new way of life. It changed my view of food and its true purposes. Food provides the required nutrients to make our bodies function. Any other uses of food are bad habits that need to be changed. Our bodies are temples of the Holy Spirit and need to be treated as such. It takes time to relearn new behaviors and change bad habits. It is said that a habit doesn't go away but must be replaced. This takes time—at least 30 days to develop a new and healthier habit.

Since it takes time to effect change in our lives, we need perseverance and determination, so we will not give up this new way of living that's healthy for us and pleasing to the Lord. In proper time we *will* see the benefits and positive results.

PRAYER

Lord, please grant me the endurance to keep making the right choices. Help me to persevere with the hope that one day I will see the rewards.

Journal: What are some ways you have used food for a purpose other than as fuel? Can you think of some ways you can prepare for a discouraging time as you change the way you use food? Who could encourage you when you grow weary?

—Roberta Wasserman

June 17

Instant Nothing

Let us not become weary in doing good, for at the proper time we will reap a harvest if we do not give up.

Galatians 6:9

Some days I feel like giving up. And today is one of them. Thankfully, God used two of my good friends to remind me of the truth found in Galatians 6:9.

When I read this verse, I often miss the phrase "proper time." We live in an instant world: instant success, instant money, instant gratification. I often look for an instant answer. Yet God says in Ecclesiastes 3:1 that there is a time and a season for everything. And in Isaiah 55:8, we hear that His ways are not our ways.

My friends recently reminded me that God is definitely interested in the end result of our journey, but the proper time will not come until the character He wants to build in us is complete. For example, if we instantly lost all the weight we wanted, would there be time for God to mold us through our nine First Place commitments into the people He wants us to be? No. Then we wouldn't be ready to keep the weight off permanently, because the character needed to do that would not be established.

If you find yourself getting discouraged by your rate of weight loss or by a situation in which you don't understand the timing, don't give up. The proper time is coming. In the meantime, we must cling to God with all our might and bind ourselves to Him through Scripture memory, Bible study and prayer. Then when the proper time arrives, we'll know because we'll be in sync with God.

Prayer

Dear God, during this time of character building, help me to take my focus off my problem and look to You instead. You are bigger than any problem I face. Help me trust You for the proper timing in my situation.

Journal: What situations is God using right now to develop your character? Are you looking for an instant answer, or are you trusting in His timing?

—Tarena Sullivan

JUNE 18

EVEN WITHOUT ROSES

Let us not become weary in doing good, for at the proper time we will reap a harvest if we do not give up.

GALATIANS 6:9

For the past several years my husband and I have helped to care for a retarded man named Don. We love him very much, and he is now a part of our family.

On the first Sunday of every month, I cook a huge meal for Don and my family. Just in the past year, Theresa, a retarded lady in Don's Sunday School class, moved in across the hall from him and began coming home with us too. Theresa loves to cook and helps to clean up.

Recently, I began feeling sorry for myself. I decided I wasn't going to do the meals anymore. As it happened, the first Sunday of the month was the next day, and I fretted all night about it. The next morning at Sunday School I didn't hear a word the teacher said because I was thinking about how unappreciated I felt.

As I left Sunday School and rounded the corner for the sanctuary, I saw Theresa and Don coming straight toward me. They had giant smiles on their faces and carried a dozen long-stemmed red roses. I said, "Wow, are those for Terry?" (Terry is their caregiver.) Theresa said, "No, Jan, these are for you. We wanted to give you something from us for working so hard on the first Sunday of the month." Needless to say, I was humbled beyond words.

Those roses lasted over a week and a half. Every time I passed by them, I was reminded that these children were God's angels. How thankful I was—and am—to be their servant!

PRAYER

Thank You for Your Word, Lord, that tells us whoever wants to be great must be a servant. Help me to serve Your special children in love and mercy today.

Journal: Make a list of people in your circle of fellowship whom you can serve. Ask God to show you ways that you can be His servant to them.

—Jan Jarrett

JUNE 19

DRESSED BY GOD

Therefore, as God's chosen people, holy and dearly loved, clothe yourselves with compassion, kindness, humility, gentleness and patience.

COLOSSIANS 3:12

This verse reminds me of my friend, Kay, a First Place associate.

Kay will tell you that if she knows anything for certain, it's that she is dearly loved by God. Kay learned this truth at a time in her life when she was dealing with some issues from way back in her childhood. Kay never felt special. Then one day God revealed, in a remarkable way, that she could let go of all those old feelings because she was *His* favorite. She realized that each child in an earthly family should be able to believe he or she is loved the most; but since that isn't always the case, she now knows that God never plays favorites and He loves each one of us the most.

Another thing I love about Kay is that she is one of the most compassionate people I have ever known. We direct many callers with questions to Kay because she is our food expert. When people talk to Kay, they always leave feeling like they have a new best friend. Kay has more *best* friends than anyone else I have ever known.

I have watched God work mightily in Kay's life since I first met her more than 18 years ago. I can truly say that when she learned that God dearly loves her, she was able to put on the clothing of compassion, kindness, humility, gentleness and patience.

All I can say is, "Kay, you're lookin' good!"

PRAYER

Dear Lord, help me believe that You love me best. I want You to develop in my life the qualities mentioned in this verse.

Journal: Write all the reasons you don't feel special. Pray over each of those areas and ask God to heal your hurts from the past.

—Carole Lewis

J U N E 2 0

HOLY AND DEARLY BELOVED

Therefore, as God's chosen people, holy and dearly loved, clothe yourselves with compassion, kindness, humility, gentleness and patience.

C O L O S S I A N S 3 : 1 2

Even knowing that we are God's beloved children, we still sometimes find it difficult to accept ourselves as "holy and dearly loved." But that is exactly what we are. God calls us holy because He has set us apart from the world. To prove that He dearly loves us, He sent His Son to die on the cross to save us from our sins.

As children, we knew that our parents loved us and protected us as much as they possibly could. Those of us who are parents now know that we love our children and would do anything we could to keep them safe. So why do we find it so difficult to believe that we are truly "God's chosen people" and to live in such a way that others will also know?

We need to learn to accept that we are beloved simply because the Bible tells us it is so. As we learn to accept this, we can then allow Him to clothe us with compassion, kindness, humility, gentleness and patience.

Learning to believe that we are loved won't happen overnight. But once we believe it and then let that knowledge transform our character, which is what Jesus desires for us, others will observe our example; and we will have opportunities to witness and win others to the saving knowledge of Jesus Christ.

P R A Y E R

Heavenly Father, help us to practice Your compassion, kindness, humility, gentleness and patience with each other as we learn to grow more like Jesus every day.

Journal: Choose two of the characteristics in today's verse to demonstrate to your family, neighbors or coworkers and ask the Holy Spirit to let them see Jesus in you.

—Wanda Shadle

JUNE 21

CHOSEN AND SET APART

Therefore, as God's chosen people, holy and dearly loved, clothe yourselves with compassion, kindness, humility, gentleness and patience.

COLOSSIANS 3:12

In order to clothe ourselves for God, we must remember our position in Christ. We are God's chosen people: He chose us! This is better than being honored as Woman or Man of the Year. It's not something you are working toward but a distinction that sets you apart.

We are holy because Christ has clothed us with His righteousness. Ephesians 1:4 reads, "For he chose us in him before the creation of the world to be holy and blameless in his sight." It is nothing that we do; it is who we are because of Christ. We are dearly loved because Christ gave His own blood and life for us.

When we recognize what Christ has already done for us, we can be clothed with His character—we can be compassionate, kind, humble, gentle and patient. All these qualities come to us from Him. We may have compassion on others because God had compassion on us. That leads to kindness as we see others as God sees them. We are humbled by the suffering of others, which reminds us of how Christ humbled Himself. We learn to be gentle with others because we see them as God's dearly loved children who still make mistakes and crave our patience with them.

The world is looking for examples of people who have these wonderful qualities. They may not yet recognize the source, but they want to know the reason for our attitudes. May we remember to share our faith as we live out Christ's character before others.

PRAYER

Lord, how awesome that I am chosen, holy and dearly loved because of You. Help me to be filled with compassion, kindness, gentleness, patience and the willingness to forgive.

Journal: Which character quality do you need to be clothed in more than any other? List some specific ways in which you would relate to others differently if this quality were more developed in your life.

—Pattie Perry

JUNE 22

A BASIC WARDROBE

Therefore, as God's chosen people, holy and dearly loved, clothe yourselves with compassion, kindness, humility, gentleness and patience.

COLOSSIANS 3:12

If on a sultry summer evening I'm going to a family fun night at the park and the plan is to play softball, I know I'd better wear old jeans and a T-shirt. The shoes I wear need to be the right ones too.

If I am going to represent the family business at a Chamber of Commerce fundraiser dinner, I know I need to wear a new outfit. I get myself a fresh haircut and get the car washed, knowing that I need to make the right impression for our business.

If I am one of God's chosen people and dearly loved, it only makes sense that I must put on those things that best represent my God. He desires that I wear compassion, so I can demonstrate His love. He desires that I wear His kindness so that others can see that part of His character. Humility should surround me like a cloak, shutting out the brazen light of pride. Gentleness and patience should flow through my speech and actions.

As a Christian, what are you wearing today?

PRAYER

Lord, help me to dress completely for each hour of the day so that I demonstrate Your character and love to those around me.

Journal: What seems to be your favorite outfit when you're "dressing" to represent Jesus to others? What other "clothing" do you think Jesus would like you to wear?

—Helen McCormack

J U N E 2 3

Dress for Success

Therefore, as God's chosen people, holy and dearly loved, clothe yourselves with compassion, kindness, humility, gentleness and patience.

C O L O S S I A N S 3 : 1 2

As women we spend countless hours trying to improve our outer appearance while the inner runs amuck. Why? In the words of a dear friend, "Because of *self*-stuff!"

First Place reminded me of God's desire that we be more conscientious about things that are eternal rather than temporal. Oswald Chambers wrote, "If Christ is to be seen, then what happened to Him must happen to us. We too, must be taken, blessed, broken, and shared."[3] Our physical bodies, however lumpy, are Christ's tools for doing His work.

Catalogs provide tips on dressing for success. But Paul supplied the *key* to true success: the virtues of Christ that we can wear in order to bring glory to God. Jesus has dressed, accessorized or completely made over those areas of my life—whether physical, emotional, mental or spiritual—that are a hindrance to the cause of Christ.

God's intervention brought a higher level of praise, prayer and Bible study; a weight loss of 125 pounds; new relationships; a fantastic group of ladies to work with; and a supportive church family. God can do a similar work in your life too.

P R A Y E R

Father of mercies, thank You for the attributes of Christ. Let my compassion have the quality of mercy, the nature of pity and the feeling of tenderness for others.

Journal: Have you inventoried your wardrobe lately? What do you need to discard?

—Pauline Hines

June 24

Learn from the Master

Take my yoke upon you and learn from me, for I am gentle and humble in heart, and you will find rest for your souls.

Matthew 11:29

I have a wonderful friend named Nancy, who works for First Place as our leadership training director.

I love Nancy so much and admire her desire for excellence. Nancy has always struggled with being what the world calls an overachiever. This is typical behavior of adult children of alcoholics. Nancy's father battled alcohol for many years; but, praise God, he came to know Christ before his death. I have teased Nancy about her pursuit of excellence but secretly have wished that a little of it would rub off on me!

A few years ago, Nancy felt that God was leading her to seriously begin memorizing Scripture. As with everything she does, she attacked this new assignment with a vengeance. She bought a flip chart of index cards and wrote the verse on one side of each card and the reference on the other. She determined to learn one verse each week and diligently practiced her verses every day while on the treadmill. I delighted in asking her to recite verse after verse to me until I finally decided that I wanted to follow her lead.

I believe God prompted Nancy to get serious about Scripture memory because He wanted First Place to give it a more prominent position in the program. It is because of Nancy and her determination that we have the Scripture Memory Music CDs as a part of First Place.

Is there something you feel called of God to do? Get determined to do it! You never know how many lives God will touch because of your follow-through.

Prayer

Dear Lord, help me start today to memorize Your Word. I want to learn from You so that I will find rest for my soul.

Journal: Write some verses that you would like to memorize and begin memorizing one each week.

—Carole Lewis

JUNE 25

THE SHEPHERD'S VOICE

Take my yoke upon you and learn from me, for I am gentle and humble in heart, and you will find rest for your souls.

MATTHEW 11:29

The most remarkable thing has happened since Nancy began memorizing Scripture! I have watched her relax more and rest more. I believe part of the change is because Nancy has not only memorized Scripture, but she has also incorporated what she has memorized into her mind and heart.

Memorizing Scripture will change the message on those distorted tapes that continually play in the back of our minds. Those tapes are lies from the pit of hell, put there by someone influential in our early lives. It might have been a family member or a teacher at school. These tapes say things like "You'll never be good enough" or "Just quit now—you'll never lose weight."

Memorizing Scripture will teach us what God is really like—and that He *is* love. It will teach you that Jesus' character is one of gentleness and kindness. When you memorize Scripture, after a while you'll find that the Scripture has not only erased the old tapes and transformed your mind, but it has also become a part of who you are.

I believe you'll like the new person you will become if you adopt this wonderful habit of memorizing Scripture.

PRAYER

Lord, give me a love for Your Word and for Scripture memorization.

Journal: Write down the times of day that you could memorize Scripture. It might be when you are driving or exercising or during your quiet time. It only takes a few minutes each day but will bring great dividends.

—Carole Lewis

JUNE 26

DON'T FIGHT IT!

Take my yoke upon you and learn from me, for I am gentle and humble in heart, and you will find rest for your souls.

MATTHEW 11:29

In biblical times, a yoke was a wooden frame placed on the backs of work animals to make them pull in tandem—one behind the other or alongside each other. Most often the yoke referred to bondage and hardship, but Jesus gave it a positive meaning. It's amazing how He always lightens our load.

When I think about people who have lightened my load, I think about my dad. As Daddy's little girl, I always helped him on the farm. Once my job was to drag the pine saplings he'd cut to the brush pile, so we could burn them later. Rushing and not listening to directions, I began pulling the trees by their tops to the nearby pile. While the sun grew hotter, I grew weary. My dad stopped his work and with twinkling eyes and a big grin explained how to properly pull the trees to their destination by pulling on the trunk end, so the branches wouldn't drag against the pulling force—*me.*

Forever wanting to do things my way, though, I continued to pull the tops. As the sun grew hotter and I grew even more tired, I never gave up my stubborn determination to show Dad my way was just as good.

Daddy just let me be and I invented a new family saying: "Don't fight it!" To this day I hate that saying because it reminds me that I'm determined to fight things—even when there's an easier, more natural or even supernatural way to do things.

With shining eyes and a kind smile, Jesus expects us to do things in tandem with Him. Then life gets easier.

PRAYER

Jesus, You make my life so much easier when I allow You to help.
Let me learn from You how to be gentle and humble.

Journal: What are you fighting that pits you against God's will? In what area(s) do you need to submit? In what area(s) do you need to walk in tandem with Jesus?

—Judy Marshall

JUNE 27

WALKING WITH JESUS

Take my yoke upon you and learn from me, for I am gentle and humble in heart, and you will find rest for your souls.

MATTHEW 11:29

When Christ is our Savior, we never travel the road alone. Jesus asks us to be yoked to Him; He desires to help us carry the load.

In life, the sins we have committed become a burden that can overwhelm us. But when we confess our sins, we receive forgiveness and the load is lightened. In sharing the load, Jesus teaches us as well. He desires our obedience and can steer us in the right direction, if our wills are yielded to Him.

When we are stubborn or proud, we bear more of the weight of the burden and do not find rest. Jesus is gentle and humble and will allow us to follow our pride until we realize the consequences and our foolishness. If we learn from Him, though, we will find an amazing inner peace along with a lighter load.

This same lesson is evident in First Place. Here we find others who are yoked to us. We have support through prayer, sharing what God is teaching us through the Bible study and even shared recipes and hints that make each day a little easier. Encouragement is another way we become yoked together and support each other in common struggles, assisting one another in overcoming them through Christ.

PRAYER

Lord, teach me to be gentle and humble so that my soul rests in You. Let me see the need in others that I may share their burden and lighten their load.

Journal: What burden is too heavy for you to bear? How has someone lightened that load for you? Does someone need you to help carry his or her load today?

—Pattie Perry

JUNE 28

LIVING FREE

So I say, live by the Spirit, and you will not gratify the desires of the sinful nature.

GALATIANS 5:16

Stephanie came to work for First Place several years ago. Stephanie is our resident computer expert and is so helpful and generous with her time. She is a young single woman who, the Lord willing, will be married to Chris by the time this book is published. I love Stephanie like one of my own children and have enjoyed watching her grow in Christ.

Stephanie moved to Houston after living her entire life in Missouri. I believe Nancy and William Taylor played a big part in coaxing her to leave her home state and move to Texas, because God had used them mightily in Stephanie's life when she was in college. Stephanie had already lost over 100 pounds when she moved to Houston, and she was happy to be able to work in a ministry that endeavors to help men and women lose weight and grow spiritually.

The reason I chose this verse to talk about Stephanie is because of the troubled childhood she endured. Multiple marriages, step-parents and step-siblings could have doomed her future. Because she met Jesus as a 12-year-old, her future was drastically altered from what it might have become.

You may know the Scripture that says that the sins of the parents will be visited on the children, even to the third and fourth generation (see Exod. 34:7). Jesus Christ can break the chain of sin in the life of any person who chooses Him as Lord.

Stephanie's precious Christian life is living proof that none of us have to gratify the desires of our sinful nature when we live by the Spirit.

PRAYER

Dear Lord, I want to give every painful memory to You today.
Cleanse my mind, heart and emotions of all my past hurts.

Journal: Make a list of all your painful memories. Go over the list and give each one to God, asking Him to set you free by the power of His Spirit.

—Carole Lewis

JUNE 29

FINALLY SATISFIED

So I say, live by the Spirit, and you will not gratify the desires of the sinful nature.

GALATIANS 5:16

I have finally learned to stop turning to food to fill the spiritual void in my heart. Gluttony and greed are both mentioned as sins in the Bible. Yet food had become an idol, and my sinful flesh and mind craved far more than I needed.

Through First Place, I learned to become more and more filled with the Holy Spirit. In this way, God has satisfied me far more than excess food ever could.

What I have learned most is this: We are emotional, mental, physical and spiritual beings. Like a table with four legs, when any one of these legs is not working properly, the table is out of balance. I had spent most of my life trying to fix the physical and emotional parts of myself without even addressing the needs of my spirit. Working on the spiritual part set me free and gave me victory over the issues that contributed to my excess weight.

PRAYER

Lord, thank You for helping me achieve balance in my life. Please show me other ways I can glorify You in my life.

Journal: To what, besides God, have you turned to find satisfaction for the cravings within? What steps could you take to live by the Spirit?

—Roberta Wasserman

JUNE 30

YOUR HOLY HELPER

So I say, live by the Spirit, and you will not gratify the desires of the sinful nature.

GALATIANS 5:16

The Holy Spirit is the key to our overcoming the temptations of this world. Jesus sent us the Holy Spirit to help us live a victorious life. When we learn this secret source of strength to overcome our sinful nature, then we need to nurture it.

Although you may have tried every different way of losing weight ever invented, try relying on the Holy Spirit and His empowerment, rather than on your own strength.

These are the skills we learn through First Place. The Holy Spirit is nourished when we memorize Scripture, which the Spirit can bring to our memory when we need to know what He desires for us. Through prayer we learn to be still before God so that the Holy Spirit may speak to us.

Learning to listen and obey that still small voice is an important skill to sharpen. We can record in our journals those times that we did hear and respond to the Spirit as well as the times we ignored it and what the results were.

Our relationship with God is built by communication over time. We need to sacrifice the time to develop this unity. Our flesh desires that we give in to its lusts. But by yielding to the Spirit, we have victory over these desires and we glorify God.

In all these pursuits we learn that the Spirit of God is truly our helper.

PRAYER

Lord, may You enable the Holy Spirit to speak loudly to me this day.
Give me ears to hear. May I rely on the strength from Your Spirit and overcome
the temptations that come at me. May this day be one of victory.

Journal: Spend some quiet time before the Lord and ask the Holy Spirit to speak to you. What did He tell you?

—Pattie Perry

JULY 1

DON'T GO IT ALONE

So I say, live by the Spirit, and you will not gratify the desires of the sinful nature.

GALATIANS 5:16

What a day! It began when I unwillingly crawled out of bed earlier than usual. I had an endless list of errands to do that day.

At 2:15 in the afternoon, I realized I had not eaten breakfast or lunch, and no water had moistened my lips. I had a headache and was grouchy. The woman at the post office was rude and a driver on the freeway cut in front of me without signaling. How dare they treat me that way! I pulled into a fast-food drive-through, ordered and sat in the parking lot to eat my calorie-laden burger and fries.

The radio was set to a Christian station, and the preacher was discussing the fruit of the Spirit. I listened as I wolfed down my food. He ended his message with Galatians 5:16: "Live by the Spirit, and you will not gratify the desires of the sinful nature."

I could barely swallow the food in my mouth. I remembered my hasty departure that morning, skipping my quiet time as well as breakfast. I had rationalized my water abstinence by telling myself I would be driving all day and could not take potty breaks.

It was a quick lesson that stuck: If the Holy Spirit is leading, I want to hear what He has to say and I will be ready to obey Him. He will help me discern between my own desires and His leading.

PRAYER

Heavenly Father, please forgive my disobedience and my unwillingness to allow Your Holy Spirit to lead me.

Journal: Have you bypassed the Holy Spirit lately? Can you see an area of your life in which your sinful nature is in control, rather than God's Holy Spirit?

—June Chapko

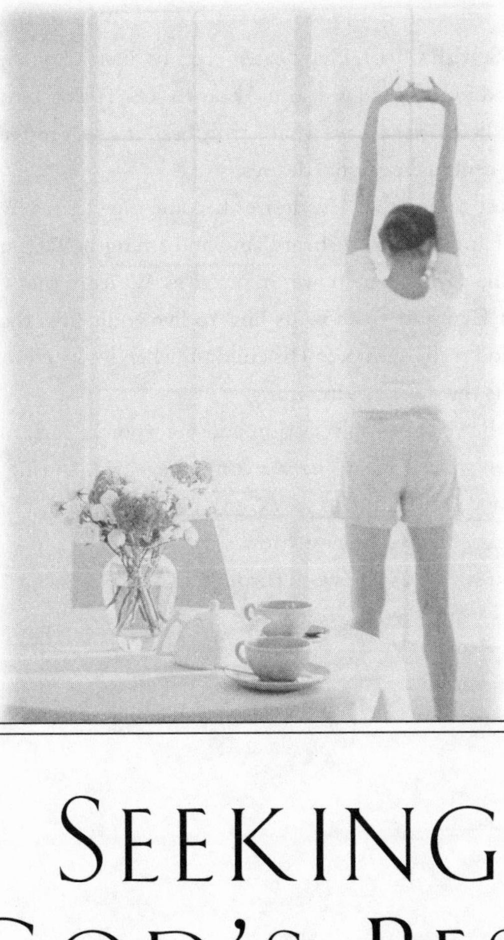

Seeking God's Best

SECTION FIVE

INTRODUCTION

Many times in my walk with Christ, I have eaten crumbs, instead of the sumptuous delicacies He has prepared for me. As I've learned how to seek His best, though, I've found that my version of the best is *not* always what's truly best. It's only my version of it, based upon my limited, self-centered personal desires.

To seek God's best means that His desires become our desires. When we seek His best, we learn to love Him with all our heart, soul and strength. We learn how to put on God's armor so that the devil has no power in our lives. We learn that God's power is all that matters and that He wants to show us how to live godly lives that are pleasing to Him. We learn that God really speaks to His children when we listen to His voice telling us the way to go. His is the way of overcoming.

If we memorize the verses in this section and incorporate each one into our daily lives, then we will learn what it means to overcome the world. During even the hardest times of our lives, if we will continue to seek God's best, then we will find ourselves able to still declare His praises to everyone we know.

My prayer for you is that as you work through this section, your life will become a praise to God—and a joy and blessing to you!

—Carole Lewis

JULY 2

God Hunger

Then Jesus declared, "I am the bread of life. He who comes to me will never go hungry, and he who believes in me will never be thirsty."

JOHN 6:35

Jesus knew the crowd was looking for another miracle. He began talking about the miracle of the loaves and fishes which He'd performed just the day before, and then He led them all into a discussion about bread.

John 6:27 is a powerful verse that would be good for each of us to meditate on today. In it Jesus says, "Do not work for food that spoils, but for food that endures to eternal life, which the Son of Man will give you. On him God the Father has placed his seal of approval."

And then Jesus goes on to tell them that the work of God is "to believe in the one he has sent" (v. 29).

Jesus, the masterful speaker, then directs their attention to the very thing He wanted to tell them from the beginning: "I am the bread of life" (v. 35). He is the only One who can satisfy their true hunger.

Are you hungry today? Is it that gnawing kind of hunger that food doesn't satisfy? Each one of us has a God-shaped vacuum inside of us that only God can fill.

As you make plans today for what you will eat and drink, give some serious thought about eating the only bread that will satisfy your inner cravings—Jesus.

PRAYER

Lord, thank You for being my food and drink. Help me remember today that spiritual food is more important than physical food.

Journal: Talk to God about areas in your life that you are using food to satisfy. Ask Him to fill you with Himself today so that you will be satisfied.

—Carole Lewis

JULY 3

SPIRITUAL SNACKING

Then Jesus declared, "I am the bread of life. He who comes to me will never go hungry, and he who believes in me will never be thirsty."

JOHN 6:35

There is a hunger and a thirst deep in our souls that call us to God. The hunger and thirst cause us to search for something to satisfy us.

When I asked God to forgive me for my sins and I acknowledged Jesus Christ as my Savior, the Holy Spirit came in to fill the emptiness. That is where my responsibility begins.

We must daily seek spiritual food for our spirit. Since Jesus is the bread of life and the stream of living water, we satisfy our hunger and quench our thirst only when we feed on the Word of God. If we satiate our spirit first, then the desires of our flesh can be brought under control because we are fueled to go the distance. On those days when we fail, we are probably "running on empty."

The great news is that we can always refuel during the day by memorizing Scripture and listening to Scripture songs. Think of it as giving your spirit a snack during the day. If we include spiritual snacks in our day, our spirits will be able to make the journey, no matter what obstacles we might face. If these habits become part of our daily walk with the Lord, then on those days when life rushes in we won't be overwhelmed.

The Bible teaches us to get our priorities straight: feed our spirits first and then our bodies.

What a way to live victoriously!

PRAYER

Lord, may You open my eyes to see what will satisfy my spirit today. Fill me with living water that will overflow into the lives of others and quench their thirst for You.

Journal: What ways can you nourish your spirit throughout the day? Just like we plan our food for the day, plan your spiritual snack too. What Scripture will you concentrate on today?

—Pattie Perry

JULY 4

TRUE WONDER BREAD

Then Jesus declared, "I am the bread of life. He who comes to me will never go hungry, and he who believes in me will never be thirsty."

JOHN 6:35

When I was a child, children were supposed to eat Wonder Bread. Remember the slogan, "Wonder Bread builds strong bodies in 12 ways"? (But I don't recall if they ever told us what the 12 ways were!)

In John 6:35, Jesus promises to "out-wonder" Wonder Bread. Of course, He wasn't really referring to physical hunger and the disciples were confused by his words. Jesus' promise in this verse is that He will satisfy the real inner needs that send us on our lifetime searches for fulfillment.

I didn't develop an eating problem because of physical hunger. Few people do. I ate wrongly for other reasons: depression, anger, loneliness. My eating often had little or nothing to do with my body's need for nourishment. There were many times that I ate to the point of discomfort, but I could never cram enough in my mouth to stop the pain in my heart.

Jesus promises in this verse that if we partake of the life He offers us, if we receive His love and wholeness deep inside, then we will finally be satisfied. He reinforces here the promise He made in the Sermon on the Mount: "Blessed are those who hunger and thirst for righteousness, for they shall be satisfied" (Matt. 5:6, *NASB*). Nothing will ever satisfy us like He will.

This spiritual food is like a buffet, but nobody—not even Jesus—is going to make you receive it. You must seek the Bread of Life and then accept Him to be satisfied by Him.

PRAYER

Dear Lord, I receive You as my Bread, as that vital necessity that nothing else can replace.

Journal: Have you ever tried to satisfy heart hunger with French fries? How can you recognize this tendency and seek to receive the only One who will satisfy your hunger?

—June-Marie Avery

More Than Enough

Then Jesus declared, "I am the bread of life. He who comes to me will never go hungry, and he who believes in me will never be thirsty."

JOHN 6:35

The more I study the life of Jesus, the more I grin at the way He taught by using everyday examples. When Jesus declared He was the Bread of Life, the crowd could still taste the bread from heaven they had received just hours earlier.

In order to get a better picture of what's going on here, let's take a trip back to the beginning of John chapter 6.

The Passover Feast is approaching and thousands have gathered on a hillside to see Jesus. The familiar story unfolds as stomachs begin to growl, but food is scarce. Jesus performs a miracle that day by feeding the crowd of 5,000 with only five barley loaves and two small fish. After all have had their fill, Jesus' disciples gather up 12 baskets of leftover bread.

The next day, Jesus invites the same crowd never to hunger again, if they will consume the true Bread from heaven—Jesus himself. Jesus not only longs to fill their physical stomachs but also their spiritual stomachs, with an overabundance of divine bread.

Some time later, during another Passover, Jesus lives out the words He speaks to the crowd in John 6:51: "If anyone eats of this bread, he will live forever. This bread is my flesh, which I will give for the life of the world."

During that Passover meal, recorded in the book of Luke, Jesus takes the bread saying, "This is my body given for you" (22:19). Later that night, Jesus is betrayed and then killed. And so His life has become the broken bread that bids us all to fellowship at God's table.

Jesus' death brings eternal life to all who will partake of His offer. And there is more than enough for each of us every day.

PRAYER

Jesus, thank You for providing me all the nutrition my hungry soul needs when I seek You. Help me never to be satisfied with anything less.

Journal: How has God satisfied your spiritual hunger? What Scriptures mean the most to you right now?

—Tarena Sullivan

July 6

Bread of Life

Then Jesus declared, "I am the bread of life. He who comes to me will never go hungry, and he who believes in me will never be thirsty."

John 6:35

Why did He call Himself "bread"?

Bread is the food the Lord gave us to keep us going and to supply our bodies with the necessary nutrients to sustain an excellent quality of life. He is also the living water that keeps us from drying up. Jesus can quench our thirst, if we believe in Him and allow Him to saturate our lives with His living water. Jesus is the ultimate thirst quencher and the bread that forever fills our bodies with the abundant life. He is our all in all!

The best thing about this heavenly bread is that we can eat all we want and never have to write it on our Commitment Record, because it's calorie free.

He is the perfect Bread of Life! You and I can keep coming back for more and more, and God is pleased with us every time we come.

Prayer

Father, I thank You for Your Son, the everlasting Bread of Life. I thank You that I can come to Your table where I will never be hungry and never be thirsty.

Journal: Do you eat too many bread exchanges? Ask the Bread of Life to help you with this commitment today. Thank Him that He will sustain us when we are hungry or thirsty.

—Beverly Henson

July 7

Willing to Be Willing

"Ever since the time of your forefathers you have turned away from my decrees and have not kept them. Return to me, and I will return to you," says the LORD Almighty.

Malachi 3:7

In December 1984, I found myself in quite a mess. I had accepted Jesus at the age of 12, but here I was, a woman over 40 years old, still wanting to run my own life.

I was at a critical juncture with God; He was pleading for me to let Him be in charge of everything that concerned me. God used terrible financial problems to show me the core problem: By not allowing Him to be the supreme boss of my life, I had really turned away from His decrees and had not kept them.

After this crisis, I heard at church a message that changed my life forever. Our pastor spoke a message about our will. He said that God was a gentleman and would not come and make changes in our lives without our permission. He said that if we weren't willing, then we needed to pray this prayer, "Lord, I'm not willing, but I ask You to make me willing."

That day, I sincerely prayed that God would make me willing—then I squeezed out a prayer asking that it wouldn't hurt too much. You see, I thought that if God had total control of my life, He would probably make my life miserable.

How foolish I was. Returning to God was the best decision I ever made.

God came close to me that day. And only because of that decision to stay close to Him, some pretty spectacular things have taken place. This is what happens when you allow Him first place in your life.

Prayer

Lord, make me willing to be willing so that You might accomplish all You want to do in my life.

Journal: List areas of your life in which you are unwilling for God to be the boss.

—Carole Lewis

JULY 8

ORDERED STEPS

"Ever since the time of your forefathers you have turned away from my decrees and have not kept them. Return to me, and I will return to you," says the LORD *Almighty.*

MALACHI 3:7

Do you realize that God *designed* you to be in relationship with Him? That is, He made you in such a way that your life does not really work right until and unless you are living in right relation with Him?

You see, God desires that His creation should acknowledge Him by living in obedience to Him. He also knows this is difficult for us, because we were given the gift of free will—the ability to do our own thing. Nonetheless, He has given us commands and decrees to follow to encourage us to walk in the path of right living.

"Obedience" is a word that's viewed so negatively in our society, yet it's such a necessary quality. Obedience means that we submit our will to a higher authority. Our human nature would rather consider our desires than God's desires. The same call to obedience mentioned in Malachi 3:7 is uttered by Jesus in John 14:15: "If you love me, you will obey what I command." In this verse, Jesus gives us the motivation for obedience: love.

As we learn this truth and obey God's Word, we submit ourselves to what is best for our health and well-being. And this applies, not just to our physical health, but to our spiritual, emotional and mental health too. As all these aspects of our being become balanced, we make progress and God is glorified. He will never ask us to do something that will cause us to fail, and He is always there to help us when we call on Him.

Be obedient out of love for God—and out of love for yourself. Ultimately, obeying God is the best thing for us.

PRAYER

Lord, thank You for being faithful in Your promises to me. I submit to You, my Lord, my Creator and Redeemer. May Your commands and decrees order my steps.

Journal: In which area of your life—physical, spiritual, emotional or mental—is it most difficult for you to be obedient to what God desires for you?

—Pattie Perry

JULY 9

STEPS TOWARD HOME

"Ever since the time of your forefathers you have turned away from my decrees and have not kept them. Return to me, and I will return to you," says the LORD Almighty.

MALACHI 3:7

How do we return to God?

We have a great example in the way the prodigal son returned home after spending his entire inheritance on wild living (see Luke 15:11-32). In this parable, the son did not know if his father would forgive him, but the son took the necessary steps to get home anyway.

I used to ask God to help me live more obediently. Then, I thought, I'd be able to sit back and live as if I answered only to myself. I expected a dramatic, magical, instantaneous change in my desires and motives. That, I have found, is not realistic.

The truth is, we tend to change gradually as we turn our focus on Him. We return home by steps. And those steps involve resisting the devil, saturating ourselves in God's Word, focusing on Him in prayer and seeking to make godly choices. Sometimes there are missteps, sometimes reversals, but eventually we grow and make progress.

Yes, God makes His power available to us. But He does not wave a magic wand and say, "You will live obediently!"

He does, however, give us a promise: "Return to me, and I will return to you."

PRAYER

Lord, teach me what obedience means. Give me Your strength to resist the devil. Remind me daily to read Your Word. May I be in constant communion with You.

Journal: How is the devil tempting you? What choices must you make to resist those temptations? How often do you read the Word? How much time do you spend in prayer?

—Helen McCormack

JULY 10

UNNECESSARY STRUGGLE

"Ever since the time of your forefathers you have turned away from my decrees and have not kept them. Return to me, and I will return to you," says the LORD Almighty.

MALACHI 3:7

The Message renders this verse: "'You have a long history of ignoring my commands. You haven't done a thing I've told you. Return to me so I can return to you,' says GOD-of-the-Angel-Armies."

Boy, does this verse nail me. I know what I should do—I just don't always do it!

The question is, Why don't I? I say I believe God has a perfect plan for my life. And yet I stumble around, ignoring His Word and making mistake after mistake. Why do I keep on stumbling?

God blessed us with free will. Unfortunately, most of the time we abuse it by choosing wrong things. We choose to eat that extra piece of cake, when we know we shouldn't. We choose to blurt out our angry words, even though we know it will cause pain. We ignore the creator of the universe whose hand is outstretched to help us as we struggle to free ourselves from the mire we've fallen in.

Why on earth would He give fools like us free will? I believe it is for this reason: If and when we finally make the decision to walk with Him, that decision to love Him is very precious to Him. The cry of His heart is, "Return to Me, so I can return to you." He longs to help us grow and learn, but He knows that until we choose Him and His ways, we won't really grow.

Our return to the Lord will come only when we realize that His way isn't just the best way—it's really the only way.

PRAYER

Father, I'm returning to You and Your ways for my life. Please return to me!

Journal: Consider the choices you make each day and make sure your choices are in line with God's ways. Are you returning or turning away?

—June-Marie Avery

JULY 11

OUR FATHER'S COMPASSION

"Ever since the time of your forefathers you have turned away from my decrees and have not kept them. Return to me, and I will return to you," says the LORD Almighty.

MALACHI 3:7

As I memorized this verse, I was reminded of one of my favorite stories in the Bible, that of the prodigal son. There is a part of this story that I absolutely love.

At his lowest point, this errant young man made a decision to turn from his sin and return to his father. Jesus tells us that even when the young man was still a long way off, his father saw him and, feeling compassion, ran out to meet him. The father embraced and kissed his returning son, welcoming him home.

Several years ago, the Lord put a love in my heart and a burden in my soul to pray for a friend who had turned away from her Christian heritage. As the story of the prodigal would describe it, she was living in "a distant country" (Luke 15:13), far from the Lord. One evening, as I was meditating on God's Word and praying for her, the Lord gave me a promise for her from Jeremiah 31:17: "Your children will return to their own land." I was so excited that I spent the remainder of the night in prayer, thanking and praising the Lord for His promise.

Early the next morning, the phone rang and I heard my friend's voice on the other end. What she said literally knocked me to my knees. She said, "I want to come home." There on my kitchen floor I wept and gave glory to God for His faithfulness in fulfilling the promises in His Word.

If you have friends or family members who are living in "a distant land" and you have been praying for their return, *don't give up*. God is lovingly waiting for them to turn to Him, so He can turn to them and welcome them home.

PRAYER

Father, thank You for lovingly and compassionately returning to us when we return to You.

Journal: Are you praying for someone to return to the Lord today? Read and meditate on God's Word, and write in your journal His promises to you.

—Pat Lewis

JULY 12

HOLY SPIRIT FIRE

Give thanks in all circumstances, for this is God's will for you in Christ Jesus.

1 THESSALONIANS 5:18

Years ago, I would have said that I could never give thanks if my husband had cancer or if we lost a child. This was before I fully understood the power that comes to us when we learn to give thanks to God no matter what our circumstance.

It is not coincidence that the verse that follows today's verse reads: "Do not put out the Spirit's fire" (v. 19).

When we accept the Lord Jesus, the Holy Spirit of God comes to reside in our hearts. If we are willing and sensitive to His leading, He keeps our lives on fire with excitement. Being thankful fuels the Holy Spirit's fire. I don't begin to understand how this is possible, but I have witnessed this phenomenon since the death of my daughter.

God has worked miracle after miracle in our lives since this tragedy happened. We didn't thank God that Shari was gone. We thanked Him because He would bring some good from this terrible event. We have all marveled as He has worked out every problem.

Giving thanks means this: I take my hands off the situation so that the Holy Spirit can work freely in my life.

PRAYER

Jesus, I don't want to put out Your Spirit's fire in my life. Thank You for the privilege of sharing in Your suffering.

Journal: List some circumstances in your own life for which you have been unable to thank God. Thank Him for each one and see what happens.

—Carole Lewis

UNSWERVING TRUST

Give thanks in all circumstances, for this is God's will for you in Christ Jesus.

1 THESSALONIANS 5:18

On a Monday in August, my husband, Ralph, and I were on our way to a week's vacation in New Braunfels, Texas. As we drove, it began to rain and I dozed on and off.

Suddenly, I felt the car swerve off the highway. I opened my eyes and thought we were going to crash into the guardrail on the opposite side of the road. I quickly closed my eyes and began to pray aloud, "Help us, Jesus! Thank You, Jesus! Thank You, Jesus!"

As I opened my eyes again, we were still traveling fast in the median on freshly mowed, rain-slicked grass. I asked Ralph, "What happened to the guardrail?" He answered, "God moved it!"

We were still riding down the median. Because we'd been taught not to use the brakes on a slick surface, Ralph hadn't used them, even though we were cruising along too fast off the highway. Ralph finally said, "I've got to do something." Then he put his foot on the brake pedal, and we slid to a stop unharmed.

Just before our vacation, I had memorized the above verse. I was learning to be thankful in all circumstances, and this was the first experience I had in which to practice the verse.

The verse tells us to be thankful *in* all things, not thankful *for* all things. It also tells us that it is the Lord's will for us to be thankful.

I found myself being thankful, not that we'd gone off the road, of course, but because He had kept us from harm in what could have been a deadly situation.

PRAYER

Lord, thank You for teaching me to be thankful in all things,
because I know this is Your will for me.

Journal: List at least two circumstances in which you have been unable to be thankful. Ask God to help you to be thankful, although the circumstances may not have changed.

—Wanda Shadle

JULY 14

GIVE THANKS

Give thanks in all circumstances, for this is God's will for you in Christ Jesus.

1 THESSALONIANS 5:18

As I read this verse I think, *Even for my broken nail? Even for missing out on that great job? Even for not getting the love of my life? Even for my own failures? I'm supposed to be thankful for all these things?*

Yes. Gratitude brings our spirit into right relationship with God. We bring everything we're going through to Him, lay it before Him and say, "Thanks, dear Father God. I know that You in Your infinite love allowed this circumstance in my life. And since I know that You cause all things to work together for my good, I can rely on the truth that this mess is good for me."

God is sovereign over the universe, so even the person who pulls in front of me in traffic is under His authority. If God allows it to happen, then He who knows the end from the beginning knows that this annoyance will work together with that frustration and sorrow for my good.

As we focus on gratitude, we focus on God; and then, like the old song says, "The things of Earth go strangely dim in the light of His glory and grace."

PRAYER

Thanks, dear Lord, for all that You lovingly provide.

Journal: What are you griping about that you should be thankful for?

—June-Marie Avery

JULY 15

THANKS IN ALL THINGS

Give thanks in all circumstances, for this is God's will for you in Christ Jesus.

1 THESSALONIANS 5:18

The phone call was a shocker. My cousin, who had been my best friend when we were growing up, had been found dead.

Although she had had health problems, no one expected her to die. Her brother wanted me to go next door to be with their 90-year-old mother, my aunt, when she was told.

Maintaining composure while waiting for the call was difficult. All I could do was pray and try to act as normal as possible. I waited until my aunt had answered the phone, and when I could tell she was being given the news, I moved to kneel by her chair. She let out a gasp. Then she was quiet. Then she asked a few questions.

As she put the phone back in the cradle, she said quietly and to my amazement, "Thank You, Father, for healing my daughter."

I saw firsthand how a godly woman found strength in giving thanks to God in all things.

Moreover, I saw how my aunt's strong faith in God carried her through the days ahead, as she adjusted to life without her only daughter.

How blessed I have been by seeing the power of God's Word at work in the life of one of His dear ones.

PRAYER

Abba, Father, hold me closer, hold me tighter, as I learn to be thankful in all circumstances.

Journal: Are you finding it difficult to be thankful in all circumstances? Tell God. He'll help you.

—Betha Jean Cunningham

JULY 16

FATHER KNOWS BEST

Give thanks in all circumstances, for this is God's will for you in Christ Jesus.

1 THESSALONIANS 5:18

When the good in our lives turns to bad, our free-flowing words of praise and thanksgiving to God can suddenly turn to grumbling and complaining. In the midst of difficult circumstances, it's easy to turn our focus from God to ourselves.

Fortunately, God does not expect us to go though any situation, whether good or bad, alone. The key to giving thanks in *all* circumstances is tucked into the last three words of this verse: "in Christ Jesus."

The apostle Paul recognized the importance of partnering with Jesus and relying on His strength to see us through the ups and downs of life. In Philippians 4:12-13, Paul says, "I have learned the secret of being content in any and every situation, whether well fed or hungry, whether living in plenty or in want. I can do everything though him who gives me strength."

When we rely on God's strength, we trust Him to take care of us. In Romans 8:28, God promises to work "for the good of those who love him." And we know from James 1:17 that "every good and perfect gift is from above."

A thankful heart understands that God is always working for our best—even when we can't see the whole picture and even when we wish He was using a different approach. Many times, we think we know what is best, only to find out God knows better.

Be encouraged: Hold on to Jesus, and practice thanking Him for saving you—from yourself.

PRAYER

God, thank You for always having my best in mind. Help me rely on Your wisdom and strength, and help me develop a thankful heart.

Journal: Spend time thanking God for the circumstances you currently face.

—Tarena Sullivan

JULY 17

EYES, EARS, HANDS AND FEET

While we wait for the blessed hope—the glorious appearing of our great God and Savior, Jesus Christ, who gave himself for us to redeem us from all wickedness and to purify for himself a people that are his very own, eager to do what is good.

TITUS 2:13-14

The longer I live, the more I look forward to Christ's "glorious appearing." The world we live in today is in such a mess. Wars are going on all over the world. People are starving in all of the Third World countries. The abortion rate is at an all-time high. America is a nation that seems to have turned her back on God.

The verse says that while we wait for the glorious appearing of Jesus, He is still working. Jesus wants to purify us and make us eager to do what is good. We are incapable of doing good works unless we are purified.

To be purified, we must give Jesus first place in all we do. Our first task is to spend time with Jesus to receive marching orders for the day. All day, every day, we are to talk with Him: about the food we eat, the places we go, what we read and what we say. When the Bible says to pray continually, this means we need to keep our hearts turned toward Him, ready to do what He says.

If we keep Jesus with us all day, we will always be eager "to do what is good." Then we will truly be glad—not afraid or ashamed—of the day of His appearing, which is nearer and nearer every day.

PRAYER

Lord, come with me today. Use my hands, feet and lips for Your glory. Before I make decisions, remind me to ask for Your directions first.

Journal: List the tasks you have to do today. Go over each one and ask Jesus to prioritize them for you.

—Carole Lewis

JULY 18

GOD OF WONDER

While we wait for the blessed hope—the glorious appearing of our great God and Savior, Jesus Christ, who gave himself for us to redeem us from all wickedness and to purify for himself a people that are his very own, eager to do what is good.

TITUS 2:13-14

Carole and I both rise early and drive a good distance to work each day. Quite often, one of us will call the other and say, "Did you see that beautiful sunrise?"

One morning I saw an absolutely breathtaking sunrise and was reminded of Titus 2:13-14, "While we wait . . . for his glorious appearing." There are times when the sky is filled with such glory that I am sure He is going to appear at any moment. We can only imagine the splendor of His beauty; nothing on this earth can compare! Think about the magnificence of our heavenly home—streets of pure gold like transparent glass, walls of precious jewels and gates of pearl. "The city does not need the sun or the moon to shine on it, for the glory of God gives it light, and the Lamb is its lamp" (Rev. 21:23).

On occasion, I witness an equally breathtaking sunset and pray that God will continue to purify me that I may serve Him in beauty and holiness while I wait for His return.

Oswald Chambers said so eloquently: "Thou art the God of the early mornings, the God of the late at nights, the God of the mountain peaks and the God of the sea, but, my God, my soul has further horizons than the early mornings, deeper darkness than the nights of earth, higher peaks than any mountain peaks, greater depths than any sea in nature—Thou who art the God of all these, be my God."[1]

PRAYER

O God, You are an awesome God, majestic in all Your ways.
Thank You for giving us just a glimpse of Your majesty in this earth. While we wait for Your soon return, let us be about the work of building Your kingdom.

Journal: How has God revealed to you glimpses of His glory?

—Pat Lewis

FAIL-SAFE COMFORT

While we wait for the blessed hope—the glorious appearing of our great God and Savior, Jesus Christ, who gave himself for us to redeem us from all wickedness and to purify for himself a people that are his very own, eager to do what is good.

TITUS 2:13-14

Not long ago, this Scripture became so much more than words for me. The reality of which it speaks hit home amid tragic circumstances.

At a Round Top retreat in March 2000, I was again challenged to begin memorizing Scriptures. At one time, I had memorized 43 scriptures but then had grown weary. Now I was challenged afresh. By the end of September, I had over 20 Scriptures committed to memory. Carole Lewis sent the "Seeking God's Best" Scripture memory cassette to all who planned to attend the October retreat. There would be a reward for memorizing all 10 verses. I hadn't tried to memorize all the Scriptures at Round Top in March; but with a head start, I was ready to do better this time.

I was pleased with my progress at first. But when I hit week four, which focused on Titus 2:13-14, it was slow going. I was two days into it when a friend called with news that my dearest friend had been found brutally murdered while delivering mail in a rural area. I was devastated. The awful news added to the difficulty of memorizing this Scripture, but I made it a personal goal in honor of my friend.

As I put this Scripture into my heart, it began to bring healing each time I said it. Despite the tragedy of my friend's death, I was able to praise the Lord for the comfort that came in knowing my friend was now purified and that no amount of wickedness can now come between her and the Father.

PRAYER

Thank You, Lord, for turning the hard things into a comfort every time I review my Scriptures. Bless my time with You today, and nourish my soul.

Journal: Write about a time when God used one of your memory verses to encourage or console you.

—Carol Moore

JULY 20

WHAT THE LORD HAS DONE

While we wait for the blessed hope—the glorious appearing of our great God and Savior, Jesus Christ, who gave himself for us to redeem us from all wickedness and to purify for himself a people that are his very own, eager to do what is good.

TITUS 2:13-14

I had been out of church for almost five years when one day, while vacuuming, something prompted me to spontaneously pray: "Please God, help me get back in church."

One day not long after, I saw a picture and article in the newspaper. First Place was starting their new session at my former church. There was a photo of a woman with whom I had at one time attended a Bible study. As I reminisced, I knew, even in my wavering state, that I had to go, that this was God's answer to my "vacuum" prayer.

I was not new to First Place. I'd been a member, off and on, for several years. Now I was back and it felt right. I remember feeling compelled to confess a summary of my sinful past to my leader, Charmaine. With love in her eyes and acceptance in her voice, she said, "Don't you think that the blood of Jesus is sufficient to cover all your sins?"

I knew from that point, my life would turn around. That was almost six years ago. Since then, I would need countless pages to convey all that Jesus Christ, my great God and Savior, has done for me. I know that I do not have to wander away from my Redeemer, who gave Himself for me to buy me back from all my wickedness and to purify me. I am His very own; and by His grace, strength and Spirit, I am eager to do what is good.

Jesus softly and tenderly called to me one day, saying, "Oh, sinner, come home." And my life began anew, with Him in first place!

PRAYER

Thank You, Jesus, for giving Yourself for me. Lord, You are great and glorious! I praise You! Thank You forever!

Journal: Today give thanks and praise to Jesus Christ, your Redeemer, for all He is and has done for you. Tell Him how you long for His return and of the hope that is within you.

—Eva Williamson

JULY 21

BREAKING FREE

The LORD does not look at the things man looks at. Man looks at the outward appearance, but the LORD looks at the heart.

1 SAMUEL 16:7

Many of us joined the First Place program because of the truth spoken in this verse. We realized that the lost world is watching us all the time to see if God has the power to change lives. We realized that even though God had given us a new heart and made us different on the inside, the world looks at our outside packaging, our body.

Just the other day, I heard a Christian woman telling that God asked her to give up cigarettes shortly after she became a Christian. She knew that God had plans for her future and that those plans didn't include cigarettes. I love it that she related how God speaks to us individually. When we get to heaven, He won't talk with us about what somebody else did. He'll only ask us what we did.

What is God asking you to do today? Jeremiah 29:11 assures us that God has a wonderful plan for our lives. Are there some habits we have that are keeping us from participating in His plan?

He is asking *something* of you because He wants to fulfill His wonderful plan in your life. He might be asking you to do something or to quit doing something. Only you know what it is.

PRAYER

Jesus, I want to participate in the wonderful plan You have for me. I give You permission to pry loose everything from my life that doesn't belong there.

Journal: Write the one thing Jesus is asking you to do or to quit doing. Look at what you've written. Are you willing?

—Carole Lewis

JULY 22

WORTH BEYOND MEASURE

The LORD does not look at the things man looks at. Man looks at the outward appearance, but the LORD looks at the heart.

1 SAMUEL 16:7

This verse changed my whole perspective on how I looked at myself. After spending a lifetime focusing on the scale and the mirror, this verse helped me see that I had the wrong focus. The world had taught me that what I weighed and how I looked was the measure of my worth. That, however, was a lie. My worth is determined by the price that was paid at Calvary for my heart.

The Lord Jesus Christ died for me. My heart is a rare jewel. It is the place where Jesus Christ resides. When the Lord looks at me, He does not see fat, ugly, gross or all the distorted lies I fed myself for years. He sees one of His most precious creations. He sees a pearl of great price.

When God looks at me, He also sees Jesus Christ living in my heart. Anything that is in my heart that does not look like Jesus Christ, God wants to heal and restore. If Jesus Christ lives in my heart, I am His chosen one.

The Lord will never reject me. He'll never reject you. We cannot base our acceptance and worth on the world's standards. What we need to do is to look at Jesus Christ and learn to reflect His beauty and glory.

Then when God looks upon our hearts, that is what He'll see—and that's what the world will see.

PRAYER

Lord, forgive me for having the wrong focus in measuring my worth. Thank You that Jesus Christ paid the ultimate price for my heart. Please help me to see myself as You see me.

Journal: To what do you look to gain acceptance? What do you use to measure your worth?

—Roberta Wasserman

JULY 23

A Gem in God's Hand

The LORD does not look at the things man looks at. Man looks at the outward appearance, but the LORD looks at the heart.

1 Samuel 16:7

Whenever I read this verse, my heart is filled with thankfulness. I feel so blessed that my heavenly Father chooses to look at the inside of me, instead of the outside.

I remember one of the first times I felt self-conscious about myself. I was leading a high school pep rally with the rest of my cheerleading squad. I knew I was overweight, but it never really bothered me until I unsuccessfully attempted a back flip. I'll never forget the taunting and laughing from the boy's basketball team. As I left the gym floor, I felt absolutely worthless.

In hindsight, I believe God used my experience to begin to direct my heart toward seeking what He wanted for me, rather than seeking the approval of others. He began to reveal new talents and aspects of my unique abilities. I began to take my focus off the ugliness everyone else saw and place it on what God saw in me—a diamond in the rough.

Now I'm continuing to let God carve away the unattractive parts of my heart, so His brilliant light can shine through the gem underneath. I know I'm not finished though, because Jeremiah 17:9 warns us the heart is "deceitful above all things." It will continue to take the skilled hands of my Father to shape and cut out in perfect formation the facets of my heart, until one day I am complete in heaven.

I am thankful that the masterful hands of One who loves me deeply are the hands that are doing the shaping.

PRAYER

Lord, thank You for Your incredible love for me. Please help me see myself through Your eyes, and continue to change my heart, so I can radiate Your light to others.

Journal: How can you begin to see yourself through God's eyes?

—Tarena Sullivan

JULY 24

INWARDLY ADORNED

The LORD does not look at the things man looks at. Man looks at the outward appearance, but the LORD looks at the heart.

1 SAMUEL 16:7

It was one of the most beautiful apples I'd ever seen. And I could taste its sweet juiciness, even before I sank my teeth past the delicate skin into the firm crispness. I could even imagine hearing the crunch and feeling the sweet juice slide down my throat and slip through the corners of my mouth. I bought the apple and planned to savor the treat.

But as I actually bit into the apple and the juice entered my mouth, I was sorely disappointed. The skin was tough and bitter, and the inside of the apple was mealy and dry. There was no juice, only a crumbling, flavorless mass. I had been too absorbed with outward appearance.

Do we as believers spend more time on outward adornment than inward beauty? While it is important that we dress neatly and properly, let us not just set our hearts and minds on what man sees.

Let us set our hearts on becoming the obedient children of God—this is what our Lord longs to see when He looks at us.

PRAYER

Lord, what do You see when You look at my heart? May I not be caught up in outward appearance, but may I be driven to become inside what You desire for me.

Journal: How much time do you spend adorning yourself outwardly? How much time do you spend in God's Word so that you may grow in obedience to God?

—Helen McCormack

JULY 25

BEAUTY INSIDE OUT

The LORD does not look at the things man looks at. Man looks at the outward appearance, but the LORD looks at the heart.

1 SAMUEL 16:7

God used this Scripture during a very difficult and emotional time in my life: I was really questioning if I should continue to be a leader of my First Place group, because I was not "at goal."

As I prayed about this, I told God I could not serve Him and be effective in this ministry until I reached my weight goal. God spoke very plainly to me and asked, "Are you willing to serve Me in the size you are now—and trust Me to change your heart and your size?"

I am so thankful that God saw my heart and not my size.

Our whole society is so caught up in outward appearances. We value the beautiful, wealthy and successful. Television and movies show slim, beautiful, expensively dressed stars. Young girls and teens worry about their weight and looks. First impressions so many times are influenced by the way a person looks.

We are of great value and worth to God. He paid the ultimate price for us. When others judge us on appearance alone, before they take time to get to know us, they miss all the wonderful changes God has made in our lives. When the Holy Spirit comes to dwell in our hearts, God's love flows through our lives and others see this love in our actions and appearance. Our obedience and willingness to learn with a servant's heart mean much more than our outward appearance.

The true blessing is that as God changes our hearts and minds, our inward beauty begins to manifest itself outwardly. And then, He helps us to change our bodies, too—to Him be the glory!

PRAYER

Lord, change my life from the inside out. May I always be willing to be focused on letting You transform my spirit into the likeness of Christ.

Journal: Are you allowing God to change your heart, attitude and character, or are you focusing mostly on outward things like weight and appearance?

—Janet Kirkhart

July 26

The Devil's M.O.

Submit yourselves, then, to God. Resist the devil, and he will flee from you.

James 4:7

As Christians, many of us live defeated lives because we have never learned the truth of this verse: If we resist, Satan *will* flee.

I have a dear friend who has struggled with being overweight her entire life. She is from Alabama and has called me many times to ask for prayer because, as she says, the devil is "messin'" with her.

When the devil "messes" with us, he usually takes something that is true, or partially true, and wraps it in a lie. He might tell us that we've had a really hard day and that we deserve that huge bowl of ice cream. Or he might tell us that the reason we yell at our children is because we had such wretched childhoods ourselves. Mixing truth with lie, he messes with our heads and tries to lead us into destructive and ungodly choices.

How did Jesus resist the devil when the devil "messed" with Him? He spoke Scripture back to Satan every time (see Matt. 4:1-11). When the devil "messes" with us and we don't know any Scripture to quote, what are we going to do?

Why not begin memorizing Scripture verses that will help you resist the devil every time he "messes" with you?

Prayer

Dear Lord, I'm tired of the devil "messin'" with me. Help me start memorizing Scripture so that I have the strength of Your Word to resist him.

Journal: Make a list of every way the devil "messes" with you. Find Scriptures that will help you resist the devil in each of these areas. Submit to God by memorizing one of these Scriptures every week so that you will be able to resist the devil's schemes.

—Carole Lewis

JULY 27

SATAN-FREE ZONE

Submit yourselves, then, to God. Resist the devil, and he will flee from you.

JAMES 4:7

Many years ago, I thought my whole world was falling apart. I was depressed about my circumstances and the way our adult daughters were living their lives. One wasn't going to church at all. The other one was attending with us, but she didn't seem to have her heart in it.

I didn't realize it then, but I was allowing Satan to drag me down, instead of allowing the Lord to lift me up. Every Sunday while our pastor was preaching a wonderful, meaningful sermon, all I could do was cry and wish my daughters were listening to it.

I didn't realize that I was continuing to look at the problem, instead of the solution—Jesus Christ.

Then I joined a First Place group, and this verse from James was one of the first ones I memorized. It took a while for me to learn that I really can resist the devil and he will leave me alone.

But by far the most important thing to learn from this verse is that we must submit ourselves to God before we *can* resist the devil. Without our submission, there can be no resistance.

Fortunately, now both our daughters are serving the Lord and are active in their churches. Although some of my circumstances haven't changed, my attitude has. Every day, I'm learning to submit myself to God, to resist the devil—and to leave the outcome to the Lord.

PRAYER

Heavenly Father, help me learn to submit myself to You in all things at all times.

Journal: Are you able to submit yourself to God in all things? Why or why not? If your answer is no, list any changes you need to make in order to say yes.

—Wanda Shadle

JULY 28

SEE SATAN RUN

Submit yourselves, then, to God. Resist the devil, and he will flee from you.

JAMES 4:7

Every believer is an enemy to the devil. He knows that he cannot have our souls, but he knows that he can steal our testimony.

I became a Christian early in my life thanks to my mother and my church family. My philosophy in life has always been to do what is expected. When I have submitted all areas of my life to God, this attitude of cooperation has served me well. To me, the word "submit" means I need to surrender to God's control all my thoughts and actions.

Many times in my life I have not been proud of my thoughts and actions, yet I could often find a way to justify those thoughts and actions. But each time, through God's grace and love, my faith has pulled me through. The very minute that I let Him regain control of my life, I could tell that those temptations were easier to control.

Yes, I have experienced consequences for my disobedient actions. But each time I returned to the Lord and submitted myself to Him—His love and acceptance are unconditional.

And Satan fled.

PRAYER

Lord, please help me not take a second look at temptation today. Help me to turn away and follow Your lead. Thank You for Your love.

Journal: What actions are you going to take to resist the devil the next time he tempts you to make a wrong choice? Write down your thoughts and commit them to God in prayer.

—Scott Wilson

J U L Y 2 9

PENICILLIN FOR YOUR SPIRIT

Submit yourselves, then, to God. Resist the devil, and he will flee from you.

J A M E S 4 : 7

God has a place of peace and prosperity for all His children to enter. The day I walked out my front door at 273 pounds and took my first steps into my promised land was the day I joined First Place.

That day I began two courses: "Submission to God 101" and "Resisting the Devil 102." Good health is part of the inheritance the Lord has for us in life, but believe me, the devil doesn't *want* us to walk in the land the Lord has promised to us. Our Father in heaven desires that we enjoy a healthy life on this earth. In order to partake in the abundant life the Lord Jesus has promised us, we need to feel good enough to enjoy it. If we don't enjoy the blessing of a healthy life, it's like waking up on Christmas morning with a raging case of the flu: You can't enjoy any of your presents because you feel so bad.

When I was so large and sitting in my Lazy-Boy recliner, I wasn't just overweight—I was in bad shape through and through. I felt tired, I didn't like people, and I didn't enjoy my life much at all. When I began to resist the devil and submit to God, I started to feel better—and with each step, I became more submissive to the Lord and more resistant to the devil.

It feels so good to be walking in the promised land of good health. I feel so good about my life that I sold that Lazy-Boy recliner. God is so good!

P R A Y E R

Lord, take my hand and teach me the way to submit to You. As an act of my own free will today, I submit my life to You.

Journal: Examine your life and the areas which you are slow to submit to God. Bring these before the Lord and ask for the strength to bring everything under His Lordship.

—Beverly Henson

July 30

Unlimited Riches

My God will meet all your needs according to his glorious riches in Christ Jesus.

Philippians 4:19

What a glorious thought: God will meet every need in my life today!

I know this promise is true because I know Jesus personally, and I have asked Him to be the boss of my life. Because of this, when God looks at my life, He wants to see the "glorious riches" of Jesus in everything I do. God wants to see me acting and talking like Jesus. When God looks at my life and sees this happening, He will meet my every need.

The question for all of us is, Are we content to keep on living the same old way we have always lived, or do we want to find out what it means to enjoy Christ's "glorious riches"? Most of us have plenty of needs. We may need more money to pay our bills. We may need to lose weight. We may need for our children to accept Jesus. We may need our marriage to be restored. We may need God to step in with healing.

This Scripture says that *all* the glorious riches we need are found in the person of Jesus Christ. If we give Him first place in everything, seeking His best for our lives, then God promises that He will meet all our needs.

How about you? Do we believe this promise to be true for your life?

Prayer

Father, I have so many needs today. Teach me about the glorious riches that are in Christ Jesus and help me to give Him first place in my life.

Journal: Make a list of every need you have. Ask God to meet these needs "according to his glorious riches in Christ Jesus." When God meets each need, return to this list and tell how God met the need.

—Carole Lewis

JULY 31

GRACE-FILLED PROVISION

My God will meet all your needs according to his glorious riches in Christ Jesus.

PHILIPPIANS 4:19

Several years ago my husband, Ralph, and I took a teenager, John Parker, his foster father and his foster grandmother out to dinner. After we left our house to go pick up our guests, we realized that we had only $7 with us. We had forgotten to go to the bank, and since it was 6:00 in the evening, the banks were closed.

We tried stopping at two different ATM machines—both of which were out of money. So we cashed a $25 check at an Exxon Station. We wanted more money, but that was all the station attendant could let us have. That gave us a total of $32 for dinner.

Nonetheless, when we picked everyone up, we told John that he could choose the place for us to eat, hoping he would choose a restaurant that accepted credit cards. Everyone decided on Furr's Cafeteria. At that time, Furr's didn't accept credit cards. Ralph and I both prayed that the Lord would take care of us by allowing us to have enough money.

As we walked into the restaurant, the above verse came to mind. Under my breath, I quoted it to myself throughout the whole meal.

When we finished, the waitress presented our bill. The total was just under $30.

I have never forgotten that evening. It has continued to remind me that God does meet all our needs, although He may not give us all we want. We have many needs other than money, of course. But no matter what, God takes care of us.

I can tell you from personal experience that He loves us and protects us in all circumstances. And He provides for us out of His great riches.

PRAYER

Father, thank You so much for always meeting my needs. Thank You especially for Your love and Your protection at all times.

Journal: How can you demonstrate that God meets all your needs? List two ways you can do this today.

—Wanda Shadle

AUGUST 1

GOD OF THE LOAVES AND FISHES

My God will meet all your needs according to his glorious riches in Christ Jesus.

PHILIPPIANS 4:19

The summer after my freshman year in college, I decided to stay in the town where the college was located, rather than go home for the break. I moved out of the dorm into a small apartment and got a job to earn funds for the fall semester.

In between receiving my first and second paycheck, there were a few days during which I had no money, no gas and no food. In my quiet time, I happened to come across this Scripture. I decided to claim this specific verse in prayer and let the Lord handle my little problems.

As an act of faith, I placed on the dining-room table a plate, silverware, a napkin and a glass of water. I sat down in the chair and said, "Lord Jesus, I'm hungry; please send food!" Then I thanked Him for the meal as if it were sitting there in front of me. I waited for 30 minutes or so, but nothing seemed to be happening.

Feeling a little foolish, I shoved the plate aside, laid my head on the table and tried to pray some more; but I quickly fell asleep.

In a short while, I was awakened by a knock at the door. Before I could answer, my friend Donnie burst through the door with a string of fish in each hand. He said, "Hey, I've been fishing all morning and caught tons of fish. I really don't have room in my freezer. Please take some!"

It was by far the best meal I've ever had, and there were plenty of fish left over to last for days. God had been so faithful to meet *all* my needs.

PRAYER

Father, thank You that before we utter a prayer, You know our need and have an answer.

Journal: Describe specific ways that God has met your needs.

—Jeff Nelson

His Love Has No Limit

My God will meet all your needs according to his glorious riches in Christ Jesus.

PHILIPPIANS 4:19

God knows my needs and in His Word He promises to provide for each one of them.

He knew my needs, for instance, on April 8, 1998, when a roaring tornado ripped through our neighborhood and demolished our home and many homes surrounding us. My friend John, who'd lived across the street for 28 years, was killed when a tree fell across him as he lay asleep in an upstairs bedroom.

Despite this tragedy, God knew the needs of Anne, John's wife. He walked with her every step of the way "through the valley of the shadow of death" (Ps. 23:4).

God met our needs as we rebuilt our home. He helped us see that our family had only lost material things, most of which could be replaced. We still had each other and our faith in a God whose love has no limit. I stand amazed that there are no boundaries to God's power and that His provision for us remains inexhaustible, regardless of our circumstances.

God was still there to meet my needs on April 15, 1999, when my beloved husband died suddenly after a month's illness. How could this happen? We had been in our new home only two weeks before his heart surgery, and we had so much we planned to do. But in my heart I knew God had provided for my needs in the past, He was present with me now, and I had the assurance that I could trust Him for all my future needs.

Truly, God is enough—He's never failed me yet.

PRAYER

Lord, I thank You that I'll never experience a need in my life that is greater than Your willingness to provide for me.

Journal: What urgent need do you have today that requires a supply of God's infinite love and grace? Open your heart to believe that He will provide.

—Irene Bonner

AUGUST 3

THE FIRST STEP

Joshua told the people, "Consecrate yourselves, for tomorrow the LORD will do amazing things among you."

JOSHUA 3:5

One of the meanings of the word "consecrate" is to solemnly dedicate. I believe Joshua was telling the people that they needed to get serious about their faith, because the Lord was going to do some pretty amazing things among them the next day.

When we consecrate ourselves, we acknowledge that there is something God wants *us* to do before *He* can do some amazing things in our lives.

We might need to get serious by making a daily appointment to show up and exercise. We might need to make a serious decision to eat only healthy food. We might need to make a serious effort to memorize today's verse.

In school, the teacher would always tell me to quit playing around. She meant that I needed to get serious about my studies. To consecrate ourselves means that we are going to get serious about giving Christ first place in everything we do.

Is there an area of your life that needs consecrating today? Why not get serious with God about your need and make the changes necessary? As the changes are being made, God will start doing amazing things in your life.

PRAYER

Jesus, I need Your help today. I want to get serious about giving You first place in my life. Help me seek Your best for my life today.

Journal: Write down specific areas of your life that need consecrating. Go over each one, asking God to take control.

—Carole Lewis

AUGUST 4

BEFORE GOD WORKS IN US

Joshua told the people, "Consecrate yourselves, for tomorrow the LORD will do amazing things among you."

JOSHUA 3:5

During a recent quiet time, I stumbled upon this verse. I believed this verse was for me, and anticipating that the Lord was going to do something amazing for me the next day kept me awake all night.

Well, several "tomorrows" passed and my weight-loss journey stayed routine. The plateau I was on did not budge and I was tired of the ordinary. I reminded God of His promise in Joshua 3:5, and although I did not expect to wake up the next morning a size 8 (I was then an 18), I truly believed that something amazing would take place. Perhaps we would discover that our church scale was reading 20 pounds over the actual weight. (Hey, it *could* happen.)

My days continued to be ordinary, and I wondered if "tomorrow" in this verse meant something different from my definition of "tomorrow." I pulled out my Bible concordance and checked the Hebrew word *machar*, which is translated "tomorrow." It's meaning is "the day following" or "a time to come." This was not helping much, but I became determined to hold God to His promise.

I waited. Nothing. Then one amazing thing did happen. I heard a quiet voice ask, "Have *you* always kept your promises to Me?"

God did do an amazing thing. He showed me how often I break my promise to "consecrate" myself, which keeps Him from doing His work in me.

PRAYER

Forgive me, Lord, for breaking my promise of obedience.
Lead me in the way I should go.

Journal: Are you waiting for God to do something amazing for you? Have you neglected to keep your promises to God?

—June Chapko

AUGUST 5

Walk Through, Not Around

Joshua told the people, "Consecrate yourselves, for tomorrow the LORD will do amazing things among you."

JOSHUA 3:5

God kept me focused on this verse for a long time. Through it, He began holding me to my promise of obedience.

When I woke up each morning, my resolve to do what is right was strong. I employed God to take away my desire for sweets, which plagued me as the locusts did Pharaoh. My days began with anticipation of success in my eating plan and ended with frustration at what I perceived as God's refusal to do that amazing thing for me.

I prayed, "God, this is not too hard for You—nothing is. So why will You not take away my desire for sweets?"

I sat rebelliously waiting for an answer. Curiously, I began thinking about a gallbladder surgery I had some years ago. The doctor described my options, one of which was getting rid of just the gallstones. He explained that it was easier than removing the gallbladder, but the stones could re-form. I opted to have the gallbladder removed, rather than deal with stones again later.

I found it amazing that in difficult situations I am prone to want the whole thing zapped for me, so I will not have to encounter even an inkling of the same sort of problem in the future.

My heart softened a bit toward God. My rebellion turned into understanding. If God took away my desire for sweets, I would not be able to choose obedience. Would I never want to enjoy something sweet?

After that, I recorded my newfound wisdom in my journal and modified my request.

PRAYER

God, help me. Strengthen me, so I can taste the sweetness of Your Son and the precious fruit You provide.

Journal: Are you asking God to take something difficult from you, rather than asking Him to help you conquer it? Have you had a rebellious attitude?

—June Chapko

AUGUST 6

No Quick Fix

Joshua told the people, "Consecrate yourselves, for tomorrow the LORD will do amazing things among you."

JOSHUA 3:5

Another "tomorrow" arrived and disappeared. I read the morning paper and noticed an ad for a new herb that promised to produce amazing weight-loss results overnight. Could God be showing me this? Was this herb the amazing thing God planned to do for me?

Then I remembered a recent sermon focused on Satan's ability to deceive. I put away the paper and opened my Bible. The verses that convinced me the herbs were not from God were 2 Corinthians 11:14-15: "Satan himself masquerades as an angel of light. It is not surprising, then, if his servants masquerade as servants of righteousness. Their end will be what their actions deserve."

I placed the newspaper in the recycle bin and recorded the day's menu on my Commitment Record.

I am a servant of God, not Satan. With my menu of healthy foods before me, I prayed for God's blessing.

And in the peace that came over me, I know I received it.

PRAYER

Lord, I am Your servant and will serve You faithfully. Thank You for Your Holy Spirit and the amazing gift of discernment.

Journal: Describe a time when you became discouraged in your weight-loss journey. What did God do to pull you through?

—June Chapko

AUGUST 7

PREPARED FOR TOMORROW

Joshua told the people, "Consecrate yourselves, for tomorrow the LORD will do amazing things among you."

JOSHUA 3:5

Today is the fourth day God has pulled me back into Joshua 3:5. "What is it You want me to see here?" I asked, rereading the verse for new insight.

"Consecrate yourselves."

Oops, where did that come from?

The first thing that came to me was that I needed to be sure I understood what "consecrate" meant. My concordance revealed that the Hebrew word for consecrate is *qadash*, which means "to dedicate, prepare, purify." I felt the Holy Spirit show me that I needed to purify myself both spiritually and physically, to prepare and purposefully dedicate myself to God, before His amazing work would show up in my weight-loss efforts. Just doing the paperwork was not what God had in mind.

The next step was to put this knowledge into action. This meant purifying myself by confessing all my acts of disobedience and asking God to forgive me. I knew that this would not be a one-time thing—purifying myself would become a daily (sometimes *hourly*) event. Spiritual and physical purification was necessary in order to consecrate myself.

Under the guidance of the Holy Spirit, I fasted (on liquids) throughout the day and used Scripture to fortify my spirit. By bedtime, I truly had a better understanding of consecration and was better prepared for what tomorrow would bring.

PRAYER

God, thank You for the wisdom You provide and the understanding You have for me. Help me to put my focus on You, not food. Please remind me to consecrate myself daily.

Journal: Are there areas of your life that need cleansing? Have you allowed the Holy Spirit to guide you? What is God asking you to do today?

—June Chapko

AUGUST 8

LASTING FRUIT

My dear brothers, stand firm. Let nothing move you. Always give yourselves fully to the work of the Lord, because you know that your labor in the Lord is not in vain.

1 CORINTHIANS 15:58

The word "vain" often means unproductive, worthless, fruitless or useless. As a homemaker, I would classify vain work as work that I have to do over and over, like cleaning the kitchen, toilet, floor, clothes, etc. That type of work has a purpose, but it doesn't last forever. Even though I've done this kind of work thousands of times, it will still need to be done again in the near future.

This Bible verse says to me that the work we do for the Lord will never be in vain. All the work we do for Him will be productive and valuable. Our work for the Lord will bear fruit that will last. When we work for the Lord, the work will be useful in the lives of people for eternity.

I believe the reason Paul is telling us to stand firm and to let nothing move us is that he knew a powerful truth that we need to learn: All the earthly things we do, even those that are necessary, do not bring us joy; joy is experienced as our lives are changed and turned to Christ.

Too often we let the good get in the way of the best. If we will give ourselves fully to the work of the Lord, we can be assured that the work we do will not be in vain.

PRAYER

Dear Lord, I want to stand firm today. Help me as I do my regular work today to make time to do some work that will last.

Journal: Make two lists. In the first list include all the things that you might consider "vain" work. In the second list include things that are work for the Lord. Ask God to help you incorporate His work into your daily life today.

—Carole Lewis

August 9

Steadfast and Immovable

My dear brothers, stand firm. Let nothing move you. Always give yourselves fully to the work of the Lord, because you know that your labor in the Lord is not in vain.

1 Corinthians 15:58

A pastor friend says that whenever we see the word "therefore" in the Bible, we need to back up a bit and see what the "therefore" is "there for." In this case, verse 57 is the reason verse 58 is at all possible. Verse 57 tells us we are victorious through the work of the Lord Jesus Christ, and that is *why* we can be steadfast and immovable.

Only if we stand on the Rock, can we be Rock-solid in all our efforts.

Standing upon the Lord, we don't need a plan B. Jesus has completed the work of salvation, and now it's high time that the fruit of this victory be seen in and through the work of the Church.

As I write this devotional, a plane has just crashed into a Queens neighborhood after take-off from a New York airport, we are at war in Afghanistan, and the economy is struggling to get back on track. And in the midst of all this tragedy, fear and anxiety, God is calling me to be steadfast, immovable and always abounding in His work, knowing that my labor is not in vain.

How?

By living and working in the bright and shining light of His victory.

Prayer

Lord, let me not be distracted by events but, rather, focused on the work You have called me to do today.

Journal: List the distractions you had yesterday. Commit each one to the Lord in prayer and ask for His perfect leading.

—Bruce Barbour

OUR ETERNAL TREASURE

My dear brothers, stand firm. Let nothing move you. Always give yourselves fully to the work of the Lord, because you know that your labor in the Lord is not in vain.

1 CORINTHIANS 15:58

I once stitched my husband's favorite saying in a cross-stitch wall hanging. He keeps it in his office at the university where he teaches. It says: "Heaven is my home. Earth is my business address."

The more I think about that saying, the more I realize how transient and temporary this time is that we spend on Earth. This is not home. The material possessions we accumulate and the awards we win will not go with us into eternity. Our favorite car or treasured jewels will not go with us into eternity either. God has given us all things to enjoy—He is so generous with His blessings and gifts. But only those things that are furthering His kingdom really matter for eternity.

A life lived in total worship of God is the only thing that matters eternally.

PRAYER

Lord, what do I treasure above You? Help me to stand firm and make all I do count for eternity. Help me to remember: "Heaven is my home. Earth is my business address."

Journal: What value do you place on Kingdom work as compared with your earthly possessions?

—Helen McCormack

AUGUST 11

GOD DOESN'T NEED A BILLBOARD

My dear brothers, stand firm. Let nothing move you. Always give yourselves fully to the work of the Lord, because you know that your labor in the Lord is not in vain.

1 CORINTHIANS 15:58

As I was driving around town, I began to notice the billboards at fast-food restaurants. I began to think of the prayer-request list in our First Place classes. I found a billboard to counteract each prayer request on our list.

We had requests for those who needed help with portion control. I saw billboards that read "All you can eat," "Combo Specials" and "Supersize your order."

Requests for their family's eating habits to become healthier were met with billboards reading "Kids Eat Free" and "Buy one Pepperoni Pizza—get the second one free."

Many had asked for help with time management, and there was a billboard advertising quick drive-thru specials.

I learned from this that after we have done all we know to do and asked the Lord for changes in our lives, we are to stand firm. We need to do this, because the world has got answers for us that are contrary to the will of the Lord in our lives. We are so bombarded by advertising that we sometimes don't see the work of the enemy as he supplies us with easy, counterfeit answers to our prayers.

Give yourself fully to the work of the Lord and stand firm. He is faithful to give you the right answer, and He doesn't need a billboard to show you the way.

PRAYER

Help me, Lord, to stand firm and know Your will for my life.

Journal: List what you sense the Lord is asking you to do in your life; then stand firm.

—Beverly Henson

AUGUST 12

A TABLE PREPARED

You prepare a table before me in the presence of my enemies. You anoint my head with oil; my cup overflows. Surely goodness and love will follow me all the days of my life, and I will dwell in the house of the LORD forever.

PSALM 23:5-6

Most of us don't have the kind of enemies that David was talking about in this verse.

Or do we? Even though David was probably talking about a human foe, we most certainly have an enemy, and his name is Satan.

I love to meditate on this verse. I think about how our enemy, the devil, must be furious when we come into the presence of Jesus each morning to sit at the beautiful table He has prepared for us. Satan hates it when we have breakfast with Jesus and he has to watch us overflow with the joy that only Jesus gives. Satan must work himself into a frenzy when God's children eat with Jesus so much that goodness and mercy just flow out of them all day long.

Have you thought about the fact that we have to die physically before we can dwell in the house of the Lord forever? I believe that because we know Jesus, He comes to dwell with us now. The question is, Do we show up at the table He has prepared?

PRAYER

Lord, forgive me for not showing up so many mornings at the table You have prepared for me.

Journal: Write down all the things that prevent you from spending time at His table. Make a promise to have breakfast with Jesus tomorrow.

—Carole Lewis

AUGUST 13

IN THE SHEPHERD'S ARMS

You prepare a table before me in the presence of my enemies. You anoint my head with oil; my cup overflows. Surely goodness and love will follow me all the days of my life, and I will dwell in the house of the LORD forever.

PSALM 23:5-6

Psalm 23 has been my comfort during a very long and difficult time in my life.

It began when my father—my hero and best friend—became very ill with Parkinson's disease. My mother was frail and not able to care for him, so I became their caregiver. This meant moving back home to the farmhouse where I had grown up and living with my parents in order to care for them, thus leaving my friends and church family an hour away.

That became a long "season of loss" for me. First, my father died. Then my mother's health continued to fail, and soon she went home to be with her Lord and beloved husband. Since that time, three close family members have passed away. The last was my mother-in-law, who died just before Christmas this past year.

I share all of this with you to tell you that being an emotional or stress eater had a dramatic effect on my personal walk in the First Place program. I gained weight. I never believed, as a mature Christian who loves the Lord with all of my heart, that I could get away from the close personal relationship with God. But I did. Nonetheless, God has been so loving, patient and gentle with me. He has kept me close, wrapped in His loving arms.

Praise God I am back where I belong spiritually, mentally and emotionally. Now He is able to work again in the physical area of my life.

I know I will see my beloved dad and mom again one day. And in the meantime, I sit at the Lord's table each day, enjoying His company and great care for me.

PRAYER

Perfect, gentle Shepherd, keep me close and guide me. Never allow me to stray away from Your protection and comfort.

Journal: Are you allowing God to be your gentle Shepherd? Are you staying in His protective loving arms?

—Janet Kirkhart

AUGUST 14

ALL YOU NEED

You prepare a table before me in the presence of my enemies. You anoint my head with oil; my cup overflows. Surely goodness and love will follow me all the days of my life, and I will dwell in the house of the LORD forever.

PSALM 23:5-6

During a long season of personal loss, God provided a banquet table for me to feast from. He used this Scripture, along with a verse from Jeremiah, to speak to me about what was going on in my life and what I needed to do.

Jeremiah 15:16 says, "When your words came, I ate them; they were my joy and my heart's delight, for I bear Your name, O LORD God Almighty." His Word has seen me through the storm and brought me back into the close, loving relationship with Him that He desires.

You see, living out here on the farm, away from my close friends and church family, I had to turn to God and search for a deeper fellowship with Him. He was all I had. He taught me so much about myself and totally changed my heart.

Today my cup does overflow with praise and joy, because of God's goodness and love. I praise Him daily that He is the Good Shepherd and He has given me yet another second chance.

As I read this very familiar verse in Psalm 23, I wrote in my Bible a statement made by Duane Miller at a conference I once attended. It always helps me when things get tough: "He is all I need when I need it all."

PRAYER

Lord, You are all I need. When no one else understands, You do.
When I feel as if no one else cares, You do.

Journal: Are you feasting on God's Word every day? Are you allowing Him to anoint you with His Holy Spirit until you are filled with joy?

—Janet Kirkhart

AUGUST 15

BOUNTIFUL TABLE

You prepare a table before me in the presence of my enemies. You anoint my head with oil; my cup overflows. Surely goodness and love will follow me all the days of my life, and I will dwell in the house of the LORD forever.

PSALM 23:5-6

The Lord has prepared for us a place precious to Him. He has tailored this precious table specifically to fit our special needs. And He does this because we are special to the Shepherd.

The Lord has prepared the table out in the open—so our enemies can see that we have a wonderful Shepherd who is mighty and strong and cares for our every need. The table has been prepared for us with, not just enough to quench our hunger and thirst, but with an overflow. There is more than we could ever imagine—only the best for His sheep.

We are somebody because the Shepherd loves us and cares for us. He cares about where we are right this very minute. He knows we have enemies, but He has made great preparation for us.

Then everyone will know to whom we belong.

PRAYER

I thank You, Lord Jesus, that You have made great preparations for my life. I come to Your table and thank You that all my needs are met to overflowing.

Journal: List your needs today and bring them to the Lord's table where all your needs will be met. Come to the table expecting great and mighty things from heaven.

—Beverly Henson

AUGUST 16

ALL THE DAYS OF YOUR LIFE

You prepare a table before me in the presence of my enemies. You anoint my head with oil; my cup overflows. Surely goodness and love will follow me all the days of my life, and I will dwell in the house of the LORD forever.

PSALM 23:5-6

"The LORD is my shepherd, I shall not be in want" (Ps. 23:1). So begins this psalm. And it ends with, "Surely goodness and love will follow me all the days of my life, and I will dwell in the house of the LORD forever" (v. 6).

There are no prerequisites to our having the Lord as our Shepherd, except to believe.

The Lord loved me just as much when I weighed almost 300 pounds as He does today, when I weigh 140 pounds. I hear those who come to class and say, "I haven't done well in my commitments this week."

Did you know that there is no condemnation to those who are in Jesus (see Rom. 8:1)? The Shepherd is our Shepherd—no matter how we did this week.

When I asked Jesus to be my Shepherd, Lord and Savior, God's goodness and love touched me like a hand on my shoulder. When I strayed from the Lord as a teenager and young adult, that "hand" never left my shoulder. It never let go when I went into bars or used foul language or was immoral. The Word tells me that God's goodness and love have been following me *all* the days of my life.

That is why I am where I am today, back at the Lord's table. Listen, friend: You don't have to wait until you are thin to partake of what the Shepherd has to offer. Take hold of it now and you "shall not be in want" (v. 1).

PRAYER

I thank You, Father, that Your goodness and love have followed me all my days. Thank You for loving me right where I am today.

Journal: Write the ways God has shown His goodness and love in different areas of your life.

—Beverly Henson

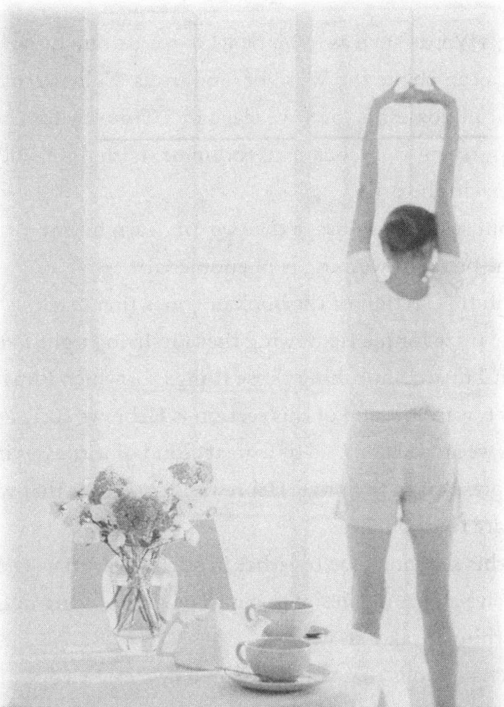

Pressing On to the Prize

SECTION SIX

Introduction

In many places in God's Word—such as in Mark 4:19—we are taught how worry and striving for material things can choke the Word of God in us. Colossians 3:14 teaches that the greatest virtue we can possess is love. We learn in 1 Timothy 6:11 that there are certain things we must pursue—"righteousness, godliness, faith, love, endurance and gentleness"—if we want to win the prize.

Behind these promises is the message that we can learn how to run the race so that we always win. And the prize for winning is phenomenal!

The Bible verses in this section of the book are ones that teach us what the prize is and how to win it. The prize for me is knowing that I'm living right in the very center of God's will for me, that I'm accomplishing those things for which I was created.

One of the verses toward the end of this section is Hebrews 12:1, a powerful verse of assurance that tells us we are surrounded by a great cloud of witnesses in heaven who are cheering for us as we press on to the prize. Hebrews 12:2 teaches that we will always win the prize—if our eyes are fixed on Jesus.

All the verses in this section come together in such a way that when you memorize all of them, you will have a burning desire to win. The prize—being in God's perfect will for us—is worth everything it takes to win it.

My prayer for each of you is that you will gain a new knowledge of what true victory means and that you will have a strong finish in your personal race.

—Carole Lewis

AUGUST 17

MORE THAN A DREAM

I press on toward the goal to win the prize for which God has called me heavenward in Christ Jesus.

PHILIPPIANS 3:14

It's been said that a goal is nothing but a dream with a time limit. I've had many dreams over the years. But the dreams I've seen blossom to fulfillment are built on attainable goals.

For instance, you might be dreaming of wearing a size 10 dress 10 months from now. If you weigh 175 pounds today, that means you might need to lose about 50 pounds in order to slip into that size 10. It's realistic to set a goal of losing five pounds a month. Fifty pounds sounds like a lot, but losing five pounds a month is an attainable goal.

What if you just dream for, say, three months about fitting into that smaller dress? Three months from now you'll have the same 50 pounds to lose, but you'll need to lose seven pounds a month to reach your goal. Add two more months of dreaming, and you'll need to lose 10 pounds per month to reach your goal.

Getting into a size 10 dress is a goal that is easier to obtain when you set a manageable time frame in which to achieve the goal. Likewise, having a treasury of Scripture is easy to attain if you memorize only one verse a week. Any goal is possible to reach, if you will start working toward it.

Losing five pounds a month means that you'll only need to lose a little over a pound a week. Memorizing in a month a passage of God's Word means memorizing only one verse a week. Why not set a small, attainable goal today and begin working to reach it?

PRAYER

Lord, I want to become a "meaningful specific," instead of a "wandering generality." Help me to set the goals You desire for me to reach.

Journal: What are some dreams you would like to see realized? Write them down, and beside each dream list small, attainable action steps that are necessary to realize that dream. Now ask God to help you pick one thing on the list to do for an entire week.

—Carole Lewis

AUGUST 18

A Higher Prize

I press on toward the goal to win the prize for which God has called me heavenward in Christ Jesus.

PHILIPPIANS 3:14

For almost 25 years, I played competitive softball with church teams. Weekly games, weekend tournaments and off-season conditioning allowed me to eat whatever I wanted without too much concern about my weight.

When I retired from softball, I realized I needed a new plan. Suddenly and for the first time, excess weight became a problem.

I remember my initial class with my First Place leader, Bob Matthews—and the shock I felt when I learned that one of the rules was "No sugar." I blurted out, "Does that include chocolate?" Chocolate and I have a long-term relationship. I once had a T-shirt that was inscribed "Chocolate: It's not just for breakfast anymore!" To me, not being allowed to eat chocolate was cruel and unusual punishment.

God encouraged me, however, through Philippians 3:14. I sensed Him saying, "Think of all the sacrifices you made over the years for softball trophies. Where are they now? Aren't you willing to make some sacrifices for the prize I offer?"

With that in mind I kept the First Place commitments. The victory was not just in losing 15 pounds or in feeling better, but the victory was also in controlling physical cravings with my eyes on a higher spiritual prize. The prize of obedience *is* more fulfilling than any trophy!

PRAYER

Lord, please help me understand that You have the "big picture" in sight. Give me strength during my times of weakness. Help me to press toward the goal to which You have called me.

Journal: What goals have you decided on, or what goals should you set, in order to do what God has called you to do? Ask God to give you strength in any difficulties you may have in reaching those goals.

—Dr. David Self

AUGUST 19

PRESS ON

I press on toward the goal to win the prize for which God has called me heavenward in Christ Jesus.

PHILIPPIANS 3:14

Achieving weight-loss victory takes time and endurance. Many times we give up because we do not see soon enough the results we desire. We want quick, if not instant, results when it comes to reversing a situation that took a long time—maybe a lifetime—to develop into the problem we now have.

It takes time to develop new ways of eating and thinking about food. In fact, it takes about 30 days to change a habit. Many times we give up before we reach that marker, not realizing that results are right around the corner—if only we had pressed on!

The picture Paul gives us in this Scripture—of someone pressing on to win a race—gives us the godly motivation to continue to persevere. It helps us to refocus on our original goal.

God wants us to have victory. Jesus Christ came to Earth that we might have abundant life. This includes overcoming obstacles in our path. Pressing on gives us more of a chance to reach our goals. Quitters never win, and winners never quit! Through Jesus Christ we can win the prize He has in store for us.

Don't give up on your race. Jesus is one of your biggest fans!

PRAYER

Lord, thank You for encouraging me to persevere. Thank You for showing me the right way to go for my reward.

Journal: How many times in the past have you given up just short of winning? Ask Jesus to help you work toward a manageable goal and persevere for at least 30 days. After one month, record how your perspective about quitting has changed.

—Roberta Wasserman

AUGUST 20

REACH FORWARD

I press on toward the goal to win the prize for which God has called me heavenward in Christ Jesus.

PHILIPPIANS 3:14

When Paul wrote Philippians, one of his last letters, he was in prison in Rome.

Paul mainly wrote to the Philippians out of his love and concern for their growth in the Lord. He wanted them to avoid the errors that plagued many of his new churches. The entire third chapter of Philippians focuses on leaving the past behind and going on with God.

In many Bible versions, a few words of Philippians are in italics, meaning they are found in some of the original copies made of Paul's letter but not in others. In the *New American Standard Bible*, which leaves out these "extra words," the verse reads as follows: "I press on toward the goal for the prize of the upward call of God in Christ Jesus."

This reading stresses what is so important as we work on the First Place Live-It plan (the choices we make to eat right): We need to forget the past and reach forward!

We can't change the past, but we can direct our lives toward a better future. Look for God's plan and reach for it; embrace it. Picture a runner stretching for the finish line. He has shaken off every burden and distraction to reach for the goal.

Okay, so you missed the mark yesterday; forget it and continue to press on!

PRAYER

Father, thank You for the power of forgetting. I choose to forgive myself, forget what I did yesterday and focus on Your plan for my life today!

Journal: What from the past do you need to forget—both the victories and the defeats? What should you be thinking about instead?

—June-Marie Avery

AUGUST 21

INNER JOURNEY

I press on toward the goal to win the prize for which God has called me heavenward in Christ Jesus.

PHILIPPIANS 3:14

Have you ever been on a long journey? You worked and worked at getting ready. You made plans, bought clothes, gathered supplies. You were committed to having a great trip. Then the day finally came for you to set out. Though there were many stops along the way, you did not give up, because you were committed to reaching your destination. That's the way most outward-bound journeys go.

First Place is also a journey, but it's not a destination. The journey has definite ongoing goals but no end, because it is, in large part, an inward journey.

When I began my First Place journey several years ago, I thought I would eat right, exercise, lose to my desired weight goal and stay there forever. How wrong I was! I did reach my goal weight, but I gained back some weight. Perhaps the main reason for my regaining weight was because I relaxed or even temporarily ignored my commitments for the journey.

Today I still run into stops and setbacks. However, even through my struggles, I have come to realize it is still a journey. I can say with the apostle Paul that I do not believe I have reached my destination. But I can bravely "press on toward the goal to win the prize for which God has called me heavenward in Christ Jesus."

As I press on toward the goals in my journey, I constantly remind myself that this journey is definitely a lifetime commitment—and follows a path well worth traveling.

PRAYER

Father, guide my footsteps today as I journey closer to You. As I look heavenward, equip me with Your strength and power, so I can keep my commitments for the journey.

Journal: What do you need to gather today for your journey? Is there anything you need to eliminate from your suitcase?

—Anita Clayton

AUGUST 22

FOLLOW THE LEADER

By faith Abraham, when called to go to a place he would later receive as his inheritance, obeyed and went, even though he did not know where he was going.

HEBREWS 11:8

I think I understand how Abraham felt—at least the "he did not know where he was going" part of the verse.

When First Place found itself in the position of seeking a new publisher after an eight-year publishing partnership came to an end, we looked totally to the Lord for guidance. Our prayer for a full year was that God Himself would pick our new publisher. There were so many that appeared to be a good fit for us, but we knew that only God knew the one that would fit perfectly. Sure enough, God led us to the most perfect publisher for us.

When we allow God to decide where He wants us to go, the ride is always sweet. God is the only One who knows all the ins and outs of every part of our particular situation. Therefore, He is the ultimate One to whom we should listen when making decisions.

If you don't have a clue where you are headed today, just hang on to God's hand and He will lead you straight to your inheritance.

PRAYER

Lord, I want to obey You and go where You want me to go.

Journal: Write down a decision you need to make. Begin to ask God to make the decision for you. Watch as He works in His own marvelous way to answer your prayer. Record the results.

—Carole Lewis

AUGUST 23

NEVER ALONE

By faith Abraham, when called to go to a place he would later receive as his inheritance, obeyed and went, even though he did not know where he was going.

HEBREWS 11:8

As I worked one morning to memorize this verse, I asked God if it would ever apply to my life. God answered, "You are going to go to the First Place conference in Utah."

Now this might not seem like a big deal to most people, but you have to understand that I'm not one to travel alone. I have never flown by myself, stayed in a hotel by myself or rented a car and driven around a strange city by myself. By the time God told me I needed to go, I also knew that no one else from my First Place group would be able to go with me.

Somehow I knew inside that traveling alone was exactly what God wanted me to do. I remember telling a friend that I could ask the whole world to go with me to the conference, and everyone would tell me no.

This was a time for me to trust God to help me through the unknown and to know that He would be with me every step of the way. What a blessing that conference was to my life. I met some wonderful people, and God gave me some great insights to ponder as well as lots of information to take back to my group.

Most important, I learned that I can trust Him with the unknown and that I don't need to fear, because He is always with me.

PRAYER

Father, thank You that when I obey and trust You, even when I don't know where I'm going and I'm unsure of myself, You are faithful to go with me.

Journal: Is there any area in your life in which you feel as if you are stepping into unknown territory? What promises has God made to you that encourage you to keep walking by faith?

—Elisa Davis

AUGUST 24

UNCHARTED TERRITORY

By faith Abraham, when called to go to a place he would later receive as his inheritance, obeyed and went, even though he did not know where he was going.

HEBREWS 11:8

Never before in my relationship with God had I experienced a call to go anywhere. But I was getting one now. Sometimes in answering our prayers, God sends us to places for indiscernible reasons.

That happened to me a few years ago when, after joining First Place, I felt a conviction that I wasn't being a witness for the Lord. I prayed that God would help me in this area. He answered a couple months later by dropping into my hands a brochure for the First Place Fitness Week in Round Top, Texas. I had never felt God calling me to a place as much as to this one.

After much prayer, I attended the Fitness Week. While pondering God's reason for this trip, I noticed that one of the topics for the week was our personal testimonies. I didn't even remember the date I had asked Jesus into my heart. All the testimonies I had ever heard had a specific date, a special prayer and sometimes even a memory of the song or hymn playing at the time. However, I knew God was faithful, and I began praying that He would remind me of my moment.

Not only did God lead me to a place where I would learn how to give my personal testimony, but He also helped me to trust Him more fully and in a new way as I followed His moment-by-moment leading.

PRAYER

Lord, may I always be sensitive to Your call. Help me trust in Your plan and believe in You, though I may not see where You are leading me.

Journal: Is God calling you out of your comfort zone to follow Him into uncharted territory? Tell Him of your fears, but commit to trust in His purpose and plan.

—Jill Jamieson

AUGUST 25

FOREVER LIFE

By faith Abraham, when called to go to a place he would later receive as his inheritance, obeyed and went, even though he did not know where he was going.

HEBREWS 11:8

I had 24 hours before the candlelight service where I would share my testimony. Although I didn't remember the date of my salvation, I wanted God to come through for me and reveal it in time for my testimony. I continued to pray during those hours, waiting for God to speak to me of my special moment. As we began the service, I purposefully sat on the far side of the room to give God a little more time.

As the woman next to me was finishing up, I pleaded, "Lord, if You are going to show me, *now* would be the time."

Instead, God chose not to show me anything. And when it was my turn, I started talking about how I was raised in a Christian home and how my family attended church every Sunday. I had been told all the Bible stories and for the most part was a good kid. But I didn't really have a faith of my own until I married. After this part of my testimony I really didn't have anything else to say. It felt awkward because my testimony felt so incomplete.

Kay Smith then said, "Jill, there are never too many times you can ask Jesus into your heart. But if you need a date, we'll give you one."

So that night, March 26, 1996, I prayed that sweet prayer and asked Jesus into my heart. I still believe I had a personal relationship with Jesus before that night. But what God gave me that night was the power of the Holy Spirit to deny Satan any ability to deceive me into thinking that I was an ineffective witness for Jesus.

PRAYER

Lord, thank You for being concerned about what concerns Your children. Thank You for the power You give us to testify of Your love.

Journal: Have you ever shared your testimony with anyone? Write it down first so that you don't allow Satan to deceive you into thinking you have no testimony. Then ask God for the power to testify for Him.

—Jill Jamieson

AUGUST 26

NEW SIGHTS TO SEE

By faith Abraham, when called to go to a place he would later receive as his inheritance, obeyed and went, even though he did not know where he was going.

HEBREWS 11:8

I had plans to fly to Houston, Texas, to attend a Christian women's conference just 10 days after September 11, 2001. I must say I was quite nervous about traveling! But I felt the Lord prompting me to go ahead with my plans. I can't describe to you the peace of God that accompanied me on that trip.

God blessed me so incredibly at that women's conference through the inspired speakers and wonderful worship. But most of all He blessed me by showing me that I do not need to be afraid of the journey. Wherever He leads me, He will come along!

Deciding to participate in First Place is certainly a journey. I remember my first session. I was terrified! Where was God going to take me? Would I be able to survive the journey? Would I get lost? Would I die along the way? Those nine commitments seemed like journeying to another world to me!

I have been on this wellness journey for eight years now, and God is still my constant companion. We have traveled over some rocky ground and up some high mountains. We even took a long dry trip through the desert, but I never grew too tired or thirsty! How exciting to think that this journey is not even over—He and I still have sights to see!

PRAYER

Lord, give me strength and courage for the journey of this day. Help me by faith to feel Your presence with me, guiding me and leading me in the way everlasting!

Journal: Has God called you to go somewhere? Ask Him to calm your fears and help you obey Him.

—Vicki Heath

AUGUST 27

Well Planted and Growing

But the worries of this life, the deceitfulness of wealth and the desires for other things come in and choke the word, making it unfruitful.

MARK 4:19

This verse is from Jesus' parable of the farmer planting seed. The seed is the Word of God. Different types of people who will hear the Word will respond in various ways. In this verse the person who hears the Word is likened to seed planted among thorns.

Many of us live in a thorn patch, yet we do not understand why our lives bear no fruit. Jesus tells us that unless our lives are planted in the good soil of His Word, we are destined to live barren lives.

By spending time with God each day, we soak up the nutrients found only in Him: peace, love, hope, joy. When we spend our lives focused on the earthly pursuits mentioned in this verse, instead of giving Christ His rightful place in our lives, we find that our lives become parched and barren.

I have an hour-long drive to and from work each day. Even though there is always a lot of traffic in Houston, I try to use those two hours to concentrate on God's kingdom. I listen to Christian music or uplifting sermons on the radio. I play my Scripture memory CDs and sing the Scriptures back to Him.

Why not find time today to let the Word of God penetrate your worries? God promises that His Word sown into our lives will always bear fruit.

PRAYER

Jesus, I want You to penetrate my life with the sunshine and rain of Your Word. Help me to put You first in all I do today.

Journal: List some worries bothering you today. Pray about each one and ask God to hold your worries while you focus on Him.

—Carole Lewis

AUGUST 28

DAILY SUSTENANCE

But the worries of this life, the deceitfulness of wealth and the desires for other things come in and choke the word, making it unfruitful.

MARK 4:19

The word "fruitful" brings to mind productivity and abundance, while "unfruitful" brings images of barrenness. Dry and barren times can cause us to grow hungry spiritually if we fail to seek the face and grace of God daily.

Strangely enough, the barren deserts of life often come after exciting mountaintop experiences when we've become so spiritually full that we think we'll never have to eat again. For some reason, it's after the best times that we become easy prey to what pinches off progress in our spiritual growth.

After mountaintop experiences of miracles in Egypt, God's people entered the wilderness. God provided manna for their sustenance but required them to gather only enough for daily use—no leftovers. God also blessed them with continuing fruitfulness as long as they were faithful to the covenant: "If you fully obey the LORD your God and carefully follow all his commands" (see Deut. 28:1).

Many hundreds of years later, Jesus prayed, "Give us today our daily bread" (Matt. 6:11). He realized His sustenance, and ours, is not from leftovers but from daily nourishment of spending time with the Father. Jesus also told us to be careful because we can be identified by our fruit (see Matt. 7:16). If we spend more time in the world than with God, our sustainer, our fruit will be much different from what He wants to produce in our lives.

PRAYER

Lord, protect me from the worries of this life, the deceitfulness of wealth and the desires for other things. Show me how I can make more time today to come to You for the nourishment and sustenance that only You can provide.

Journal: What are some things in your life that choke the Word, making you unfruitful? How can you effectively rearrange priorities in your day to allow more time with God? God doesn't give you leftovers; what fresh thing is He providing to you this day?

—Judy Marshall

AUGUST 29

A Proper Focus

But the worries of this life, the deceitfulness of wealth and the desires for other things come in and choke the word, making it unfruitful.

MARK 4:19

When my son was six months old, he crawled behind a chair one day and discovered an electrical cord. When I caught him in the act, he had just decided that it made a perfect teething toy.

I picked him up and brought him to another area, distracting him with a toy. My husband and I then went on with our work. Almost immediately, though, my son headed back to that spot behind the chair where he'd found this new "toy."

Again we picked him up, brought him to another area and distracted him with a toy. When we went back to our work—you guessed it—almost immediately he made his way back to that area of the room, looking for that cord.

One evening, during a brief lapse in our attention, he found a lamp plugged in and proceeded to repeatedly pull the plug out and push it back in. Not knowing how to hold it properly, he received a small shock. It did not really hurt him, but it stung enough so that he never tried it again.

Sometimes a one-track mind is a good thing and sometimes it is not. With our mind focused on the Lord and His Word, there is fruit. When we are distracted from Him by the worries of this life, by wealth or by the desire for other things, then there is no fruit.

What are you focusing on today?

PRAYER

Lord, let me not be distracted by the temptations of this world but be drawn to Your Word, for in it there is fruit. Build a one-track mind in me that is focused only on You.

Journal: What distracts you the most? Worries about your children? Finances? Food? Clothes? TV? Shopping? What would be the equivalent of touching a live electrical cord in any of these areas? How could you begin to focus more attention on God's Word?

—Helen McCormack

AUGUST 30

DON'T WORRY ABOUT IT!

But the worries of this life, the deceitfulness of wealth and the desires for other things come in and choke the word, making it unfruitful.

MARK 4:19

It was 2:00 A.M. when I slipped out of my young son's hospital room to spend the remainder of the night in the waiting room. Tim had just broken his neck in football practice; the prognosis was uncertain. Hospital rules would not allow me to stay with him through the night.

As I entered the waiting room, my good friend was sitting there. She knew the hospital rules and didn't want me to be alone when it was time to leave the room.

I had always been a worrier. I worried about my children and anything else I could think of. Once, laughingly, I told Carole that I even worried about her children since she didn't. In the wee hours of that morning, Carole asked me a profound question that would dramatically change the course of my life: "Pat, did you ever think to worry about whether Tim would break his neck?"

After I pondered her question, I said I'd never thought to worry about that. She remarked, "Well, it happened anyway."

It was a simple observation, but God used that moment to show me the futility of worry. Worry says we do not trust in God's faithfulness to protect and provide for His children.

Tim is now the father of four wonderful children. Today I pray for my children and grandchildren, instead of worry about them, knowing that I can entrust them to God's care.

PRAYER

Lord, I am so grateful that You are God and there is no worry in this life that is beyond Your divine power. Thank You for Your abundant love that provides for our every need as we trust You with our lives.

Journal: List the things you are worried about, and ask God to help you trust Him with each one of them.

—Pat Lewis

AUGUST 31

The Down-Filled Virtue

And over all these virtues put on love, which binds them all together in perfect unity.

COLOSSIANS 3:14

Paul tells us, in Colossians 3:12, that we are to clothe ourselves with the virtues of "compassion, kindness, humility, gentleness and patience." All of these qualities create a blanket that is similar to the soft blanket I sleep under each night. It is warm without being heavy. It is light and has a soft covering of cotton. I can snuggle under it and rest perfectly.

In Colossians 3:14, Paul tells us something that is equally important: If we will place on top of this blanket of virtues the down comforter of love, our lives will reflect perfect unity.

Sometimes I wake up and don't feel rested because my sleep has been interrupted. My mom is 89 and lives with us; but because of her health condition, I sleep with a baby monitor in my room. Sometimes Mom wakes up and needs attention. Sometimes the cat needs to go outside. Every time I have to get up, I come out from under my warm blanket for a little while.

The virtues mentioned in Colossians 3:12 must stay wrapped up in the comforter of love for us to feel truly rested in spirit.

How can we show compassion, kindness, humility, gentleness or patience without God's love covering us? Life is so *daily.* To live it victoriously, we must spend time with Jesus, the One who is love.

What kind of blanket do you sleep under? Is it the scratchy wool blanket of anger or bitterness? If it is, you are most likely going through the day exhausted.

PRAYER

Lord, I want You to clothe me with Your virtues. I'm exhausted and tired. Cover me with Your love today.

Journal: Write down things that keep the virtues named in Colossians 3:12 from shining through. Ask God to cover each one of those things with one of the virtues Paul mentioned.

—Carole Lewis

SEPTEMBER 1

The Power of Love

And over all these virtues put on love, which binds them all together in perfect unity.

COLOSSIANS 3:14

Above all, put on the ultimate attribute—the ultimate prize of Christ—love. It is said that love is our most powerful ally in our battle against a self-destructive lifestyle.

As an equipping agent of Christ, the First Place Wellness Program has taught many believers like me that Christlike selfless love comes through prayer—not a "gimme, gimme" kind of prayer, but a prayer request that will enable others to comprehend the all-embracing love of Jesus Christ.

Why is that so important? Only when we forgive ourselves and others can we truly pursue an intimate relationship with Him through prayer. Our relationship with Jesus becomes more and more intimate through prayer; and this is what brings balance, stability and nutrition for the mind, body, heart and soul—*total wellness*.

I feel so much excitement when I see "new things" in the lives of dedicated men and women of God. Need an encouraging example? How about a month-long churchwide fast called by our pastor? Loving, caring friends? Or the addition at a public school of a First Place class through which one of our new members lost 103 pounds.

Yea! Go, God, go!

PRAYER

Lord, thank You for expressing Your heart through infinite love. I'm praying that as we press on to the prize You will fill each of us with power through the Holy Spirit.

Journal: One of the best ways that you can love others is to pray for them. For whom have you prayed lately?

—Pauline W. Hines

PERFECT COOKIES

And over all these virtues put on love, which binds them all together in perfect unity.

COLOSSIANS 3:14

One day my husband and I were having a cookie-baking marathon. We were puzzled when we pulled away from the oven a pan of baked chocolate chip cookies much flatter than we'd ever expected. This recipe was tried and true, so we puzzled over the problem and went over the list of ingredients, trying to determine the reason for the disaster.

Then it dawned on us. We'd made a double batch and we'd doubled everything—except the flour. Obviously, an adequate amount of flour was necessary for those cookies to hold together! When we added more flour to our dough, the other ingredients were bound together in unity and the usual chocolate chip cookies baked up just fine.

The same is true of love. There are several godly characteristics (virtues) that should be growing in the life of every Christian. This verse says that love binds them all together in perfect unity. When we add love to our lives, it binds other virtues together and produces the kind of life that is pleasing to the Lord.

PRAYER

Lord, help me grow in all those virtues that You desire in my life. Most of all, let me grow in love, that I can be best used in worship and service.

Journal: How could you add more "flour"—more love—to encourage unity among your family, friends, coworkers and church members? Do any specific names come to mind?

—Helen McCormack

SEPTEMBER 3

GET MOVIN'!

And over all these virtues put on love, which binds them all together in perfect unity.

COLOSSIANS 3:14

You may be the kind of person I am. If I don't love something and have a heart to do it, it is next to impossible for me to do it. As I began to participate in the First Place program, I knew I needed to exercise, but I literally hated to exercise. I was the master of excuses when it came to exercise. I would go out of my way not to do it.

As the Lord led me through the First Place Bible studies, I began to realize that the key to my getting out of "fat prison" was through exercise. I prayed and told the Lord that I had changed a lot of things in my life. I had changed my diet; I had changed my habits; I had even changed my mind about some other things. But the one thing I didn't have the power to do was change my heart about exercise. I needed a heart transplant. I needed to develop a love for exercise.

To make a long story short, I have now walked 7,482 miles. In the past, when I went on vacation, I used to plan in advance where I was going to eat; now when I go on vacation, I plan where I can work out.

God gave me a love for exercise to replace my dread of it. God can change your heart too and give you a love for the areas in your life you formerly avoided. The result will be more balance and unity in your life.

PRAYER

Father, I need a heart transplant. I don't know how to change my heart and give myself a new attitude, but You do, Father. Today I give You permission to change me within.

Journal: Once you have your new heart, the enemy has plans to make you reject the transplant. But you can keep rejection from occurring if you start moving. Ask the Lord to help you get moving today!

—Beverly Henson

SEPTEMBER 4

JUST ADD LOVE

And over all these virtues put on love, which binds them all together in perfect unity.

COLOSSIANS 3:14

The first time I memorized this verse, I saw a mental picture of "all these virtues." I imagined them contained inside myself and saw myself putting on a T-shirt with "Love" written on it, bonding all the other virtues together in perfect unity. This image helped me to learn the verse.

We have so many of these virtues, but practicing them without love does not bring perfect unity. I make dinner most every night; but last night I "put on love" and made something for my husband that he really, really likes. It took a little more time, but it brought such joy to him.

When the children were growing up, I called the special things we did "making memories"—but really it was just adding love to the everyday virtues of life.

How hard is it to do the good things I do with more love? I'll put more love into my prayers for people on my list today. I'll put more love into grocery shopping and see it as loving my family. I'll love my Lord, myself and my family by putting in a good workout on the treadmill today and find more joy in it. As I put on more love, God uses that love to bring unity in my family and in the Body of Christ.

PRAYER

Lord, help me to see ways I can add love to everything I do today. Help me to do this for my loved ones; but, Lord, I also want You to help me do this for the people and the tasks I do not like. Teach me how to put on love for everyone and everything.

Journal: What tasks face you today? How can you add love to those tasks?

—Carol Moore

IN PURSUIT OF THE RIGHT THINGS

But you, man of God, flee from all of this, and pursue righteousness, godliness, faith, love, endurance and gentleness.

1 TIMOTHY 6:11

In his first letter to Timothy, Paul tells the younger man that "the love of money is a root of all kinds of evil" (1 Tim. 6:10). In the next breath, he tells us that instead of pursuing money, we are to pursue the spiritual virtues that last.

Sometimes it takes a crisis to help us recognize the goals that really are worth pursuing.

There was a time, back in 1984, when we had absolutely no money. We had lost our business and almost everything we owned except our home and its contents. This tragedy helped us take a long, hard look at our lives.

I found that my life was sadly lacking in the godly virtues of today's verse. I had sought after earthly pleasures and ended up bankrupt in more ways than one.

I finally hit rock bottom and confessed to God that I had made a huge mess of my life. I told Him that I didn't have a clue about how it could be fixed. He came in that very minute and took control; then He taught me some of the most valuable lessons I have ever learned.

One thing I learned is that my lack of money isn't a problem for God. Since He owns everything in the world, it is no problem for Him to give me whatever I need, if I will only pursue Him, instead of money.

When it comes down to it, this verse is talking about our *priorities*. Daily we need to ask ourselves, *Are my priorities in order or am I in a bankrupt condition?*

PRAYER

Dear Lord, help me to give You first place in my life. My priorities are misplaced and I need Your help.

Journal: Think about your life and list specific things from which you need to run. Give God permission to gently take each one from you and replace it with Himself.

—Carole Lewis

SEPTEMBER 6

Courage to Flee

But you, man of God, flee from all of this, and pursue righteousness, godliness, faith, love, endurance and gentleness.

1 TIMOTHY 6:11

In *The Message*, Eugene Peterson renders this verse: "Run for your life from all [worldliness]. Pursue a righteous life—a life of wonder, faith, love, steadiness, courtesy." The intended implication is that we are in danger if we do not flee.

We need to remind ourselves of this command to flee the next time we're tempted. We need to stop pausing to consider the disobedient thing we're being tempted to do; we need to quickly move on. We need to turn our face away from anything that keeps us from moving toward "righteousness, godliness, faith, love, endurance and gentleness."

"Flee" has another aspect to it. When we're fleeing, say, from a burning building, we don't have time to stop and grab all our treasures and valuables. We leave all baggage behind to escape with our very lives.

I love this verse because it reminds me that at times of temptation there is no time to stop and think—no time to figure out how much I can obey God and how much I can get away with.

I just need to flee.

PRAYER

Lord, I pray You will keep evil from me today. Keep my thoughts on Your righteousness and godliness. Strengthen my faith, love and endurance. If I am in an uncomfortable situation today, give me courage and wisdom to turn toward You and Your ways.

Journal: What areas in your life do you need strength or courage to flee? What can you do today to pursue a life of faith, love, steadiness and courtesy? What is most wonderful about Jesus, Lord of lords, today?

—Judy Marshall

SEPTEMBER 7

TAKE OUT THE GARBAGE

But you, man of God, flee from all of this, and pursue righteousness, godliness, faith, love, endurance and gentleness.

1 TIMOTHY 6:11

In just a matter of weeks after I had started participating in First Place in 1995, friends were commenting on the noticeable difference in me: I truly was a new person! I was reading the Bible daily, doing my Bible study and filling my mind with Christ. According to my friends, it showed.

In large part, I know it was because I was no longer taking in the garbage of the world. Instead, I was feeding my soul on the Word of God.

I've come to realize how important it is to monitor what we take in during our daily routines. What kind of books do we read? What are we listening to on the radio? Who are our friends?

In this verse, Paul commanded Timothy to "pursue righteousness, godliness, faith, love, endurance and gentleness." We must surround ourselves with these things to be able to actually live them.

In a sense, we are like sponges, because what we "soak up" each day is exactly what will come out when the pressure is on. Sure, it's easy to put on godliness when life is going our way. But when we get a little stressed or pushed about, how do we react? If we've truly pursued the traits listed in 1 Timothy, godliness and love will naturally pour out during life's ups and downs.

Remember: Positive In = Positive Out. Fill yourself to overflowing with the Lord, and others will see the light of Jesus all around you!

PRAYER

Lord, help me to cover myself in Your righteousness and godliness so that others will see You in me. May I live my life as a true example of the love You have for us all.

Journal: What are you filling your mind with each day? Do you need to monitor what you, as well as your family, are watching on TV or listening to on the radio? What, if any, garbage do you need to throw out?

—Terri Richardson

SEPTEMBER 8

HOLY ENDURANCE

But you, man of God, flee from all of this, and pursue righteousness, godliness, faith, love, endurance and gentleness.

1 TIMOTHY 6:11

Awhile back, I was riding my mountain bike on a trail when I made a bad move. In a second, I was flipping backward down a hill, with my bike on top of me. When I finally came to a resting place, I slammed to a halt and continued to lay there and shake for a few moments. I thanked the Lord for being with me through the fall. He brought to my mind the importance of developing endurance—and that it is a process.

Four years ago, when I weighed almost 300 pounds, any fall would have been tragic due to my weight and the poor condition of my bones and joints. I have been working out for four years now—a long process that has developed in me the endurance to even ride a bike. And I now have the muscular and cardiovascular endurance to survive a fall.

Likewise, four years ago when I began First Place, I didn't have the spiritual endurance to take the ups and downs and falls that I can take today. Staying in the Word, doing my Bible studies and attending meetings have gotten me in the best spiritual shape of my life. This too was a process that helped me to endure and get from point A to point B.

Many times, we become weary in doing what is right, and we give up much too easily. We need to ask God to give us some of His holy and anointed "stick-to-it-ness"—otherwise known as *endurance.*

PRAYER

I thank You, Father, for how far You have brought me. I thank You for how far we are going to go together. I thank You, Father, that I am not where I used to be. Father, throughout this journey You and I are on, give me holy endurance.

Journal: How is your endurance today? Begin your process toward spiritual strength by asking Jesus to help you keep keepin' on!

—Beverly Henson

SEPTEMBER 9

RUN TO WIN

Do you not know that in a race all the runners run, but only one gets the prize? Run in such a way as to get the prize.

1 CORINTHIANS 9:24

I was once asked to speak at a church in the suburbs of Dallas. I arrived on a Friday afternoon sick with a fever. A First Place leader had come with me in the event that I was too sick to speak when the time came.

That evening, God gave me the strength to speak. In fact, my fever broke the minute I finished speaking, and I found myself soaking wet with sweat as I talked with the people at the end of the banquet.

The next morning the church sponsored a three-mile Fun Run. Having been sick the day before, I started the race fearing that I would finish in last place. I pushed myself harder than I ever had before and finished the race with a time of 27 minutes! This was the fastest I had ever run three miles, and I was astonished to win a medal for my age division. (I should tell you right now that I was the only woman in the 50+ age division, so that's the reason I won!)

I treasure my little medal because I ran hard enough to win the prize.

Are we running hard today, or are we barely shuffling through life? Do we find that life is running right by us because we've lost hope and are discouraged? If so, let's get back in the race today. Jesus wants to run our race for us, if we will only give Him permission.

PRAYER

Lord, help me to get back in the race You have set out for me.

Journal: List the reasons you have quit running your race. Place each thing you wrote at the feet of Jesus and ask Him to pick you up and help you get back in the race.

—Carole Lewis

SEPTEMBER 10

EYES ON THE FINISH LINE

Do you not know that in a race all the runners run, but only one gets the prize? Run in such a way as to get the prize.

1 CORINTHIANS 9:24

The First Place program is a training ground to run the race to weight-loss victory. This program provides all the tools needed to succeed.

As runners, we must first set our minds on the goal—our eyes must be on the finish line. Then we must enter into training. To train, we invest time, energy and determination to do what it takes to win the race. We practice daily so that we learn the right way to run to win.

Only one thing guarantees not winning—and that's *quitting*. If we decide that quitting is not an option, then we will win. If we choose to train and stay in the race, we will win!

God is on our team. He wants us to win. He is at our side all the way to the finish!

PRAYER

Lord, thank You for teaching me how to run the race. Thank You for seeing me through to the finish line.

Journal: What is your goal in this race to physical and spiritual wellness? Can you imagine the finish line? Are you willing to go into training to run in such a way as to win?

—Roberta Wasserman

SEPTEMBER 11

WILLING TO RUN

Do you not know that in a race all the runners run, but only one gets the prize? Run in such a way as to get the prize.

1 CORINTHIANS 9:24

I really needed to win this time. It was August 1993, and I was defeated. I lived each day with shortness of breath, hypertension, a serious abdominal disorder and 100 pounds of excess weight. I was a Christian, a pastor, a husband and a father; but as a believer, I was defeated.

I had often tried to gain self-control on my own, attempting every diet and health plan presented to me. I had invested years of my time and hundreds of dollars. If I was going to try again, I really needed to win this time.

Someone introduced me to First Place, a Christ-centered health program. Although I was skeptical, I soon realized that First Place provided a way to succeed that I had never considered. Winning the prize of renewed health and a renewed spirit would not be because of me but because of Him.

When I entered the race for my health again, it was clear I was entering a marathon. My only qualifications were my willingness to run the race, my love for Jesus and my desire to be acceptable to Him. Soon, with improved health and a restored testimony, I began to see myself as a winner in Christ.

That was nine years ago. Now I am 80 pounds lighter, my health problems are under control, and I am walking three miles a day.

I want to be more like Jesus every day. I want Him to be in first place in my life. This makes me a winner already!

PRAYER

Father, when I grow weary and the finish line seems so far away, help me to realize that the prize is worth the race and I need to keep my eyes focused on You.

Journal: Winning athletes say the goal has to be worthy of the commitment. Today, renew your commitment to the goals you have set.

—Jim Clayton

SEPTEMBER 12

CHECK YOUR RUNNING SHOES

Do you not know that in a race all the runners run, but only one gets the prize? Run in such a way as to get the prize.

1 CORINTHIANS 9:24

The Olympic torch relay recently came through my hometown on its way to Salt Lake City. As the torchbearers carried the flame through the streets, I noticed the sense of pride etched on their faces. This was a historic moment, because they were part of a worldwide event.

We, too, have the chance to take part in a race of tremendous proportion and eternal significance.

In this spiritual race of life, our sights are set on the prize to which God has called us: knowing more of Him and sharing His love with those we meet along our path.

Just like every Olympian, we need the right equipment and a strict training regimen. Fortunately, running doesn't require much, except a good pair of shoes. Ephesians 6:15 says our spiritual foot protection comes from God's Word; and Psalm 119:105 tells us God's Word is a lamp to our feet and a light for our path.

If we daily set our feet on the terrain of God's Word, we will train our hearts and minds to know more of God and desire to share Him with others.

Our eternal prize awaits us at the end, but we can taste the sweetness of victory now. So let's lace up our running shoes and run the race, not for Olympic glory, but for God's.

PRAYER

Lord, thank You for revealing Yourself to me through Your Word. As Hebrews 12:1-2 says, help me to run my race with perseverance and keep my eyes fixed on the prize, which is You, Jesus.

Journal: How can knowing more of God be considered a prize? Do you need to take your training to the next level? What will be your next step?

—Tarena Sullivan

SEPTEMBER 13

THE WINNER'S CIRCLE

And when the Chief Shepherd appears, you will receive the crown of glory that will never fade away.

1 PETER 5:4

I won a little bronze-colored medal with a red, white and blue ribbon attached. I received this medal for being the winner in my age division in a three-mile race.

It didn't matter to me one bit that I was the *only* woman in my age division. So I won by default—so what?! I had great plans for that ribbon. I would frame it in a shadow box, so the world would know about my accomplishment.

Well, I never got around to doing anything with it, and it has been laying in my jewelry box for 10 years. The medal is now tarnished and wouldn't look very nice in the elaborate shadow box I had planned for it.

How comforting to know that the spiritual race I am running today will produce a crown of glory that will never tarnish or fade away.

As a child I often heard the phrase, "Only one life, 'twill soon be past; only what's done for Christ will last." I didn't understand the truth of that statement until I started my adult race with Christ. All He asks me to do is to keep running. It doesn't matter if I feel weak or insignificant. Whatever I do in obedience to Him makes me a winner.

PRAYER

Jesus, help me keep running the race for You. I look forward to receiving that crown of glory from You that will never fade away.

Journal: If you've stopped running your race, think about what made you quit. Write out exactly what happened. Ask Jesus to help you get back in the race again.

—Carole Lewis

SEPTEMBER 14

YOU ARE ROYAL

And when the Chief Shepherd appears, you will receive the crown of glory that will never fade away.

1 PETER 5:4

Whenever I read this verse, somewhere in the back of my mind I can hear Bert Parks singing, "There she is . . ." It makes me realize that when Jesus comes on the scene, I will receive a crown of glory that won't ever go away.

I remember that when I was a little girl, I watched the Miss America pageant; and after I saw the crown placed on the new Miss America's head, I wished I had a crown like that on my head. I knew the reality of that happening was next to nonexistent. I knew that I would never be Miss America. So many of us grew up with low self-esteem, which contributed to our becoming overweight.

The good news is this: When our Chief Shepherd appears, we *will* all receive a crown. I know that Jesus has made numerous appearances in my life, and each time I've felt His presence, He has made me feel like Miss America.

The good news about the crown Jesus places on your head? It won't mess up your hair. And you will hear the angels singing, "There she is . . ."!

PRAYER

Thank You, Jesus, that I am "somebody" because You love me!

Journal: All the dreams we missed out on in childhood can be fulfilled by Jesus, if we will trust Him and have faith in Him. How have your dreams changed since you became a child of the King?

—Beverly Henson

TODAY'S REWARDS

And when the Chief Shepherd appears, you will receive the crown of glory that will never fade away.

1 PETER 5:4

We've had some nice victory celebrations for my First Place groups during the last five years. I've even joked that I wish I could give them all brand-new cars for the outstanding jobs they have done. But those cars wouldn't hold a candle to the Chief Shepherd's awards that will never fade away. Even if I could give away cars to my special people, the tires would wear out and the cars themselves would become eyesores after a while.

This is not so with the awards handed out by our Chief Shepherd!

One of the secrets of being successful in First Place is collecting our awards daily and learning to take great joy in what we can do now. We can learn new things, change our eating habits, exercise and honor God with our bodies.

Remember, we don't have to wait for all of our awards. Yes, we will have to wait for those that never fade away; but the better health, feeling better able to serve the Lord, the pure joy that you can do this—those awards can be yours today.

PRAYER

Lord, help me to collect my awards today for the things that I can do now, as I prepare for Your awards that will never fade away. I desire to receive a wonderful crown of glory to lay at Your feet on that day.

Journal: What awards will you collect today—for instance, filling out your Commitment Record, exercising or having your quiet time?

—Carol Moore

SEPTEMBER 16

BRASS KEY OR GOLD CROWN?

And when the Chief Shepherd appears, you will receive the crown of glory that will never fade away.

1 PETER 5:4

Years ago, I joined one of the major nationally known weight-loss groups. When I joined, they promised that if I lost weight and reached my goal, I would receive a bright shiny brass key. I love shiny things, so I decided to go for it!

When I reached my weight goal, the leader presented me with my key, which symbolized my status as a lifetime member. I assumed that meant I would successfully stay at my goal for a lifetime!

Recently, I came across that key and was rather disappointed to find that it was faded and discolored—how fitting. After receiving that key, I had also gained and lost weight more times that I would like to admit. The tarnished key reminds that what I earned back then was merely a temporal prize, which quickly lost its glory.

Unlike my prior attempts at weight loss, my First Place journey has encouraged me to pursue discipline in my physical and spiritual life.

One discipline that has changed my life is Scripture memory. The memorized Word has changed my attitudes, broken down strongholds of fear and has forever changed my entire thought processes.

Brass keys and trophies will all fade away one day. But when God's Word changes your life, the change lasts forever!

PRAYER

Lord, thank You for forever changing my life through Your Word. Thank You that the crown I will receive from You one day will last forever.

Journal: List the spiritual disciplines that you have been struggling with and commit them to the Lord.

—Nancy Taylor

SEPTEMBER 17

OUR CHEERING SECTION

Therefore, since we are surrounded by such a great cloud of witnesses, let us throw off everything that hinders and the sin that so easily entangles, and let us run with perseverance the race marked out for us.

HEBREWS 12:1

My good friend Martha Norsworthy had just memorized this verse while participating in First Place when tragedy struck her life. Her only child, Carol, and Carol's husband, Bryan, were killed by a drunk driver. God kept the verse before Martha the entire time she was reeling from shock.

I couldn't have imagined how God would use this verse in my life, too. But when my daughter Shari was killed, He did. As I write these words, it has only been six short weeks since Shari went to join Martha's daughter and son-in-law in that great cloud of witnesses.

When I find myself thinking about all the things Shari will never see or do again, I immediately transport my thoughts to heaven. When I see her in that great cloud of witnesses who no longer see "through a glass, darkly" (1 Cor. 13:12, *KJV*) as we do, I am filled with joy for Shari and wouldn't want to call her back.

I want to run my race in such a way that nothing hinders me, certainly not the sin that so easily entangles. I want to run with perseverance because of that great cloud of witnesses who have gone on before me. They are standing beside Jesus, cheering me on.

PRAYER

Help me press on with perseverance the race marked out for me. Thank You that You don't call me to run anyone's race but my own.

Journal: Write the things that hinder you today from running the race God has marked out for you. Ask Jesus to fill you with His power so that you can reach the finish line.

—Carole Lewis

ELBOW DEEP IN DONUTS

Therefore, since we are surrounded by such a great cloud of witnesses, let us throw off everything that hinders and the sin that so easily entangles, and let us run with perseverance the race marked out for us.

HEBREWS 12:1

Countless times I had succeeded in passing the bakery counter at the grocery store where I shopped. But one day, I decided it was okay to cave in to temptation. Long before I reached the actual place of temptation, I had convinced myself that having "just one" after so many weeks of doing without was not going to hurt me.

Wouldn't you know, as I approached the counter I saw her out of the corner of my eye—one of the ladies from my former First Place class. She waved as she approached me—actually catching me red-handed in the bakery line.

"Hi," she greeted me. I returned her greeting cordially, thinking, *Darn my luck.*

"Are you still in the First Place class?" she asked.

"Yes, I am," I stammered.

"Oh . . ." she replied, looking confused—and maybe somewhat suspicious.

I then confessed my intentions and walked away. Had it not been for her witnessing the event, I probably would still be elbow deep in chocolate donuts.

That day I also gained some insight as to what it means to persevere and why it is important to remember at all times that people are watching and noting our weight-loss success and our failures in First Place. With so many other diet programs out there, other people, like us, are seeking the perfect program. I believe God uses our transformed lives as a witness to His glory, not our own.

PRAYER

Lord, help me to be worthy of watchful eyes so that I may point them to You, that You would indeed be glorified by my continued success and perseverance.

Journal: What are some of the things that hinder or entangle you personally? Are you up to the challenge—ready to persevere regardless of circumstance?

—Danna Gilmore

SEPTEMBER 19

LIFE'S HURDLES

Therefore, since we are surrounded by such a great cloud of witnesses, let us throw off everything that hinders and the sin that so easily entangles, and let us run with perseverance the race marked out for us.

HEBREWS 12:1

As the participants of the high hurdle started the race, my grandson wanted to know what they were doing.

"What kind of race is this?" he wanted to know.

I explained that each time they knocked a hurdle down, points were taken away from their score. My husband, who had been on a track team, patiently corrected me. "No, they don't take any points away. It just might hurt a little and slow you down, so you won't win the race."

Hebrews 12:1 came to my mind as I watched runners knocking down the hurdles. I considered Joe's explanation of the rules and thought, *God, that is one of the reasons You gave us a list of witnesses to help us run our race with the best speed and without so much pain.*

The lives of men and women of faith help train us to leap the hurdles. They show us how to get back up after we fall. David can be such a great example of someone who totally messed up but was completely forgiven and restored (see 2 Sam. 11–12). Peter's restoration, after denying Jesus three times (see John 18:15-18,25-27; 21:15-19), encourages us to come back to God after any failure or disobedience.

My husband's explanation also reminded me of God's grace. God doesn't subtract points; He just wants me to be able to leap over the hurdles and not suffer the bruises. Learning from the examples of such great witnesses as David and Peter is God's training for my life.

PRAYER

Thank You, God, for the Bible, my training handbook. Give me a passion to know Your Word. Allow the Holy Spirit to reveal to me Your truth and give me Your wisdom to apply it in my life.

Journal: Write some of the ways you have leaped over hurdles without bruises, because of God's grace.

—Kay Smith

SEPTEMBER 20

STILL RUNNING THE RACE

Therefore, since we are surrounded by such a great cloud of witnesses, let us throw off everything that hinders and the sin that so easily entangles, and let us run with perseverance the race marked out for us.

HEBREWS 12:1

Excitement was in the air as I awoke to a beautiful winter morning on December 22, 1993. It was Wednesday, and my daughter, Carol, and I had to get Bibles and Christmas gifts ready for 50-plus children.

After getting the presents in order, we started back to town. Suddenly, my daughter exclaimed, "I see the rainbow."

I couldn't believe my eyes. There had been no rain and the sun had been shining all day, yet arching across the sky was a beautiful stream of color! The sight of it filled us with joy and prepared us for our van trip to pick up and drive children to our midweek prayer service.

We completed our Wednesday night van route. What a wonderful day it had been. I said to Carol as she left, "See you at the restaurant about 9:30." I didn't know these would be my last words to her.

Not long afterward someone came to me and said there had been a very bad car wreck. It involved Carol and her husband, Bryan, in the church van. Driving to the site only one mile from the church seemed to take forever. As I watched the van burn, God said to me, "You have been surrounded by such a great cloud of witnesses, and Carol and Bryan have joined that crowd."

My Scripture memory commitment that week was Hebrews 12:1. God has used this verse continually to bring healing to my grief-stricken heart and mind.

PRAYER

Father, today I seek to throw off everything that hinders and the sin that so easily entangles. I seek to praise You for the work You are doing in my life.

Journal: What do you need to throw off that is hindering you? What sin has so easily entangled you? Ask your Father to help you throw off these things today.

—Martha Norsworthy

SEPTEMBER 21

No Excuses

Therefore, since we are surrounded by such a great cloud of witnesses, let us throw off everything that hinders and the sin that so easily entangles, and let us run with perseverance the race marked out for us.

HEBREWS 12:1

Holidays are often celebrated with too much food and often with too little meaning. Having an excess of unhealthy food that has no nutritional value is a double-whammy disaster.

As I read Hebrews 12:1, I reflect on the holiday excesses that become hindrances I can easily throw off. I am determined to do my holiday shopping differently from now on. For instance, no more chocolate bunnies, jelly beans, chocolate hearts, candy corn or candy canes. I don't need them and neither does my family. Buying these things—even as decorations—only makes it easy for sin to entangle me.

In a recent edition of the popular "Cathy" cartoon in our local paper, Cathy's mom bought Cathy a cinnamon roll at the bakery. Her mom had second thoughts, realizing that Cathy would be tempted, then eat it and hate herself later. Being a "good mother," she ate it before leaving the bakery, so Cathy wouldn't suffer because of her. On her way out the door, tossing the bag into the trash, Cathy's mom justified her actions by telling herself she's still gaining "baby weight"—even though she gave birth to her baby some 30 years ago!

How hard do we try, really, to throw off *every* weight that hinders and entangles us? How many times do we set ourselves up for failure and then rationalize our behavior?

PRAYER

Lord, help me quickly to realize any rationalizing I do and let it, instead, become my prayer for Your help. Give me a clear picture of what You would have me do about the unhealthy areas in my life.

Journal: Are you setting yourself up for failure in any choices you're making today? Tell the Lord about your poor choices and ask for His guidance.

—Judy Marshall

SEPTEMBER 22

THE EYES HAVE IT

Let us fix our eyes on Jesus, the author and perfecter of our faith, who for the joy set before him endured the cross, scorning its shame, and sat down at the right hand of the throne of God.

HEBREWS 12:2

Ironically, the only way I am going to be able to finish the race set out for me is if I take my eyes off the race. I must learn to fix my eyes on Jesus, instead of the race I am running. I need to set my eyes on Him, because He is the One who helps me run the race.

As most of us know, life is hard. But Jesus tells us in Matthew 11:29 that if we take His yoke upon us and learn from Him, He is gentle and humble and will give rest for our souls. Pressing on means that we don't have to bear the heavy load of this world, because Jesus bears it for us. He endured the cross so that we don't have to press on alone. He sits at the right hand of God, cheering for us every time we overcome temptation. He gives us strength to bear up under the difficulties of life and to walk in victory through each one.

Whatever you are facing today, Jesus can miraculously step in with great power and work mighty miracles in your life.

By fixing your eyes on Jesus, instead of your circumstances, you can learn what it means to have your faith perfected.

PRAYER

Jesus, help me today to fix my eyes on You, instead of on my circumstances.

Journal: Write down some of the circumstances of your life today. Thank Jesus that because He was willing to die for you, you are able to share in His power.

—Carole Lewis

SEPTEMBER 23

THIS IS FOR YOU, LORD

Let us fix our eyes on Jesus, the author and perfecter of our faith, who for the joy set before him endured the cross, scorning its shame, and sat down at the right hand of the throne of God.

HEBREWS 12:2

Accepting God's gift of salvation was the easy part, wasn't it? The Christian life involves work—sometimes hard work.

When I became a Christian at age nine, my war against sin had hardly begun. As an adult, I discovered there were areas of my life, such as taking care of my body, that required discipline I did not want to practice. I would rather eat high-fat and high-sugar foods than healthy foods. I would rather lay in bed than exercise. I've learned that I can only win this war against my flesh when my eyes are fixed on Jesus.

My prayer as I tie my laces to go for a long walk often is, "I don't think I can do this, but God I love You enough to try." My prayer as I say no to a donut usually is, "Lord, You know I want this donut more than I want to be thin, and this *no* is a sacrifice to You."

As I put any of my sufferings up against the backdrop of the Cross, though, they instantly shrink. Jesus was able to endure the pain of the cross and the shame, because He was going home to "Daddy." As I look to Jesus, He gives me an example of how to endure the trials of this life.

PRAYER

Jesus, thank You for Your sacrifice. Thank You for Your example, a life I can daily fix my eyes on for instruction, strength, comfort, forgiveness and love.

Journal: Look back through your prayer journal and estimate the time you have spent alone with God in the past month. Highlight the answered prayers.

—Kay Smith

SEPTEMBER 24

PERFECT IN CHRIST

Let us fix our eyes on Jesus, the author and perfecter of our faith, who for the joy set before him endured the cross, scorning its shame, and sat down at the right hand of the throne of God.

HEBREWS 12:2

If you asked the average woman how she felt after looking through a fashion magazine, she would probably say "Depressed!" I know I find it frustrating to look through a magazine or watch television and be constantly assaulted with pencil-thin women.

These celebrities and fashion models we are trying to emulate are not even real! Many of these photographs are airbrushed to achieve that fabulous "flawless" look. Real people don't look like that! What we feel envious of are unreal images.

I have also been guilty of looking at others and their weight-management success and have found myself feeling envious or even resentful of their progress or achievement.

The apostle Paul so gently warns us of the danger of this and encourages us to "fix our eyes on Jesus." If God designed me, then who better than Him to know how to "perfect" me—to help me become all He wants me to be. God desires for me to become more like His Son, Jesus. He wants me to look like Him!

So I am learning to fix my eyes on Him, not on others around me. I have a ways to go—no one has recently mistaken me for Jesus—but I am thankful that He is in charge of the perfecting process. And I love the changes He is taking me through.

PRAYER

Lord, help me to have a grateful heart for who I am and the unique ways You have formed me. Help me, not to compare myself to others, but to stay clearly focused on Jesus—the author and perfecter of my faith.

Journal: Talk to God about one specific area in your life, one that needs your attention retrained so that your eyes fix on Jesus.

—Vicki Heath

SEPTEMBER 25

A Happy Ending

Let us fix our eyes on Jesus, the author and perfecter of our faith, who for the joy set before him endured the cross, scorning its shame, and sat down at the right hand of the throne of God.

HEBREWS 12:2

A visiting minister to our church shared a story about a little boy who was taken to the pet store to pick out a new puppy. After the boy selected the scraggliest-looking one, his dad asked him why he picked this particular pup. The puppy's tail never ceased its wagging, and the boy replied, "Because he has a happy ending."

As we think about our Jesus and the pain and suffering He knew He would endure on the cross, how could He have joy set before Him? In Matthew 26:38, Jesus said, "My soul is overwhelmed with sorrow to the point of death." How could He go from being overwhelmed with sorrow to having joy set before Him? As the author of our faith, He knew there was a happy ending.

By His pain, suffering, death and resurrection, He paid our price and conquered death so that we might have eternal life. By believing in Jesus and accepting Him as our Savior, our happy ending is a glorious beginning of life everlasting.

No matter what battle or burden you are facing in this life, fix your eyes on Jesus. Remember, we are not victims or even just victors—we are more than conquerors with Him. Praise His holy name!

PRAYER

Father, help me keep my eyes on You today.

Journal: Name some specific ways you could more closely fix your eyes on Jesus today.

—Mary Etta Jackson

SEPTEMBER 26

LIVING YOUR LEGACY

Let us fix our eyes on Jesus, the author and perfecter of our faith, who for the joy set before him endured the cross, scorning its shame, and sat down at the right hand of the throne of God.

HEBREWS 12:2

The week ahead was going to be hard for me because it would be my first birthday without my daughter, Carol, and her husband, Bryan. We had survived Christmas and New Year's, and now this hurdle stood before me.

I was not working at the time and decided to go through some more of Carol and Bryan's things. My husband, Jerry, stayed home with me, so we could do this together. The pain of their deaths was still fresh for us both. We decided to start with Carol's car. There were many college books and papers in it.

As we took the last of the books out, including her book bag, we found Carol's and Bryan's First Place notebooks and prayer journals. We took them in the house, not knowing if we should open them and read them. We decided to wait and continued our packing project.

Several nights later, we were both drawn to those First Place materials. We sat down together and looked through the Bible study lessons and then the prayer journals.

Words cannot adequately express the blessing these journals contained for us. What a legacy of joy and comfort they were. We knew that Carol and Bryan were Christians, but we didn't realize the strength of their faith, the depth of their commitment or the character being formed in them as they faced struggles with God's help. We know it now.

This is the kind of legacy you too can create as you follow God in daily obedience to His will.

PRAYER

Father, I commit all my grief and pain to You today. Thank You for the comfort You give me through Your Word. Help me to run with perseverance the race You have marked out for me until You call me home.

Journal: As you read Hebrews 12:1, what comfort does God seek to give you through these words? What will your legacy be?

—Martha Norsworthy

SEPTEMBER 27

THE FRAGRANCE OF GRACE

See to it that no one misses the grace of God and that no bitter root grows up to cause trouble and defile many.

HEBREWS 12:15

If we belong to Christ, Satan knows that he will never lay claim to our souls.

He also knows, however, that if he can keep us defeated, we won't be responsible for bringing any other people to Christ.

Years ago, a friend got mad at me. She believed that she had been slighted, and she let a bitter root grow in her heart. She made a point not to speak to me when we saw each other. I prayed for her every time this happened and asked God to heal this root of bitterness in her heart.

One day I spoke to her and she actually spoke to me. We talked together for a few minutes, and since that time, it's been quite obvious that she decided to forgive me. Prayer releases God's power in the lives of those around us.

Many years ago, a good friend told me I needed to "stop becoming a part of other people's problems." We need to become part of the answer. One way to do this is to pray about problems, instead of worrying about them. When we pray, our lives exude the sweet fragrance of the grace of God. It is grace alone that overcomes bitterness.

See to it that no one who touches your life in any way misses the grace of God. You can do this by praying for each one, even those who don't like you, on a daily basis.

PRAYER

Jesus, thank You that Your grace is the balm You use to heal our hearts.

Journal: Is there someone you don't like? Write his or her name in your journal. Even if you believe you are justified in the way you feel, choose to forgive this person so that no bitter root grows in your heart.

—Carole Lewis

SEPTEMBER 28

WEED-PULLING EXPERT

See to it that no one misses the grace of God and that no bitter root grows up to cause trouble and defile many.

HEBREWS 12:15

One Saturday morning, I set out on a weed-pulling mission in my backyard. As I was crouching over the flowerbed, I noticed this about weeds: Some have weak, shallow roots, which make them easy to pull. Others have very long strong roots which make them extremely hard to remove.

In that moment, God reminded me that we must remove any thoughts of bitterness before they take root. The longer we allow bitter thoughts to stay in our minds, the deeper the bitterness grows and the harder it is to remove.

After witnessing an unfortunate incident in our First Place class, a member came to me and said, "You do not deserve to be treated that way!" She was very upset with the person whom she felt had treated me badly. Hebrews 12:15 came pouring out of my mouth in response to her words. It was as if the Holy Spirit directed my every word: "Let's give him the benefit of the doubt. I am extending God's grace to him. Would you do the same?"

Later that week she called to thank me for sharing the verse and for directing her to truth. I had pulled a weed!

Let's set out on a weed-pulling mission by pulling weeds of bitterness and extending God's grace to everyone who crosses our paths.

PRAYER

Lord, show me if I have allowed any roots of bitterness to grow in my heart and, by Your grace, help me to remove them. Thank You for Your grace and forgiveness. Empower me to extend that same grace and forgiveness to others today.

Journal: Has someone hurt you? Choose to extend God's grace to that person today. Write this commitment in your prayer journal as a memorial to one weed pulled!

—Nancy Taylor

SEPTEMBER 29

A HEART WITHOUT DANDELIONS

See to it that no one misses the grace of God and that no bitter root grows up to cause trouble and defile many.

HEBREWS 12:15

Every spring a certain yard captures my attention. At first, it looks beautiful, with the first sign of green grass after the last winter snow. Within a few weeks though, the lush green is dominated by a carpet of bright yellow dots—the dandelions!

They literally take over, until all you see is yellow. Then, a few weeks later, the dandelions go to seed and turn the yard into a dingy white color as the seeds are whisked off in the spring breeze to take over another unsuspecting yard.

God recently showed me how this yard reflected my own life. I had let the bitter root of unforgiveness anchor itself in the fertile soil of my heart. Instead of immediately digging up the root through reconciliation, I let the root grow deeper and deeper.

I tried to "mow over" this spiritual weed by offering momentary forgiveness. But this weed kept returning, each time leaving a darker stain on my heart, just the way a dandelion leaves a stain on your hand. Then it took over my heart, and I let the flowers go to seed through gossip, sowing dandelions in the hearts of others.

Finally, I let Jesus, the master gardener, dig the dandelions up by their roots. Only then did the green grass of my heart return.

PRAYER

Dear Lord, please forgive me for letting this bitter root take hold of my heart. I need Your help, because I'm too weak on my own. Help me to rely on Your strength to lovingly confront through reconciliation any bitterness.

Journal: Are you just mowing over the "dandelions" in your heart, or are you digging them up with Jesus' help? Do you need someone to hold you accountable?

—Tarena Sullivan

SEPTEMBER 30

APPLE-CHECK TIME

See to it that no one misses the grace of God and that no bitter root grows up to cause trouble and defile many.

HEBREWS 12:15

Each fall we are privileged to be able to pick apples at the family farm. Some years the apples are bountiful. We make applesauce and pies, and we take them to work in our lunches for several months.

Sometimes, however, we're caught off guard. We've learned to keep checking our store of fresh-picked apples, just in case one has gone bad. Occasionally, we'll find that one apple has spoiled beyond recognition. Then we have to sort through the whole box to see how many others that one bad apple has affected and caused to rot.

The same can be true with relationships. Bitter roots in a person's heart, just like spoiled fruit, can affect everyone near and "defile many."

It is important for us to ask God to search our hearts. He can spot the attitudes spoiled by unforgiveness and bitterness.

PRAYER

Is there bitterness in my heart, Lord? Is it affecting others and causing trouble? Please uproot that bitterness so that I may demonstrate Your grace, rather than defile many.

Journal: If there is bitterness in your life, what do you need to do to get rid of it?

—Helen McCormack

OCTOBER 1

YOUR MOMENT IN TIME

See to it that no one misses the grace of God and that no bitter root grows up to cause trouble and defile many.

HEBREWS 12:15

Over the course of 20 years, I have tried every diet in the world. Joining First Place was my moment in time—the moment when God extended His grace to me to accomplish His will in my life.

I have now lost 147 pounds, and I have kept it off for over four years.

Do you know that I could have missed my moment in time? I could have excused myself and remained seated in my Lazy-Boy recliner, wondering, *Why me?* I would have become even fatter and more bitter in my misery.

I could have missed my breakthrough moment by sitting around waiting for something to happen. But there are no "drive-thru breakthroughs." God gives us the Scriptures and the tools we need, and He extends His loving grace to us to accomplish the task at hand. It is totally up to us whether or not we take Him up on His moment in time.

This is your day. Just as Jesus asked the man at the healing pool of Bethsaida, "Do you want to be made whole?" (see John 5:1-15). He is asking you the same question today. If your answer is "Yes, I want to be whole," then Jesus says, "Get up and walk."

Today is the day to get up and walk in the grace God is extending to you.

PRAYER

Lord, thank You for Your mercy and grace offered to me through the blood of Your Son, Jesus. Father, I do want to take advantage of Your grace, and I acknowledge that this is my moment in time. Help me to be a good steward over the task You have entrusted to me.

Journal: Do you want to be made whole? Do you have a problem getting up to walk every day? Ask Jesus to change your heart about exercise.

—Beverly Henson

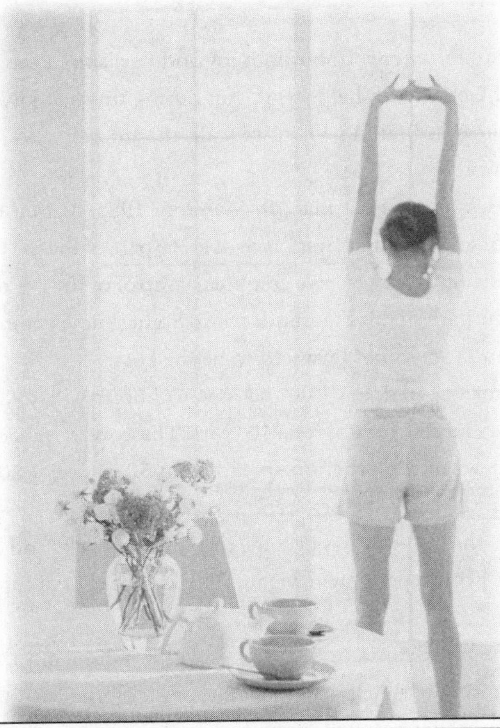

Pathway to Success

SECTION SEVEN

Introduction

On this pathway called life, we encounter both joy and hardship. Learning how to walk on the level ground of God's truth helps us to run during times of joy. God's truth also keeps us from stumbling and falling when we walk the uneven, and sometimes steep, surfaces of pain and trouble.

I joined the first session of First Place in March of 1981. At that time I was introduced to the concept of giving Christ first place in every part of my life. I played with the concept for a few years, not willing to give complete control of my life to Christ. During those years, I walked the path of double-mindedness. Sometimes I wanted Christ to have first place in my life, and sometimes I wanted to be the boss.

When I finally surrendered my life and my stubborn will to Christ's control, I walked the pathway of success for a joyous 10 years. These were years of growth for the ministry of First Place, when the program spread from 50 to over 1,200 churches. The pathway was smooth and I savored every step.

The last four years the pathway has become increasingly rocky and has grown steeper than I ever dreamed I could possibly navigate. This has been true for personal as well as professional reasons.

This section of the book contains verses that will, when memorized and incorporated into our minds and hearts, help us to joyously walk on the pathway to success.

My prayer for you is that you will come to know that whatever pathway you are walking today, whether painful or sweet, it is made better when you walk it with Christ.

—Carole Lewis

All Things Are Possible

Where there is no revelation, the people cast off restraint.

PROVERBS 29:18

I talk with many men and women who have "cast off restraint" where their eating is concerned. Most of them have very little or no revelation of God's character or the extent of His love for them. They have no hope that anything will ever change enough that they will be able to lose weight and keep it off.

"No revelation" means that even though God has revealed Himself in His Word, we are unable to believe and act upon the truths found there. Sometimes there is a reason for this. It could be that we had an earthly father who never kept his word. We might have lost a parent in childhood through death or divorce, and now we suffer from feelings of abandonment. There could be many reasons we don't believe in the core of our being that God has the power He says He has.

The apostle Peter tells us, "His divine power has given us everything we need for life and godliness through our knowledge of him who called us by his own glory and goodness" (2 Pet. 1:3). Let those words soak in for just a minute. *His power has given us everything we need?* It is my belief that until we understand and believe how much power God really has, He can never reveal Himself fully to us.

If you are a person who continually casts off restraint by binge eating or practicing some other compulsive behavior, cry out to the One who has the power to make the necessary changes in your life.

PRAYER

Father, I saw myself in today's devotional. Teach me how much power You have to change my life.

Journal: Write down the main reason you are unable to trust God. Write out 2 Peter 1:3 and begin to memorize it. Read or say it every day until you begin to see positive change.

—Carole Lewis

October 3

Be Thou My Vision

Where there is no revelation, the people cast off restraint.

Proverbs 29:18

When I discovered that to perish means to suffer a violent or untimely death—to pass from existence—my pre-First Place life of dieting immediately flashed before my eyes. Both definitions accurately describe all the unhealthy years I had spent desperately trying to attain someone else's vision of the perfect size that each diet program promised. This was so frustrating, unrealistic—even impossible!

On the verge of perishing, with my heels digging trenches in the sidewalk leading to my church, I reluctantly joined a First Place session. My preconceived vision was that of familiar failure because I had so many times before proven that diets don't work.

I soon learned that what works in First Place is not the what but the *who.* I love Proverbs 29:18 in its entirety: "Where there is no revelation, the people cast off restraint; but blessed [happy] is he who keeps the law."

The reason First Place works for me is because *God works,* and the image of Him working powerfully on my behalf is now my vision. The Live-It food plan and First Place commitments are the simple restraints, or laws, that we keep so that we will be happy.

I no longer perish or suffer, because Christ is my vision. He is in my sight at all times, and I am truly blessed and happy.

Prayer

Lord, thank You for the vision I have now in You. From past experiences of failure in dieting, I realize that You are my revelation in all areas of my life. With Your help and constant presence, I am able not to cast off the commitments that lead to the discipline I need.

Journal: What vision do you have of yourself? Is it different from God's vision of you?

—Judy Marshall

OCTOBER 4

A LIFE WELL READ

Where there is no revelation, the people cast off restraint.

PROVERBS 29:18

Most of us start out life waiting for a particular event to happen so that our lives can really begin. We couldn't wait to be a teenager, to be sixteen, to graduate from high school and college, and finally to marry and have children and/or work in our chosen profession.

Solomon was aware of the fact that most human beings live without a vision for their lives, so he wrote about this and many other truths in the book of Proverbs. Having a clear vision of what we want to achieve in the future helps us keep moving forward with hopeful diligence. Solomon encourages us to look to God because God is always forward looking.

What are you looking forward to now?

For a long time I didn't think I had anything left to look forward to in the future. I married the man of my dreams, worked in my chosen profession of nursing for many years and raised two lovely daughters who are now adults. Although one daughter still lives with us because of several back injuries, in many ways my children do not need me anymore. So I had to ask myself, *What am I looking forward to now?*

My answer was to continue seeking, finding and doing the Lord's will for my life. As long as He leaves us here on Earth and hasn't yet called us home to heaven, He is not through with us yet, and we need to keep being His witnesses to the rest of the world.

Remember, you may be the only Bible the people around you know. What are they reading from your life?

PRAYER

Lord, help me to see You as my "vision." Help me to continue to look forward to what You have planned for me.

Journal: List three things you can accomplish today to show yourself and others that your vision is eternal, rather than temporary.

—Wanda Shadle

OCTOBER 5

FORK IN THE ROAD

Where there is no revelation, the people cast off restraint.

PROVERBS 29:18

I was about to begin my third session with First Place—but I knew I was at a fork in the road.

I had already shared my concern with my leader: I was struggling with the program. At the highest point, I had lost 24 pounds. I had also begun a more regular prayer time and an in-depth Bible study. I had started a prayer journal and gained knowledge about food. I was enjoying the subtle changes in my body. I had also begun to make a connection between Scripture and my dependency on food.

But I felt I wasn't progressing quickly, and I felt ashamed as I fluctuated on the scales. The first Scripture memorization for session three was Proverbs 29:18. I knew I wanted to receive more revelation and I didn't want to lose what I had learned by "casting off restraint."

Realizing this, I was able to decide to stay the course and not give up.

I believe First Place is where I will continue to receive the Word of God in a manner that is applicable to being overweight. It is where those who serve us are living testimonies to the rewards of obedience.

If you are at this same fork in the road, I encourage you to continue on and receive revelation as the Lord plants the seeds of change in your heart.

PRAYER

Lord, continue to reveal to me the areas in which I need restraint,
and strengthen all areas, which are under Your control.

Journal: List the areas in which the Lord has planted seeds of success and you see changes taking place in your life.

—Anne Marenko

OCTOBER 6

YOUR POWER SOURCE

May he give you the desire of your heart and make all your plans succeed.

PSALM 20:4

The deepest desire of my heart is to become a godly woman. I prayed this prayer for many years before I fully understood what I was praying.

The apostle Peter says, "His divine power has given us everything we need for life and godliness through our knowledge of him who called us by his own glory and goodness" (2 Pet. 1:3).

What is the deep desire of your heart today? Do you find that all your plans succeed? If not, it could be that you are functioning under the false idea that you have some power of your own to make your plans work.

God tells us so many times in His Word that He is the One who has the power to change lives. When we walk on the pathway to success, we learn that each step forward is because of God's power working in us.

I have become so aware of the power of God while writing these devotionals. Right now, because of the death of my daughter just six weeks ago, I find that I don't have the creative energy to even think, much less write. God has supernaturally infused me with His power as I have written each one.

Draw from His power today, and you will come to know the God of power. Then He will give you the desire of your heart and make all your plans succeed.

PRAYER

Lord, You know the deep desire of my heart today. Teach me about Your power so that my plans might succeed.

Journal: Write down the deepest desire of your heart. Ask God to work in your life, by His power, to give this desire to you and to make your plans succeed.

—Carole Lewis

The Desires of God's Heart

May he give you the desire of your heart and make all your plans succeed.

Psalm 20:4

According to biblical scholars, the phrase "the desire of your heart" is subject to two possible interpretations: (1) God will give you what you really want; or (2) God will change what you want.

Based on other Scriptures, I believe the second interpretation is the more accurate one. God is not the great candy store in the sky. He desires us to come into agreement with Him and His plans.

When you make plans based on God's promises and line up your desires with His desires for you, you know that your plans will succeed. Until that is done, there is no guarantee that your plans have any hope of success.

There is a big bonus to letting God place the desires in your heart: you will find yourself surrounded by the peace of God. Isaiah tells us, "[God] will keep in perfect peace him whose mind is steadfast, because he trusts in you" (26:3). This assures us that when we have our focus right, God will keep us in perfect peace that only God can give.

True success is found in making the right plans—the ones that God gives you—and allowing Him to lead you to success.

Prayer

Lord, give me the desires of Your heart and make them mine.

Journal: What are your most dearly held desires? Are they based in God? Write a prayer and ask God to reveal to you His desires and to make them yours.

—June-Marie Avery

WHOSE PLAN IS IT?

May he give you the desire of your heart and make all your plans succeed.

PSALM 20:4

We all want to have our desires fulfilled. We all want to be successful. But how do we determine when we have achieved fulfillment and success?

The usual response to that question is "When I get what I want." Sometimes, however, getting what we want turns out to be unsatisfying.

What we really need to do is figure out what we really want and how our wants and desires are directed and determined.

We need to ask ourselves, *Do my desires stem from a heart governed by self and my sinful nature, or do they stem from a heart saturated by God's Word and filled with His grace?*

As we pray and claim this verse, let us always remember that God's ways are best. We need to be sure that the desires of our hearts are governed and controlled by a life saturated with His Word, with prayer and with accountable relationships with other believers. If our plans are His plans, then we will really have the desire of our hearts. Then *our* plans will succeed and we will find fulfillment.

PRAYER

Lord, guide me to know Your plans for my daily life. Teach me from Your Word that You may establish the desires of my heart.

Journal: Are your heart's desires fed and saturated by Scripture reading and prayer? If you need more nourishment in this regard, take in the meat of His Word and meditate on His desires for your life. What did you discover?

—Helen McCormack

Hold the Chili Cheese Dog!

May he give you the desire of your heart and make all your plans succeed.

Psalm 20:4

For years, my favorite food was a foot-long chili cheese dog at my favorite drive-thru restaurant. Whenever I was on one of my "diets," I knew I could not have the foot-long chili dog. But when I lost all of my weight, I would be able to eat one or two.

In the meantime, I would drive by that restaurant and just smell that greasy food cooking and say to myself, "When I lose all my weight, I will be there eating a foot-long chili cheese dog." Getting that chili cheese dog was my goal.

Then I came to First Place. I dived headfirst into the Scripture and began to find out what Christ meant by the abundant life. As I lost weight, I began to look at life differently.

I also noticed that God had begun to work in my heart. My plans had changed. I no longer wanted to just lose weight. My plan was to become healthier, and through the power of God, I was becoming a success. The day came when I rode by the chili dog restaurant, inhaled the greasy smell and wanted to shout for joy. I no longer lusted after food. I didn't even want a foot-long chili cheese dog any longer.

God gave me new desires in my heart. Not only did He change my heart, but He also gave me a little extra bonus—He changed my taste buds.

Prayer

Thank You, Father, for making Your plans my plans and giving me desires in my heart that are Your desires for my life.

Journal: Think about the changes in your lifestyle and build an altar to God's faithfulness by writing about it.

—Beverly Henson

OCTOBER 10

A Godly Mind-Set

Love the LORD your God with all your heart and with all your soul and with all your strength.

DEUTERONOMY 6:5

Our family has a history with God. We have this history because my mom and dad made the decision to trust Jesus when I was five years old. Since that time, our extended family has come to know and love Jesus. We're all at different stages of growth, but we're all on the pathway to success.

I recently received a note from my precious niece, Julie. Julie is the daughter of my only sibling, Glenda, who went home to be with Jesus over seven years ago. Julie and my daughter Shari were just 10 days apart in age and were as close as sisters.

In the note, Julie told me that over a year ago, Shari had called and asked her to pray for me as I cared for Mom. Shari let Julie know that Mom thought the medicine she needed to take was going to kill her, so we really needed Julie and her family to pray for our situation. Julie's suggestion had been to keep Mom surrounded with Scripture and Christian music. Shari told her, "Why don't you call Momma and tell her yourself?"

Julie said in her note: "Well, here I am a year later, telling you this." The amazing thing is that even though Julie didn't call, God sent her message to us through Deborah, the Christian lady who cares for Mom during the day. God has taught us that Mom's fears are greatly diminished if she only watches inspirational Christian videos and listens to Christian music.

When we focus on the Lord—His goodness, mercy, faithfulness and love—then the anxiety and fears that so often plague us dissipate and lose their power in our lives.

PRAYER

Lord, I need balance in my life in every area. Teach me the importance of living a balanced life so that I can have victory, even in the difficult times.

Journal: Is there something God wants you to give up or start doing that will bring more balance into your life? Write about it and ask God to give you the strength to make the necessary changes.

—Carole Lewis

OCTOBER 11

HISTORY WITH GOD

Love the LORD your God with all your heart and with all your soul and with all your strength.

DEUTERONOMY 6:5

Why do some of us find it easier to love a dog with all our heart, soul and strength than to love God that way? Maybe one of the reasons is that we're more sure about the unconditional love of our dog than we are about the unconditional love of God.

First Place helps people learn what this verse really means. If we are ever to walk the pathway to success, it is imperative that we learn how to love God with our body, soul, mind and spirit.

Because God has taught me how to balance my life, He has taught me, not how to endure, but how to walk in victory these four years since my husband, Johnny, was diagnosed with cancer. I am able to walk in victory even though I am watching my 89-year-old mom, who lives with us, slowly lose the mental faculties that have been so much a part of the mother I have known and loved. Because God has taught me how to love Him with every part of my being, I know that in the years to come, I and my entire family will walk in victory, even after the devastating loss of our daughter only weeks ago.

How can I write these words? Because our family has a history with God. He has proven Himself faithful in the good and the bad times.

PRAYER

Lord, I want to learn what it means to love You with all my heart, soul, mind and strength. Teach me how to live a balanced life.

Journal: Write down the greatest need in your life today. Is it for patience, love, endurance or compassion? Ask God to meet this need with His power and love.

—Carole Lewis

OCTOBER 12

CLOSE TO THE KING

Love the LORD your God with all your heart and with all your soul and with all your strength.

DEUTERONOMY 6:5

Whenever I grumbled or complained about my circumstances, I had to ask myself why I did, but as a Christian, I knew the answer: Something was wrong with my relationship with Jesus.

I have been a Christian for over 50 years, and I always thought I was doing the best I could to live the way the Lord wanted me to. But now I know I was swept along for many years in the current of active church attendance and service. Much of the time I was doing, not only what I thought I should do, but also what *others* thought I should do.

Then about 20 years ago, I became really miserable with my weight and the circumstances of my life. Fortunately, I learned about a total health program that was coming to our church and that eventually became First Place. When I saw how the Lord was changing me during my participation in the first session, I joined the second session to continue my new journey with Jesus Christ. I eventually lost 41 pounds.

By then, the weight loss had become secondary. I finally had a true, satisfying relationship with God through Jesus Christ.

PRAYER

Lord, help me always to give You first place in my life as You continue to show me how to love You with all my heart, soul, mind and strength.

Journal: What can you do to demonstrate that you are trying to put Christ first in your life? Make a short list of things you know you can accomplish today.

—Wanda Shadle

October 13

All of You

Love the LORD your God with all your heart and with all your soul and with all your strength.

Deuteronomy 6:5

Science can supply us with many facts regarding our flesh and bones—but humankind's greatest struggles are matters of the heart.

The heart is the most inward part of our being. The heart is the seat of motive, intellect, emotions and will. Therefore, our heart is the seat of our belief system. It has been said that we act on what we believe, not on what we know.

Our bodies also house our souls, or personalities. Our personalities make us unique, allow us to interact with each other and give us identity.

Our strength is easy to see with human eyes. Yet do we recognize where we put our spiritual might? Do we recognize that if we are God's children that we are warriors for His kingdom? Are our motives pure, centered on Christ, or are they sinful, centered on self?

Our lives are played out in full view of the King of kings. Keeping our heart, soul and strength pure allows us the peace that passes all understanding.

Prayer

Lord, show me myself that I may begin to love You with my heart, motives, emotions and will. Lord, let my personality reflect the characteristics of Christ when dealing with others.

Journal: What activities has God asked you to take out of your life? Tell Him how you need His power to change your life.

—Denise Peters

OCTOBER 14

UNTOLD WEALTH

Love the LORD your God with all your heart and with all your soul and with all your strength.

DEUTERONOMY 6:5

When I was a young woman, one of my favorite books was *The Richest Lady in Town* by Joyce Landorf Heatherly. Joyce shared great examples of why she thought of herself as the woman in the title—even though she had gone through some very hard times in her life and marriage.

As I read Heatherly's book, I realized how much richer I was because I hadn't gone through anything approaching the terrible circumstances she had endured. When I realized how rich I truly was, I began to enjoy my circumstances more.

Today—after 35 years of marriage, with two grown children and my first grandchild and with a very rewarding ministry in First Place—I realize I'm still the richest lady in town. And I must thank this author because she helped me as a young woman to learn the secret road to riches: "Love the LORD your God with all your heart and with all your soul and with all your strength."

Oh, yes, I've had some hard times but nothing like the times I would have had if I had not become in spirit the richest lady in town.

Riches are a wonderful asset in times of trouble. Feel free to store up your godly wealth.

PRAYER

Lord help me to love You with all my heart, soul and strength today.
And, Lord, help me to see how I'm the richest lady (or man) in town.

Journal: Write down all the ways in which you are rich today (if you have just come to know the Lord, you are rich because you now have eternity with God). Go ahead and brag about your wealth—God wants to enjoy it with you.

—Carol Moore

OCTOBER 15

No Fiery Darts Here!

Put on the full armor of God so that you can take your stand against the devil's schemes.

EPHESIANS 6:11

Today I would like for you to get your Bible and turn to Ephesians 6 and read verses 14-16. These verses tell us what kind of armor we need to put on so that we aren't tripped up by the devil's schemes.

God didn't cause a drunk driver to strike and kill our daughter Shari, although He welcomed her home because she knew Him. He is also able to work mightily and help each of our family members recover from this loss because we understand what it means to be protected by His powerful armor.

I vividly remember standing in the shower the morning after Shari died. It hit me like a bolt of lightning that Shari's death was another one of the devil's schemes sent to defeat us. I told the devil out loud, "If you think this one will do it, you are sadly mistaken. Your scheme will not do anything but fuel us."

Weeks later, I am able to see that on that morning, God had me totally covered in His armor of love, grace and peace so that the devil's lies couldn't penetrate my mind and heart.

We learn to put on the full armor of God by spending time with Him and learning about and memorizing His Word. We develop a close friendship with Him and, on a daily basis, we talk with Him about everything.

PRAYER

Father, teach me today what it means to walk through each day covered in Your armor so that I can take my stand against the devil's schemes.

Journal: Write in your journal the pieces of armor that you are not wearing on a daily basis. Is it the belt of truth found in God's Word? Is there some sin that keeps you from putting on the breastplate of righteousness? Ask God to remove anything from your life that keeps you from wearing every piece of His armor.

–Carole Lewis

OCTOBER 16

STAND WITH THE ARMOR

Put on the full armor of God so that you can take your stand against the devil's schemes.

EPHESIANS 6:11

There was a time when everywhere I turned, Satan had a scheme to render me helpless. I was so busy dealing with health issues, family problems, financial difficulties and church issues, that my spiritual life began to decline. When I memorized this Scripture, its truth hit me like a ton of bricks: Satan was working against me.

I also realized how I'd reacted to the attacks I was under. The hour I had set aside for quiet time and Bible study diminished, and my prayers became shorter. I found less time to grow relationships with friends and my class members, and even the quality time in my marriage was hindered.

When I memorized this verse and meditated on it, I saw that I needed to put on the *full* armor of God, not just part of it. When I neglected one part, that was where Satan hit me the hardest. I came to understand that the devil's schemes will not cease. But when I put on His full armor, I can stand against them while God fights the battle.

With the full armor of God intact, I began keeping my morning appointment for quiet time. God gave me a deeper understanding in studying His Word, and my prayers took on a new dimension. I once again could feel the power of the Holy Spirit within me.

PRAYER

Father, thank You for providing Your armor. Help me to remember I need each piece to enable me to have full coverage against Satan's schemes. Thank You, Lord, for fighting the battle and giving me victory.

Journal: Have you discovered all the parts of God's armor and learned how to put them on? Start with the helmet of salvation and then check the rest of the pieces listed. Which piece do you need to put on today?

—June Chapko

OCTOBER 17

UNCOVERED FACES

Put on the full armor of God so that you can take your stand against the devil's schemes.

EPHESIANS 6:11

Costume parties were always fun when I was young. I would spend all afternoon getting every detail taken care of, saving the mask for the very last. As long as the mask was off, I was still myself; but when my face was covered, I became another person.

The full Christian life may be masked and never seen. Some masks we wear are pride, deceit, false humility, discontentment, the devil's schemes, unconfessed sin. We must daily peel off our masks and replace them with the full armor of God.

Only when our human masks are shed and we don God's armor can we stand against the devil's schemes. This means we must put on the belt of truth and the breastplate of righteousness, and we must fit our feet with readiness that comes from the gospel of peace. It means we must be strong to hold up the shield of faith, the helmet of salvation and the sword of the Spirit. Most of all, we must learn to stand our ground in prayer (see Eph. 6:14-18).

What pieces of God's armor do you need?

PRAYER

Lord, thank You for the armor with which You provide me. Only with Your preparation for my soul can I stand against the devil's schemes. Make me aware of when I put on a human mask to hide my weaknesses and help me quickly to replace those weaknesses with Your armor.

Journal: What human masks do you wear? In what area do you need to take a stand today? Read Ephesians 6:10-18. What are you struggling against today?

—Judy Marshall

October 18

Tailor-Made Armor

Put on the full armor of God so that you can take your stand against the devil's schemes.

Ephesians 6:11

When I was little, I memorized this verse with my mom. At some point during our recitation, she shared with me a thought that stuck in my young mind. She said, "When you have on the armor of God, Satan can't tell whether it's you in there or whether it's Jesus."

When I think of putting on armor, I am reminded of David and Saul (see 1 Sam. 17:37-39). Back in the days when Saul was still nice to young David, Saul offered David his own armor to wear while fighting the giant Goliath. Can you imagine how clumsy and awkward the boy David must have felt in the mighty warrior Saul's armor? I'm sure he was weighed down and stumbled over everything.

David refused the armor and instead took his stance on a bold faith declaration: The Lord would be with him and deliver him from the hand of Goliath. David had all the spiritual armor he needed—the presence of God Himself.

If David had worn Saul's oversized armor when he went against Goliath, the enemy would have laughed at the sight and immediately seized the opportunity to destroy him. It's like that with Satan. He's just waiting for the right opportunity to destroy us.

But if we are perfectly outfitted in the armor of our God, Satan won't know what to do. He won't know who's in there—you or Jesus. Then he will flee in fear.

Prayer

God, help me to become comfortable with wearing Your armor. I pray it will become a part of me, so I can take my stand against Satan. Help me to tailor my life perfectly to Your armor.

Journal: Read Ephesians 6:14-17. What does each part of God's armor represent? How can you begin to tailor your life to fit this armor perfectly?

—Tarena Sullivan

DON'T LEAVE HOME WITHOUT IT

Put on the full armor of God so that you can take your stand against the devil's schemes.

EPHESIANS 6:11

I live in a climate that becomes very cold in the winter; therefore, it's necessary to plan what to wear. I purchase warm coats, gloves, hats and boots and have them ready for the day when the cold weather arrives.

Whenever I go out during the winter months, I wear these items of clothing so that I can stand against the cold. If I am going to travel a long distance by car, I take extra clothes along, in the event the car breaks down or there is a travel delay. I need to be this vigilant about preparation so that I am ready for any trouble that might come. My life may very well depend on being prepared.

In the same way, I must prepare for the trickery and schemes of Satan by putting on the full armor of God. There is action expected on my part. I must learn what the armor is for and how to use it. Then I need to put it on so that I can stand against the devil's schemes—because those schemes will come.

My life—and yours—may very well depend on our preparedness.

PRAYER

Lord, teach me about the armor You have placed at my disposal. Teach me how to put it on and how to use it. Teach me how to stand against the devil.

Journal: Do you know what armor you need and how to wear it? What schemes of the devil are unfolding in your life that you need to stand against?

—Helen McCormack

OCTOBER 20

MERCIFUL GRACE

His divine power has given us everything we need for life and godliness through our knowledge of him who called us by his own glory and goodness.

2 PETER 1:3

Every word of God is true—but sometimes we're unable to live in the truth because we're lacking knowledge of God's power, glory and goodness.

Since my daughter's death, God has hammered the truth of this verse into the minds and hearts of my family. *He is our power, our glory and our goodness.* He will continue to supply everything we need for life and godliness. Why? Because we know Jesus, and He is our friend.

My oldest granddaughter, Cara, lost her mom the November night we lost our daughter. She was 19 and planning to leave home for the first time to attend college. We fervently prayed for Cara as she made decisions about roommates and courses—that God would provide for her every need. He has

- given Cara a Christian roommate and two Christian suitemates;
- made sure these girls were members of the church Cara needed to attend;
- caused Cara to run into many of her old high school friends every day so that she doesn't suffer from too much loneliness.

God *has* the power. All we need to do is trust Him and obey.

PRAYER

Lord, I need to learn more about Your power, love and goodness. Teach me today.

Journal: Write about whatever you have need of today. Ask God to fill your need with His power.

—Carole Lewis

October 21

Basic Ingredients

His divine power has given us everything we need for life and godliness through our knowledge of him who called us by his own glory and goodness.

2 Peter 1:3

My mom can make a five-course meal with just a handful of items. I look in my refrigerator and pantry and declare, "We have nothing to eat!" But my mom looks in the same refrigerator and pantry and sees the ingredients for a creative dinner party! Although we both see the same ingredients, we see two different solutions.

The same can be said concerning our pursuit of godliness and wellness. The Lord has provided all the ingredients needed for each of us to live a life pleasing to Him. We can either believe this truth by seeking to apply His Word to our lives, or we can murmur and complain that we just don't have what it takes to be successful. Attitude is everything!

The nine commitments in the First Place program are the ingredients for success as you seek to put Christ first in every area of your life. *Attendance* gives us support. *Encouragement* gives us friends. *Prayer* gives us faith. *Bible reading* gives us truth. *Scripture memorization* gives us a weapon. *Bible study* gives us wisdom. The *Live-It plan* gives us health. *Commitment Records* give us discipline. And *exercise* gives us strength.

All these ingredients combined will provide you with what you need to succeed in putting Christ first in every area of your life. You have the ingredients for a very creative and godly life!

Now what about your attitude?

Prayer

Lord, thank You for providing everything I need for life and godliness. Help me today, not to complain but to rejoice in all that You have given me.

Journal: What ingredient are you overlooking, or which of the First Place nine commitments do you need to start applying to your life today?

—Nancy Taylor

OCTOBER 22

DAILY BREAD

His divine power has given us everything we need for life and godliness through our knowledge of him who called us by his own glory and goodness.

2 PETER 1:3

I have been a Christian for a very long time and I've seen God's hand of provision in many different areas of my life. But never have I seen His provision more clearly than when Jeff Nelson and I began to compose the music and melody for the First Place Scripture memory series.

I have been a songwriter for 30 years and would like to be able to take all the credit for these musical compositions. But I know all too well that there was a divine hand guiding us through the writing of every song.

Please understand that when Carole first asked me if I could put these Scriptures to music, I said, "No problem." Once the reality of writing 80 songs sank in, I knew I would have to trust God for a serious amount of help. That's also when I realized I was going to need another person with different gifts.

God provided Jeff Nelson to collaborate and engineer. Looking back, I can't tell you how many times Jeff and I would look at one another with amazement at the ease with which melodies and chords fell from the sky. I remember telling Carole how well things were going, and she would be quick to remind me of how many people were praying for us. The Scripture memory series has served to remind Jeff and me, once again, of God's awesome power.

God really has given us everything we need to accomplish the task He has called us to do—whatever that may be.

PRAYER

Lord, I see that there is no end to Your divine provision and power. Help me to remember in times of need that You have called me by Your own glory and goodness and, because of that fact, You will always provide for me. Thank You, Lord.

Journal: What do you truly need from God today? Whatever it is, write it down in prayer form and believe in the promise of His Word that He will provide for all your needs.

—Rick Crawford

OCTOBER 23

TRUST THE PROMISE GIVER

His divine power has given us everything we need for life and godliness through our knowledge of him who called us by his own glory and goodness.

2 PETER 1:3

I must have come out of my mother's womb a worrier. When I was growing up, it seemed my assignment in life was to worry. My mother often said that if I didn't have something to worry about, I would find something.

I have learned that worry creates fear; and what we fear, many times, creates worry.

When I began establishing a quiet time alone with the Lord, He began to convict me about worry. When we worry, we activate the devil. When we pray, believing, we enlist the help of God.

By staying in the Word and on my knees, I have learned to claim God's promises. He will take care of everything. Worry only causes me to take my eyes off Him and to be distracted from the work He has called me to do.

Keeping a journal is another way I found strength and freedom from worry. Writing is a tangible way of taking the concerns of my heart and handing them over to Him.

Someone once said that a Bible that is worn out is usually owned by someone who is not. Studying God's Word sustains me and gives me courage to trust. Trusting allows Him to meet my every need.

Give God your worries, for He is faithful!

PRAYER

Lord, today I want to walk in holiness, and I can't do that unless I seek You and Your power. Give me courage to let go and let You take care of all my needs for today.

Journal: What are you worried about today? What are the "what ifs" you need to hand over to God?

—Carolyn O'Neal

YOUR EVERY THOUGHT

Search me, O God, and know my heart; test me and know my anxious thoughts. See if there is any offensive way in me, and lead me in the way everlasting.

PSALM 139:23-24

In Jeremiah 17:9, God says through the prophet, "The heart is deceitful above all things and beyond cure. Who can understand it?" The memory verse for this week tells me that only God can help in the area of my emotions, because He knows my heart completely.

Anxious thoughts spring from our hearts. They first creep into our minds where they take root. Aren't we glad that God knows our hearts, even when we don't? He knows our anxious thoughts and will deliver us from them, if we will only ask.

My 89-year-old mom is losing her ability to think. Even though she is unable to reason, her emotions are still active. On any given day she might decide that her food is going to make her sick or that her medicine is poisoning her. Some days my heart becomes anxious too, and I start thinking that we won't be able to keep her at home much longer.

I have marveled at how God comes in to help her and us, when we ask Him. When we take our anxious thoughts to God, He comes through in power and might.

I don't know what the future holds. But I know God has held Mom in the past, and He holds her today. I am confident that He will hold her until He leads her "in the way everlasting."

He'll do the same for you and me if we will ask Him.

PRAYER

Lord, You know my anxious thoughts today. Cleanse me of anything offensive and lead me in Your way.

Journal: Write down the thoughts that are making you anxious today. Ask God to help you rest in Him.

—Carole Lewis

OCTOBER 25

SEARCH PARTY

Search me, O God, and know my heart; test me and know my anxious thoughts. See if there is any offensive way in me, and lead me in the way everlasting.

PSALM 139:23-24

God already knows everything about me—so why should I ask Him to search me?

Though God may know all about me, I have areas in my heart that I have hidden from myself—secrets I don't even tell myself.

Have you ever said, "I just ate a whole package of (fill in the blank) and I have no idea why"? When you stuff yourself numb with food, God knows the emotion you are trying to bury under food. It grieves Him for us to deal with our pains and problems without Him.

When God searches us with our permission, He gently shows us the pain and the way to healing at the same time. If we are hurting ourselves, He shows us the right path, "the way everlasting."

If you find yourself engaging in the very behaviors you hate the most, ask God to search you, and then accompany Him as He explores your heart. When you go with God on the journey, He can heal the hurts and change your ways at the same time.

PRAYER

Search me, O God, and know my heart; try me and know my thoughts. Point out anything in me that offends You, and lead me along the path of everlasting life.

Journal: Plan and then write down how you can open yourself and allow God to search your heart.

—June-Marie Avery

OCTOBER 26

UNFAILING LOVE

Search me, O God, and know my heart; test me and know my anxious thoughts. See if there is any offensive way in me, and lead me in the way everlasting.

PSALM 139:23-24

As God's creations, we are designed to be fully known by Him. Yet even in our most intimate human relationships, we find it difficult to express our deepest thoughts and failures, let alone confess them to a holy and perfect God.

Let me encourage you with Psalm 51. Here we see King David, after committing adultery with Bathsheba, begging God for mercy. David asks God to take away his sin according to God's unfailing love and great compassion. David knew the Father would not turn from His love for His child, even when David had committed such an offense.

Obviously, David found forgiveness and restoration with God, because he also penned Psalm 139. In the first 22 verses of that psalm, David describes what it's like to be known intimately by God. He describes God as knowing all of our ways, what we will say before the words leave our lips, what our days will hold, as creating our inmost being, and thinking about us constantly.

What great love! God knows *everything* about us, and He still loves us. In fact, God loves us so much, He longs for us to trust Him with everything, even our anxious thoughts and offensive ways.

The more you know Him, the more you will trust Him and find that His love for you never changes.

PRAYER

Dear God, help me know You and trust You enough to feel comfortable presenting You with my anxious thoughts and offensive ways. Please remind me that even when I have to confess sin, You look upon me with unfailing love.

Journal: What areas of your life are you hiding from the searching eyes of God? Why?

—Tarena Sullivan

OCTOBER 27

GOD OF THE MESSY CLOSETS

Search me, O God, and know my heart; test me and know my anxious thoughts. See if there is any offensive way in me, and lead me in the way everlasting.

PSALM 139:23-24

Did you ever receive a surprise call that unexpected overnight company would arrive at your house in one hour? How many things were stuffed in closets just to get the clutter out of the way?

While a few people do have everything in perfect order in all cupboards, drawers and closets, at all times, I think most of us would admit there are some areas in our homes that we don't want our company to see.

Our verses today invite God to search our hearts—to know our hearts, even in the dark corners and private closets that we protect and cherish. These verses invite a thorough inspection.

How willing are we to expose the messy areas of our lives to the eyes of almighty God? It's not as if God would be surprised by what He sees, for He already knows everything. However, we sometimes live as though we think we have secrets from Him. We do things or act a certain way because "no one" is looking.

Now we're instructed to yield to His inspection and guidance. If we are going to live obediently, we must open every aspect of our lives to His inspection.

PRAYER

"Search me, O God, and know my heart; test me and know my anxious thoughts. See if there is any offensive way in me, and lead me in the way everlasting."

Journal: What areas of your life are you keeping secret? What areas do you need to yield to God?

—Helen McCormack

OCTOBER 28

THE FATHER'S EYES

Search me, O God, and know my heart; test me and know my anxious thoughts.
See if there is any offensive way in me, and lead me in the way everlasting.

PSALM 139:23-24

In the first three verses of this psalm, David states: "O LORD, you have searched me and you know me. You know when I sit down and when I rise; you perceive my thoughts from afar. You discern my going out and my lying down; you are familiar with all my ways. Before a word is on my tongue you know it completely, O LORD."

David goes from a positive statement—acknowledging that God knows every thought, action and emotion before anything happens—to praising God for creating him. And at the end of the psalm, he willingly invites God to improve on His creation! What faith!

As I focus especially on the above verses, I know there are anxious moments and offensive ways in my life—but do I want to have them pointed out to me? I have to confess that the thought of having that happen is not comfortable.

A great preacher once said that when we're in difficult situations, we need to pray, "Lord, I'm not willing, but I'm willing to be made willing."

PRAYER

Father, forgive my lack of faith and my failure to ask if there are any anxious thoughts or offensive ways in me. I must ask You if I'm to be the person You need me to be.

Journal: Ask God if there are any anxious thoughts or offensive ways you need to turn over to Him. Are you willing to be made willing?

—Betha Jean Cunningham

OCTOBER 29

GET OVER IT

Everyone born of God overcomes the world. This is the victory that has overcome the world, even our faith. Who is it that overcomes the world? Only he who believes that Jesus is the Son of God.

1 JOHN 5:4-5

In years past, I would attend conferences and hear speakers tell how God had helped them overcome terrible trials. As I listened, I would always think about how fortunate I was that I hadn't faced such awful things. I probably had just a little bit of spiritual pride, thinking that God loved me so much that He wouldn't allow me to suffer. The last four years, as God has allowed me to share in the sufferings of Jesus, I have learned the truth of what those conference speakers were saying.

The world around me is difficult; but God says that because I believe in Jesus, I *will* overcome it. Jesus does His best work when my faith is weak or wavering. As believers, we can call out to Him right now because of the truth of this verse.

My husband, Johnny, loves country music. He frequently writes words that he thinks would make a good country song. The other day he handed me a piece of paper with these words written on it: "What you don't get over will get all over you." I thank God today that I have the power to "get over" my circumstances because of the shed blood of Jesus.

PRAYER

Thank You, Jesus, that in You I can overcome the world.

Journal: Write about the trials in your life. Give them to Jesus and ask for His power to overcome each one.

—Carole Lewis

OCTOBER 30

THE FATHER'S ARMS

Everyone born of God overcomes the world. This is the victory that has overcome the world, even our faith. Who is it that overcomes the world? Only he who believes that Jesus is the Son of God.

1 JOHN 5:4-5

When I was seven years old, my father said he wanted to teach me an important lesson. He stood by our front porch and told me to jump into his arms. I was reluctant to jump, but I knew Daddy would catch me, even though I was afraid he might drop me.

I finally jumped—and of course he caught me.

Then he explained that was what faith is like. As long as I stayed on the porch and didn't jump, I really didn't have faith that he would catch me. When I jumped into his arms, it demonstrated my faith.

In the same way, if we are to demonstrate our faith in the Lord, we have to live in such a way that our actions prove to those around us that we truly believe Jesus is the Son of God. We may have never thought of ourselves as overcomers, but that is exactly what this verse tells us we are. Our faith is the victory.

The question is, What are we going to do with this knowledge? Now that we know we are overcomers, what changes are we going to make in our everyday living?

The measure of faith we have will determine what we accomplish in our lives. What we are called to accomplish will be different for each of us. But with the Lord's help we *can* do all He wants us to do (see Phil. 4:13).

PRAYER

Lord, increase my faith through the First Place Bible studies and memory verses, so I can truly be an overcomer.

Journal: List several changes you can make on a daily basis to behave like the overcomer you are.

—Wanda Shadle

OCTOBER 31

VICTORY IN JESUS

Everyone born of God overcomes the world. This is the victory that has overcome the world, even our faith. Who is it that overcomes the world? Only he who believes that Jesus is the Son of God.

1 JOHN 5:4-5

The Message renders the above verses this way: "Every God-begotten person conquers the world's ways. The conquering power that brings the world to its knees is our faith. The person who wins out over the world's ways is simply the one who believes Jesus is the Son of God."

Are you a conqueror or the conquered? The choice is yours. No one else can decide that for you.

God provides us with all the weapons we need to conquer. In fact, Paul calls us "more than conquerors" in Romans 8:37 (*KJV*)! Why are we "more than conquerors"? Because Jesus has done all the conquering. All we have to do is take hold of the victory He has already won for us.

We overcome by our faith—that is, faith in the victory of Jesus Christ who has already won our battle with the horrific price of the cross. When we waver or let the enemy jerk our faith away, we are not considering the amazing sacrifice Jesus made for us.

We must pick up that precious faith we have dulled with our fears and failures and turn it toward the all-conquering One. When we use our faith as a weapon of our warfare, it will soon be gleaming again.

PRAYER

Beloved Lord, thank You for giving us the victory.

Journal: Are there areas in your life in which you have allowed the devil to steal your victory? How can you take your victory back?

—June-Marie Avery

N O V E M B E R 1

THE OVERCOMERS' CLUB

Everyone born of God overcomes the world. This is the victory that has overcome the world, even our faith. Who is it that overcomes the world? Only he who believes that Jesus is the Son of God.

1 JOHN 5:4-5

To a person who has been in bondage to food, words like "overcome," "overcomers" and "victory" all deal with diets and food.

Whether or not I feel victorious has to do with whether I have been "good" or "bad" this week. Underneath it all is the hope that, miraculously, I will have this thing beat one day and become a conqueror.

This is nothing more than the "diet mentality." When you think this way, you are unwittingly giving in to a demonic stronghold. As long as you think losing weight is the *only* way you can be an overcomer, you will be shadow-boxing for the rest of your life.

When I weighed almost 300 pounds, I was an overcomer. The Word doesn't say anything about overcomers being an elite club of thin people. It tells me that if I am born of God and believe that Jesus Christ is the Son Of God, then *I am an overcomer.*

When you come to the realization that being an overcomer is a starting point, not a finishing line, then Jesus can begin to do that work in your life you so desire.

Welcome—right now, this minute—to the overcomers' club!

P R A Y E R

I thank You, Father, that without doing anything except believing in Your Son, I am an overcomer in Your eyes.

Journal: Write a love letter to Jesus to thank Him for His work on the cross and for your membership in the overcomers' club.

—Beverly Henson

NOVEMBER 2

On Your Worst Day

Everyone born of God overcomes the world. This is the victory that has overcome the world, even our faith. Who is it that overcomes the world? Only he who believes that Jesus is the Son of God.

1 JOHN 5:4-5

There are days when I feel strong and able to take on the world. Then there are days when I feel weak and worthless. It is during the latter that I usually get in trouble, because I start trying to make something happen by my own efforts and I mess things up.

We get into trouble when we live by our feelings, using how good or bad we are doing as a gauge for our standing with our Father in heaven. At times I find myself thinking that when I eat a cupcake or a bag of chips, I blow it. I imagine that God is up in heaven frowning down on me, saying, "I don't think she's ever going to get it."

But then I read this encouraging Word that to be an overcomer, all I have to do is have faith and believe that Jesus is the Son of God.

On my worst day and through the very nastiest of circumstances, I always believe that Jesus is the Son of God. So guess what? Without doing good or bad, I am automatically a victorious overcomer.

Once you understand that you are an overcomer, always in good standing with God, then the door of your heart is open for the restoration of your temple—your body.

PRAYER

I am Your child, chosen and called by Your name. Thank You, Father, for making me Your child and for giving me a new life.

Journal: If you feel like you've blown it today, renew your mind by meditating on and writing about today's Scripture. Remember, there is no condemnation to those who are in Christ Jesus.

—Beverly Henson

FINELY TUNED HEARING

Whether you turn to the right or to the left, your ears will hear a voice behind you, saying, "This is the way; walk in it."

ISAIAH 30:21

In the time since Shari's death, our family has experientially learned the truth of this verse.

My son-in-law, Jeff, has called out to God for help—to show him how to finish raising his three teenaged daughters. I have called out to God for help in writing these devotionals during this time of grief and mourning. We have experienced the truth of this verse as we walk on the uncertain path of loss. And for His part, God has worked miracle after miracle because we have trusted Him to meet the needs of each day.

I used to struggle with how to know God's will for my life. I have learned, mostly through pain, that if I spend quality time with God in the morning, He will take care of the circumstances on the path I walk today. It is impossible to get out of the will of God, if we would only crawl up into His lap, snuggle down and rest.

A good friend of mine says, "*Being* comes before *doing*." When will we learn that God desires to be with us so that we are listening when He shows us what to do? Most of us are so busy doing things *for* God that we don't take the time to *be with* God.

The big question for today is, Will we walk in the direction God is pointing?

PRAYER

Lord, teach me to hear Your voice when You speak to me. After I hear Your directions, help me to heed them.

Journal: Is God telling you to do something today? Write about what God is telling you to do and ask for His power to do it.

—Carole Lewis

NOVEMBER 4

THE ONLY VOICE

Whether you turn to the right or to the left, your ears will hear a voice behind you, saying, "This is the way; walk in it."

ISAIAH 30:21

After I got in my car to come to work this morning, I had not traveled far when I heard a man's voice speaking intermittently.

Since I had not turned on my radio or cassette player, I looked at the cars around me and saw nothing unusual. It was not long before I discovered that the voice belonged to none other than Buzz Lightyear, a toy that talks, and I remembered that my granddaughter had left him in the car the previous evening.

I didn't recognize this voice, because it wasn't a familiar one. By the time I reached my destination, I was more familiar than I wanted to be with Buzz, because I couldn't reach him to turn him off. Listening to Buzz all the way to work, I couldn't hear anything else, because he was the focus of my attention.

I wonder how often we allow other voices to drown out the voice of God. I often hear people say they never hear God speak to them. Could it be because we allow the many voices of this world to drown out His still small voice?

Jesus knew the voice of his Father. He said in John 12:50, "Whatever I say is just what the Father has told me to say." He could hear God speak because He spent time with Him and was familiar with His voice.

God wants to speak to us today. And we will hear Him, if we will turn off the other voices that dominate our thoughts and listen only to His voice.

PRAYER

Father, how I pray that You would dominate my thoughts and my attention until all the other voices are diminished and I can only hear Your voice. Let me become so familiar with Your voice that I recognize it instantly when You speak.

Journal: Make a list of all the familiar voices within your circle of friends, family and acquaintances. Ask God to help you turn off those voices that distract you from becoming familiar with His voice.

—Pat Lewis

NOVEMBER 5

IN GOOD HANDS

Whether you turn to the right or to the left, your ears will hear a voice behind you, saying, "This is the way; walk in it."

ISAIAH 30:21

On September 11, 2001, I walked down to the mailbox and there was a letter from First Place, offering me an opportunity to write a devotional for this book. The events of that morning, however, overshadowed my desire to write anything uplifting.

For some time I was unable to write. With the deadline looming, one night I went outside to speak with God and ask Him to put some measure of peace back in my life. As soon as I had prayed, I looked up and saw a shooting star, complete with a sparkling trail following it across the sky. This would not seem too unusual except that I'd seen a shooting star in exactly the same spot in the sky where I'd seen one the night before! Twice, when I hadn't expected it, I had seen light in the darkness.

Why is this important? Although I am not blessed with audible voices from our Father, that night I was very sure He was telling me that despite chaotic events on Earth, He is still in control of the whole universe.

Laughing, I thanked God and came back into the house to see if He would lead me to a verse. Of course He did. In Isaiah 30:20, God tells us that even in times of adversity, He will send us teachers to show us the way. Then, in the verse for today, He tells us that in no matter what form the "teacher" appears, the voice will be His.

As I consider this great promise, I can picture my Father saying that it doesn't matter which way I turn—He will always be behind me to tell me which way to follow His light.

PRAYER

Father, thank You again for reminding me that You are still in control.

Journal: Are there people in your life that God has put there in order to teach you? Has God put a burden on your heart to teach others? Whose names come to mind?

—Dee Brewer Strickland

NOVEMBER 6

Get the Grit Out

Whether you turn to the right or to the left, your ears will hear a voice behind you, saying, "This is the way; walk in it."

ISAIAH 30:21

As I started my walk today, I was blissfully happy to get my heart-rate monitor up into the optimal zone. But the more I walked, the more I became painfully aware of a little rock in one shoe. It kept sliding around and would get under my toe where I couldn't feel it and then slide back to my arch and then to my heel. It was very irritating, but I didn't want to stop, because it would knock me out of the optimal zone on my heart-rate monitor.

The more I walked, the bigger the rock seemed to become. Finally, I could stand it no longer. I took off the shoe and shook it violently. To my surprise, the tiniest piece of grit fell out. How could that small particle have caused me so much irritation and stolen the pleasure from my walk?

As I continued my walk, I realized that I didn't notice this problematic grit when I was sitting in the car but only when I began to walk.

Our enemy loves to keep us in a sedentary position. Why? Because when we're seated—out of action—we can't feel the uncomfortable grit in our lives. Only when we try to enter into life will we encounter the imperfections and irritations that trouble our lives.

PRAYER

Lord, You are the rock of my salvation and I thank You that You have taken the grit of my life and made me a clean vessel filled with Your grace and used for Your glory.

Journal: Are there "little pieces of grit" in your life that are robbing you of the joy and pleasure of walking with God? Ask God to show you what the irritations in your life are and ask for His help to shake them out of your life today.

—Beverly Henson

NOVEMBER 7

FOLLOW THE LEADER

Whether you turn to the right or to the left, your ears will hear a voice behind you, saying, "This is the way; walk in it."

ISAIAH 30:21

As children, we played a game called Follow the Leader. We would get in line behind the child who was the leader and imitate his or her silly actions and movements.

As an adult who was caught up in the diet rat race, I sometimes felt as if I were I child again, playing Follow the Leader. I took pills, followed liquid diets and tried grapefruit diets, always imitating silly actions and movements on the command of someone I didn't even know. I felt like a diet-industry puppet, in bondage to their ideas and plans.

First Place showed me a different way to think. Isaiah 30:21 tells us that we don't have to be in bondage. We have *freedom* to proceed through life with the Lord behind us, coaxing and encouraging us that we are on the right track. *We are on His track.*

When we're on God's track, it makes no difference if we turn right or left; He is right behind us, telling us in His still small voice, "This is the way; walk in it." No more following a leader and wondering if we're "doing it right."

Walk with the Lord today and hear His precious voice tell you, "Welcome to My track. Now let Me help you walk in it."

PRAYER

Thank You, Father, for getting me out of the diet rat race and onto Your track.

Journal: Express your thankfulness for the freedom you have to make good choices and for the leading of the Holy Spirit to teach you how to make those choices.

—Beverly Henson

NOVEMBER 8

HOLY BANK DEPOSIT

Guard the good deposit that was entrusted to you—guard it with the help of the Holy Spirit who lives in us.

2 TIMOTHY 1:14

When I make a deposit into my bank account, I am exhibiting trust that the bank will guard the deposit and I won't have to worry about writing a bad check.

God has deposited His Holy Spirit into my whole being—mind, heart, soul and body—because I have accepted the sacrifice of God's Son on the cross. And Jesus should never have to worry about whether or not I will guard that deposit.

Why is it then that sometimes God "writes a check," hoping to draw on the deposit He's made in me, only to find that the check "bounces"?

Unconfessed sin in our lives means that we have ceased to guard God's deposit, quenching the Holy Spirit. First John 1:9 tells us, "If we confess our sins, he is faithful and just and will forgive us our sins and purify us from all unrighteousness."

God desires only good for us. He wants to be able to use us mightily for His kingdom work. When we hang on to sin and refuse to give it up, we are in essence saying to God that our account with Him is closed.

As we confess our sins, God fills His account in us so full of the Holy Spirit that He is able to write as many checks as He desires, knowing they will be covered.

PRAYER

Dear Lord, I have some things to confess to You today. Help me remember each and every thing that keeps me in a bankrupt condition.

Journal: Write down every sin that is keeping God from using you. Ask for His strength to turn from each one so that you can once again guard what the Holy Spirit has deposited in you!

—Carole Lewis

N O V E M B E R   9

SHARED SUCCESS

Guard the good deposit that was entrusted to you—guard it with the help of the Holy Spirit who lives in us.

2 TIMOTHY 1:14

When I first began the First Place program, I weighed 273 pounds. It wasn't until six moths later that I began a very regimented walking program to jump-start my slow metabolism caused by years of yo-yo dieting. I was very much our of shape, and it was extremely difficult and painful for me to walk.

I told Jesus that because He had carried that cross for me up the hill to Calvary, I knew I could do this for Him. But I also knew I couldn't do it on my own. So I told Him He was going to have to help me and walk with me. I made that commitment and prayed that prayer every day. And every day He walked every step of the way with me.

One year and one month later, I have lost 147 pounds. I know I couldn't have done this without the help of the Holy Spirit. But I also couldn't have done it without the prayers and support of my First Place group. They cried when I cried; they felt much joy with me as I lost the weight. Each week I looked forward to going to class to see them. I worked hard, because I felt they were anticipating each class just as much as I was.

As a result of out sowing a "good deposit" of prayer into each other's lives, we all had significant weight loss as a group that year. Every member also said their exercise habits changed too. I will never forget my First Place group. To this day my heart fills with joy to think of these God-friends.

P R A Y E R

Thank You, Father, for the people who faithfully pray for me. May I be just as faithful to encourage and pray for others.

Journal: Name the people who have supported you the most in your weight-loss journey Just as you have been encouraged by them, call one or two people today and sow the seeds of encouragement in their hearts.

—Beverly Henson

NOVEMBER 10

SPECIAL LOVE REMINDERS

Guard the good deposit that was entrusted to you—guard it with the help of the Holy Spirit who lives in us.

2 TIMOTHY 1:14

When my daughter, Stef, was three, she made me lots of special cards—cards for Father's Day ("You are the best daddy"), birthdays ("Have a super day") and just special days ("You are my best friend"). I kept these cards in a file, and over the last couple of years I've been bringing them out to share with Stef, who is now a senior in college.

Each card was a special creation that meant something to both Stef and I and can never be taken from us. Even when we were at odds, even when we had seemingly impossible ground to cover to get back together again, each card was a special reminder to me of a unique love and a special relationship that only Stef and I shared.

Throughout the year, God blesses us with an abundance of good things for which we are grateful. Above all else though, never forget the good news of the risen Son—a "good thing" we can keep before us, by the power of the Holy Spirit, as a reminder of the unique love relationship we have with the Father.

PRAYER

Lord, grant me the grace and mercy to draw near to You today and embrace the power of Your Word to keep me in Your light every moment.

Journal: Make a list of the good things God has committed to you this past week and thank Him for each blessing.

—Bruce Barbour

NOVEMBER 11

Upgrade and Download

Guard the good deposit that was entrusted to you—guard it with the help of the Holy Spirit who lives in us.

2 TIMOTHY 1:14

I spend a lot of time working at the computer, and I'm aware of continuous offers for upgrades to my online service provider. The Internet companies do not rest on their laurels; they offer new versions of their software soon after the original is less than a year old. Internet service providers are intent on serving their clients in the best possible way.

While waiting for my Internet service provider to download its latest version, I thought about 2 Timothy 1:14 and how God has gifted me with certain abilities and skills to communicate, encourage, counsel and teach. Certainly, the levels of those abilities are not the same as they were 20 years ago. I have felt many times quite inadequate and questioned my leadership capabilities. I have asked God, "Are you sure I'm the one you want? Look at all the mistakes I've made, Lord."

This verse has helped me to understand, first, that it is not *my* ability but the power of the Holy Spirit that sustains me. Second, God has shown me that my mistakes will enable me to reach others who have made them as well.

It is my responsibility to build on the foundation of my gifts by using the basic skills I have. But when I need help to go beyond my own abilities, I look to where the power is. That power comes from the Holy Spirit who lives in me. If I follow His leading, I will succeed.

PRAYER

Jesus, thank You for the gifts with which You have provided me and the constant upgrades I receive when I ask. Help me to always download my strength from You.

Journal: Have you matured in your faith, grown in your abilities and sharpened your skills? In what area(s) could you use an "upgrade"? Ask the Holy Spirit to download into your life what He knows you need.

—June Chapko

NOVEMBER 12

OUR ROYAL FAMILY

You are a chosen people, a royal priesthood, a holy nation, a people belonging to God, that you may declare the praises of him who called you out of darkness into his wonderful light.

1 PETER 2:9

William, the oldest son of England's Prince Charles, was chosen at birth to become that nation's future king. As he has grown into a young man, the magazines and tabloids are full of pictures and articles about everything he says and everything he does. The world we live in loves to know everything about England's royal family.

As Christians, *we* are part of a royal family. We were adopted into the royal family of God the minute we accepted Jesus as our Savior. The world loves to watch us to see if we are living up to our royal heritage.

Aren't we glad that reporters aren't present to catch everything we say and do? Would we want our picture on the front of a magazine telling the world about our personal lives? Well, reporters are present all the time and their names are "lost world."

They watch us when we lie. They watch us lose our tempers. They watch as we manipulate them to get what we want. I've heard it said that there are only two reasons that people don't become Christians: they don't know any Christians, and they do.

Read today's verse again. Our King is pleading with us to act like His chosen people—royal in the truest sense.

PRAYER

Lord, I have been content to live as a pauper ever since You adopted me into Your royal family. Help me learn what it means to be holy.

Journal: Confess to God some of the things present in your life that keep lost people from coming to Christ. Today ask Him to forgive you and help you act like His son or daughter.

—Carole Lewis

N O V E M B E R 1 3

LIVE GOD'S DREAM FOR YOU

You are a chosen people, a royal priesthood, a holy nation, a people belonging to God, that you may declare the praises of him who called you out of darkness into his wonderful light.

1 PETER 2:9

Aunt Rose continually encouraged Sonny, her hydrocephalic son, and assured him that he was special and gifted. She worked with him day after day, despite the doctor's pessimistic prognosis. He recommended institutionalizing Sonny, but Aunt Rose's deep love and belief in her son motivated her never to give up on the dream she had for him—the dream of a healthy and happy life.

I am happy to say Aunt Rose's determination paid off! Sonny went on to graduate from high school, marry and raise a family of his own. He believed what his mom told him and lived out the dream.

God, the creator, formed you in your mother's womb. He chose you for His very own, to be His child. You are a child of the King. He has declared that you are holy and set apart for His pleasure.

The world often says you are not smart enough, pretty enough, rich enough or good enough to meet their requirements for success. Don't believe the world's prognosis. Choose instead to believe that your heavenly Father loves you and has plans for your success (see Jer. 29:11).

Believe what He says, and become the person you have been called to be.

P R A Y E R

Lord, I choose to believe the truth today. Thank You for choosing me and calling me out of darkness, making me a part of Your royal family through the blessed name of Jesus Christ, my redeemer.

Journal: Have you been living like a chosen, royal, holy child of God? What must you do to live out the plans God has for you? Write out a prayer of thanksgiving to God for choosing you and for all the ways He has blessed you.

—Nancy Taylor

NOVEMBER 14

HIS WONDERFUL LIGHT

You are a chosen people, a royal priesthood, a holy nation, a people belonging to God, that you may declare the praises of him who called you out of darkness into his wonderful light.

1 PETER 2:9

Early one morning, I sat with a coffee cup warming my hands, waiting to see the first light of dawn. The dark sky appeared to hold the promise of a bright clear day. I closed my eyes, meditating, praying in the quietness.

My eyes opened to the first hint of morning light, foretelling a beautiful sunrise. Wisps of Ozarks mist soon moved across the entire scene. In minutes, the mist turned to a deep fog. Like a gray engulfing blanket, the darkness wrapped its mood around my thoughts.

Reaching for a light switch, I decided to find a warm, lit, secure corner of the house for continued meditation. A single shaft of sunlight streaking across the leaden sky caught my vision. Like a restless, mischievous child, I wanted to get away. But for some reason, I sat again and watched.

In only minutes, more shafts of sunlight joined the first one and danced with the slightest breeze to drive the fog away completely. The sun burst into view on a beautiful day. Its light changed me instantly.

How often have I missed God's creative, powerful light because I felt lost in the gray reality of hopelessness? His light promises that I am His chosen, beloved child. He has called me out of this world's rush, clatter and darkness to watch His Son's light rise in me daily.

PRAYER

Lord, it is difficult to believe that I am chosen, royal and holy. But You have invited me to be Your beloved, a person belonging to You. Let the light of that fact declare Your wonderful praises through me.

Journal: Write down five painful, dark aspects of your life right now. Match them with Scripture promises that shed His light on your journey.

–Nan Olmsted

NOVEMBER 15

WHO WE REALLY ARE

You are a chosen people, a royal priesthood, a holy nation, a people belonging to God, that you may declare the praises of him who called you out of darkness into his wonderful light.

1 PETER 2:9

"I'm just a housewife."

"I don't have any important gifts."

"I'm no good at anything."

"Someone like me will never amount to anything."

Most of us make statements like these all the time. They are full of false humility, searching for a compliment and missing the fact that we are wonderful creations planned and molded by God.

Nothing is ours. All we have and are is a gift from Him. We must not criticize God for what He has made; we must seek His will as good stewards of what He has given us.

This verse by the apostle Peter says wonderfully unbelievable things about those who are Christians:

- We are a chosen people.
- We are a royal priesthood.
- We are a holy nation. The Church is His!
- We belong to God. We can always run to His arms!
- We were called out of darkness into light. We don't need to stumble in darkness!

How should we respond to these rousing words of Peter? We are to declare the praises of God. We do this by praising Him each day with our thoughts, actions, words and choices.

When we see ourselves as He sees us, when we live out who we really are, our lives become a praise to Him.

PRAYER

Lord, may I see who I am in You. May it not fill me with pride but the realization that it is all because of You.

Journal: If you picture yourself as royalty, how does that affect how you live? Do you praise God as you should? How can you worship God in all of life?

—Helen McCormack

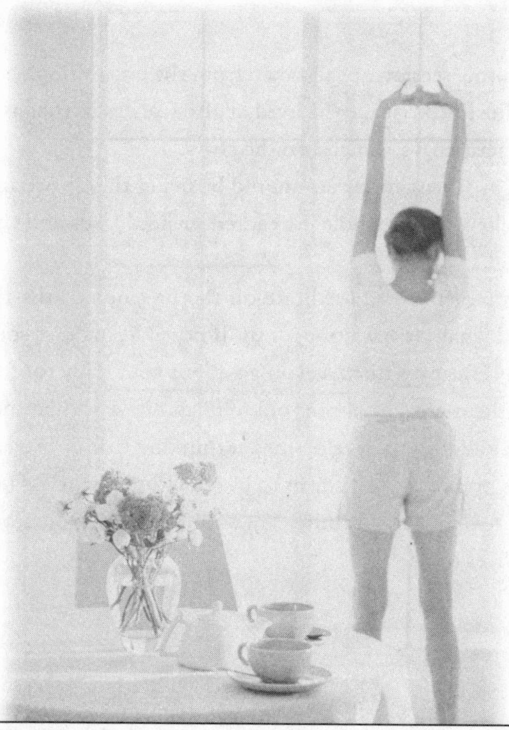

Living the Legacy

SECTION EIGHT

INTRODUCTION

The 10 verses found in this section are all taken from the book of Ephesians. Each verse teaches us about how life in Christ is to be lived. It also teaches us that as believers we are a living legacy of the sacrifice Jesus made on the cross.

Our primary aim as Christ followers should be living the Christian life. From seasoned saints to new believers, our whole life centers around Jesus and the abundant life found in Him.

Take time to savor each verse. Meditate on the precious truths the words reveal about who Jesus is and what He has done for us. If possible, make it your goal to memorize each verse. Then reflect on them as you go about your daily routine. Memorizing verses will reprogram the messages of the "old self" and its world-bound thinking with new messages of hope and joy—to develop in you thinking that is heaven-bound.

Each of the verses points the way for us to live holy and blameless lives full of grace, peace, love, righteousness, light and unity. These things can be ours because of God's Holy Spirit who now lives in us.

—Carole Lewis

NOVEMBER 16

HERE TO HELP

He chose us in him before the creation of the world
to be holy and blameless in his sight.

EPHESIANS 1:4

All of us love to be chosen. As children, we loved to be chosen to be the classroom monitor. As teenagers, we longed to be chosen for the lead part in a play or for a spot on the cheerleading team. As young adults, we dream of being chosen to attend the college of our choice or to be someone's future husband or wife.

Do we really believe that God chose us, before the creation of the world—and that He chose us to live in the mess some of us find ourselves in today? If we know Jesus personally, we can be assured that He is quite aware of our circumstances. He is the only One who can help us live holy and blameless lives when life presents constant difficulties.

What do you need today? Love for a rebellious teenager? Peace about whether God has a mate for you? Hope for your troubled marriage? Self-control in regard to your weight or money? Comfort to face a debilitating illness? Patience at work? Kindness to your family members?

Jesus, the One who chose us before the creation of the world, is also the One who can fix the messes in our lives. Whatever we need, Jesus is always the answer. He is the fixer of broken dreams and lives, because we belong to Him.

If we want to find the way through and out of our troubles, we can—if we relinquish control of our situations to Him.

PRAYER

Jesus, my life is difficult in so many areas. Some of the mess is because of choices I have made and some of it is by Your design so that I might grow in Your love and grace. Today I want to take my hands off my mess because You chose me for greatness.

Journal: List every difficulty in your life. Beside each one, write "Jesus wants to fix this mess."

—Carole Lewis

NOVEMBER 17

CHOSEN BY GOD

He chose us in him before the creation of the world to be holy and blameless in his sight.

EPHESIANS 1:4

Do you know what it's like to be chosen? Do you know what it's like to be left out?

As an overweight child I found that many others were often chosen before me. Sometimes I'd be the last in line. There were special times, too, when I won certain contests based on my abilities or talents; but they were earned events, and I was "chosen" based on what I could do.

With God, we were chosen for His purpose before we were even born—chosen not for what we can do but because of who we are. He sees us as we are destined to be as we live in Him.

As I struggled with excess weight, I didn't feel too holy or blameless; it was more like guilty and ashamed. But when God touched me through the Holy Spirit in the First Place ministry, He transformed me to be the person He had created me to be: holy, blameless and precious in His sight. As I grew to understand that reality more clearly, my self-destructive choices lessened. I began to treat myself more honorably, because of the new reflection God gave me through His Holy Word.

With God's help and grace, I have chosen to be for me—just as He is for me.

PRAYER

Lord, thank You for choosing me. Thank You for seeing me through Your eyes and revealing my true identity to me through Your holy Word.

Journal: How did it feel to be chosen or picked by others? Do you believe God has chosen you? Are you ready to see yourself as God sees you?

—Roberta Wasserman

CHOOSING TO OBEY

He chose us in him before the creation of the world to be holy and blameless in his sight.

EPHESIANS 1:4

If God chose every one of us to be His children, holy and blameless—then why isn't everyone a Christian?

This question arose as I was learning this memory verse. Then I learned the answer: Though He chose us, He also gave each of us the free will to either accept or reject Him. God's plan was to have every man and woman inherit His kingdom. Sadly, many reject Him and in doing so choose to be disinherited.

When Eve chose to disobey, she set forth a series of events leading to her and Adam's expulsion from the Garden. Likewise when I choose to disobey, I will suffer the consequences. First Place gives me many choices with the Nine Commitments. I can follow the program, make the right choices and receive the rewards of good health; or I can make poor choices and see no progress in the areas of weight loss, spiritual closeness to God or memorization of Scripture.

Now it's clear: God chose me. He reached out to me and made a way for me to be called his very own. Now it's up to me to choose that way—faith in Jesus Christ—and live for Him.

Only then will I receive the inheritance He has in store for me.

PRAYER

Father, I thank You for loving me and choosing me as Your child. Help me to live each day in accordance with Your will for my life.

Journal: Select an area (such as prayer, Bible reading, Scripture memorization) with which you are having trouble. What stops you from keeping this commitment?

—Martha Rogers

NOVEMBER 19

HOPE FOR HOLINESS

He chose us in him before the creation of the world to be holy and blameless in his sight.

EPHESIANS 1:4

We are to be holy and blameless in God's sight!

When I read this, it makes me freeze. How can I offer a life to God that is perfect and fit—when God *is* perfection? Nothing that I can ever bring will satisfy the perfection of God. I can never earn or deserve the approval of God. No one can.

So does this mean we are without hope? No! But the first step toward being a holy offering is to realize that we can't do it. We must realize the battle is too great to win alone.

How thankful I am that God has made provision to cover our imperfections. First Peter 1:18-19 tells us we are bought with the precious blood of Christ. Jesus sits at the Father's right hand, and His blood allows us access the Father's presence. We can petition the Father for mercy and grace to help us with our needs. In fact, the Father longs for us to approach Him. He purchased this access at a great cost—the life of His only Son.

Daily fellowship with our Father is vital. Whatever we are feeling and wherever we have been, Jesus understands and He is our way of escape.

All we need to do is show up—and then let God demonstrate His love and faithfulness.

PRAYER

Lamb of God, thank You for laying down Your life and bridging the gap between perfect God and sinful man. Cover my transgressions with Your precious blood and forgive my sins.

Journal: In what ways are you attempting to be perfect? List them and then surrender each one to God, allowing grace to work in you what pleases God.

—Becky Sirt

NOVEMBER 20

BUILDING A LEGACY

He chose us in him before the creation of the world to be holy and blameless in his sight.

EPHESIANS 1:4

God chose us and He wants us to be His. He sees our faults and He knows our potential. His love existed for us before creation. God longs for us to approach Him, so He can lavish His love upon us. As Frederick Faber once said, "How thou canst think so well of us, and be the God Thou art, is darkness to my intellect, but sunshine to my heart."[1]

Ephesians 1:3 says God has blessed us "with every spiritual blessing in Christ." The word "blessed" in this verse means "good things spoken." God Himself has spoken good things over us.

Think about what this means! By His spoken word, light separated from darkness. Stars were flung across the universe. A living soul was created. God's spoken word has power and nothing can stand against it. He has spoken good things over each one of us—individually. He has given each of us exactly what we need to become Christlike. It is not a future state, waiting to be created, but a condition in us that exists today!

In Christ, we are building a legacy that we are going to pass down to every life that is connected to ours. What we allow to be poured into to our hearts, minds and bodies will be poured out on others.

We must daily allow God to fill us with His love and healing so that we can leave a precious legacy to those coming after us.

PRAYER

God, thank You for choosing me, even before You began creating the world. Help me to live my life in the freedom of this truth and to begin to comprehend what this means.

Journal: What choices have you made this week that glorify and please God?

—Becky Sirt

BELONGING TO HIM

By grace you have been saved, through faith—and this not from yourselves, it is the gift of God—not by works, so that no one can boast.

EPHESIANS 2:8-9

Most parents delight in giving gifts to their children. Even in the poorest of homes, parents do without things they want in order to buy the things their children want and need.

Our three children were very different, so the gifts we gave them were very different. Lisa is our competent, organized, oldest child, who can handle most situations by herself. She never asks for much and is always content with what she has. Even though Lisa is strong, she knows that we are and always will be there if she does have a need. Shari, our middle child, found it easy to ask for what she needed. Many times, the middle child has needs just because of his or her middle position in the family. John, our baby and only boy, never needed to ask for much because his dad would give him gifts before John knew he even had a need. None of our children ever had a need that we as parents didn't try to fulfill. There are probably more things we would have given if they had only asked.

God wants to do far more for His children than we could ever do for ours. He has given us His free gift of salvation, just because we asked for it.

Our children would never dream of boasting about the things they were given as children, because they know they didn't work for any of them. May we never boast about what we receive from God. His gifts to us have absolutely nothing to do with how hard we work.

As His children, we are blessed, just because we belong to Him.

PRAYER

Thank You for Your free gift of salvation. May I never boast, except in Your love.

Journal: List the many gifts you have received from God. Then thank Him for being such a loving Father.

—Carole Lewis

NOVEMBER 22

Relying on Him

By grace you have been saved, through faith—and this not from yourselves, it is the gift of God—not by works, so that no one can boast.

EPHESIANS 2:8-9

It never seemed to fail. Whenever I would diet and begin to approach my goal weight, I would do an about-face.

It seemed that whenever I started feeling so good—so proud—about my weight loss, I would sabotage my hard work and effort. Before I knew it, I was falling off my diet and quickly regained the weight. In fact, it always came back on far easier than it went off. *Why does this happen to me?* I wondered.

I now know what my problem was: I had always been counting on my own willpower alone. As I began to see results, I would then let it go to my head and feel that I could relax my hold a little. The result was a quick ride down a slippery slope! Self-will just wasn't—and isn't—enough.

God wants us to fully rely upon Him. That's why He gives us His grace, His unmerited favor. There is nothing we do to earn God's grace—and nothing we do to lose it. Grace is a gift that is given regardless of who we are, where we've been, what we do or why we do it. Grace comes to us because of who *God* is. All we have to do is believe in Him and receive His blessing.

This truth touches every area of life. If we rely on ourselves, we will eventually fall into the pride of boasting in what we've accomplished. If we rely on God and His gift of grace, we will humbly follow His way and receive lasting weight loss as His gift. We will have an attitude of gratitude and only boast in the Lord.

PRAYER

Lord, please forgive me for ever boasting in myself. Thank You for the gift of grace and for helping me achieve weight loss and victory in my health concerns.

Journal: Are you ready to accept God's grace to help you in your time of need? Write a prayer of praise, thanking Him for His gift of grace.

—Roberta Wasserman

NOVEMBER 23

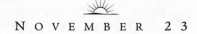

AMAZED BY GRACE

By grace you have been saved, through faith—and this not from yourselves, it is the gift of God—not by works, so that no one can boast.

EPHESIANS 2:8-9

Although I've heard these verses most of my life as a Christian, I never really considered what they meant until a few years ago. At that time I'd become involved in numerous activities at church, including being a First Place leader. I listened to the praise from others as to what a great job I was doing and was pleased when they asked how I could do so much. The compliments fed my ego and made me feel good because I thought it pleased God, and they motivated me to do even more—for the wrong reasons.

Then these verses came up during our Bible study. As I read them, the realization of what my life had been became clear. Rather than giving praise to God for His grace and mercy, I had been boastful and proud of my accomplishments, taking all the credit.

His amazing grace is a free gift. We don't have to work for it to prove ourselves. All we need to do is serve Him with our whole heart and have faith in His promises.

What aspect of God's grace do you need to count on today?

PRAYER

Lord, help me to remember my salvation is a free gift of grace and mercy from You.

Journal: Make a list of the things you have in your life because of God's grace and mercy. Then write a prayer thanking God for His free gift of salvation.

—Martha Rogers

NOVEMBER 24

SEEING THROUGH GRACE

By grace you have been saved, through faith—and this not from yourselves, it is the gift of God—not by works, so that no one can boast.

EPHESIANS 2:8-9

God is Love. For this reason, sin is a crime—not against *law*, but against *love*. It is possible to atone for a broken law, but it is impossible to make atonement for God's broken heart. Only an act of forgiveness by the grace of God can put us back into a right relationship with Him.

We will never *earn* God's forgiveness. We can only accept the special gift of grace from Him. What is grace? Grace has been expressed as God's righteousness at Christ's expense. Grace is getting something we don't deserve, and mercy is not getting what we do deserve.

Through Christ, we find abundant grace. He came and brought hope as He broke sin's power over us. My mom taught me that when someone loves us and we love them, this love causes us to see good things about ourselves we didn't even know existed. We find that our capacity to be our best is stretched and even defined by that relationship we have with another. The company we keep easily defines our future potential.

So it is when Christ becomes our Lord. Good things come from our hearts and souls that we didn't know existed there before. We are made in God's image. We are created to walk in love and fellowship with God.

Only with Christ in our life can we hope to experience such favor.

PRAYER

Father, I know my sins break Your heart. Against You alone have I sinned. Please forgive me and extend grace and mercy to me. Help me remember Your forgiveness is a special gift and I can never earn it. Let me spend time in Your company and let me be known by the company I keep.

Journal: Is it possible to be good enough to please God, and how much is enough? Do you work hard to prove yourself worthy of God's forgiveness? Do you understand the extravagance of His gifts of grace and mercy? Are you known by the company you keep?

—Becky Sirt

NOVEMBER 25

COMMITTED TO GRACE

By grace you have been saved, through faith—and this not from yourselves, it is the gift of God—not by works, so that no one can boast.

EPHESIANS 2:8-9

Bible historians tell us Ephesus was a city ruled by sin. Yet, despite all of the abominations, God chose to bring the Ephesians His message of love and salvation.

It is very fitting that God chose this place to explain that it is by His grace we are saved. It is a gift of God. Nothing we do can ever be good enough to earn salvation. The word "grace" in this verse means "to bestow with special honor, to make accepted."[2]

Our society today does not differ very much from ancient Ephesus. As Christians, it is overwhelming to see all the darkness that fills our world. Yet God promises us, in Romans 5: 20, that "where sin increased, grace increased all the more." It is a law, just like gravity. You can't see gravity; yet, you know that if you jump off anything, you will fall because gravity is there.

So it is with grace. When you are fixated on sin, you can't see grace. But if sin shows up in full force, then grace will be there in greater force. All we have to add to the battle is a little bit of faith. Faith means to believe, commit and put our trust in Jesus.

How can we take hold of the kind of faith we need to give us the spiritual backbone to trust God in all things? Think of the nine commitments in First Place, in particular the commitments about reading the Bible every day, coming to class to hear God's Word and learning the memory verses. Romans 10:17 says that "faith comes from hearing the message, and the message is heard through the word of Christ."

Are you listening?

PRAYER

Father, Your salvation is freely given to everyone who will receive it. Never allow my focus to remain on darkness or my failures. Give me a heart that always looks for Your grace in all circumstances. Help me extend Your grace freely to others in my life. Anoint my ears to hear Your Word and give me faith to trust You in all things.

Journal: Do you stay in the Word, so your faith continues to grow? Are you quick to accept God's grace, or do you waste time placing blame for your failures? Are you quick to extend grace to others?

—Becky Sirt

NOVEMBER 26

No More Walls

He himself is our peace, who has made the two one and has destroyed the barrier, the dividing wall of hostility, by abolishing in his flesh the law with its commandments and regulations.

EPHESIANS 2:14-15

We understand barriers. As babies, they kept us safe so that we didn't fall down stairs or get into cabinets containing poison. As teenagers, we had curfews, which were barriers meant to keep us from getting into trouble by staying out too late.

Before we came to know Christ, there was a barrier between Him and us. Jesus, by His death on the cross, tore down the dividing wall of hostility that separated us from Him.

I have learned the powerful truth of this verse during the last few years. Because Jesus is my peace, I can be at peace, even though my husband has cancer. I have peace about having my 89-year-old mom, who is losing her mental capacities, living with us. I even have peace about God calling our daughter Shari home to be with Him.

Is it possible to have the peace in myself? Absolutely not! My peace is possible because of the peace of Christ residing in me.

As believers, we have two choices: We can choose to live behind the wall of hostility, which once separated us from Christ, or we can trust Him to become our peace. As we allow Jesus to methodically tear down the wall of hostility that once separated us, we become truly free.

This wall of hostility will be torn down as we are able to trust Jesus to do what He says He will do in our life.

PRAYER

Jesus, tear down every wall of hostility keeping me from experiencing the peace that only You can provide.

Journal: Make a list of the circumstances in your life that need Christ's peace. Ask Him to tear down any wall that is keeping you from experiencing His peace.

—Carole Lewis

NOVEMBER 27

FREEDOM IN PEACE

He himself is our peace, who has made the two one and has destroyed the barrier, the dividing wall of hostility, by abolishing in his flesh the law with its commandments and regulations.

EPHESIANS 2:14-15

When it came to dieting, I found the plans were always laid out for me; and if only I could follow them perfectly, I would reach my goal weight. There was only one problem. I couldn't seem to follow the plan perfectly—and sometimes not at all.

What I needed was God's help and power. This Scripture speaks of the dividing wall of hostility that separates us, and I can truly relate. I found that through my relationship with the Lord, the more I overate, the less I felt God near me. It was as if eating too much food separated me from God and His presence. My smallest slipup was a dividing wall of sorts.

I had to come to terms with the fact that I did not have the power to overcome on my own. That meant coming into agreement with God about my failures. Scripture speaks of gluttony as a sin, and I had to accept that fact. Gluttony, as well as all the other broken commandments in my life, separated me from God.

I began to discover through the study of God's Word in First Place and through times of eating healthy, that being close to God was far more satisfying. I felt complete and whole. I felt fulfilled when He was near. As this reality surfaced through my walk with God, I desired less and less to indulge in excess food.

Now I want more and more to be close to the Lord and to know this Prince of peace.

PRAYER

Lord, please forgive me for all my choices that place a dividing wall between You and me. Thank You for granting me peace with my concerns about food and weight.

Journal: Do you sense the times when God is near and the times when He seems far away? Do you believe that sin separates you from God? Are you willing to change?

—Roberta Wasserman

WALKING THROUGH WALLS

He himself is our peace, who has made the two one and has destroyed the barrier, the dividing wall of hostility, by abolishing in his flesh the law with its commandments and regulations.

EPHESIANS 2:14-15

Have you ever felt as if there were a wall between what you want to do and what you actually do?

Many times, those of us who have been slaves to our weight and body size have felt the presence of this wall in our lives. We buy a treadmill fully intending to walk on it every day, but we end up using the treadmill as a clothes hanger. We want to walk on it, but we can't make ourselves do it.

Somewhere inside ourselves, a wall runs right down the middle. Things never seem to line up together because of these strongholds in our lives.

This is where Jesus steps in. His purpose was to create in Himself one whole new person out of the two, thus making peace. He gave His life to abolish that dividing wall in life and bring the two together, so you can experience peace.

Jesus knows of the walls inside you that keep you stuck. He knows the pain you feel because you just can't seem to get it together. Mark 16:14 tells us that Jesus literally walked through a wall in a room where His disciples were eating.

Today, give Jesus permission to walk through any of your walls to resolve what is bothering you. When He destroys those barriers, then you will feel like a complete person, full of peace.

PRAYER

Father I thank You that You sent Your Son to break through the walls in my life. I thank You, Father, for the abundant life I live through the shed blood of Your Son, Jesus. Today, I invite Jesus to walk through my walls.

Journal: The walls and strongholds in our lives are oftentimes blanketed by excuses the enemy has dropped in our minds to blind us. Today, ask the Lord to give you eyes to see the walls and barriers in your life and the desire to have Jesus remove them and bring unity into your life.

—Beverly Henson

NOVEMBER 29

PEACEFUL PURPOSE

He himself is our peace, who has made the two one and has destroyed the barrier, the dividing wall of hostility, by abolishing in his flesh the law with its commandments and regulations.

EPHESIANS 2:14-15

Some days we find ourselves just going through the motions of life, don't we?

We have rules and regulations and schedules we follow. We are so bound to life as usual that we sometimes forget to do things with purpose.

For so many years everything in my life revolved around becoming thin—diets, food, diet food, when I was going to eat, how much I was going to eat. That single purpose drove me on a daily basis. I felt that if I could just become thin, all of my problems would be solved. How wrong I was. How many years I wasted in frustrated, futile effort, focused on myself and my eating.

Our enemy, the devil, would love to keep you in this thought pattern. But when you change your purpose in life, Jesus can go to work on restoring your soul and making you strong enough to escape the traps of futility that Satan sets.

Through First Place I was able to walk free of the spiritual trap of a dieting mentality because I discovered a new purpose. I was no longer fixated on losing weight. My new purpose was to become a physically fit citizen of the kingdom of God.

Jesus has a specific purpose for you. Go through life with a new purpose and you will begin to see those diet strongholds come miraculously crumbling down.

PRAYER

Father, give me new purpose in my life. Change me to align with Your will for my life.

Journal: Ask the Lord to give you a new outlook on life with Jesus as your specific purpose.

—Beverly Henson

NOVEMBER 30

FAMILY TIES

Know this love that surpasses knowledge—that you may be filled to the measure of all the fullness of God

EPHESIANS 3:19

My parents loved me a lot. Both of my parents accepted Jesus when I was five years old, so I had the advantage of growing up in a family who loved Him.

My mom never worked outside the home, so she was always available to meet my wants and needs. When I was a teenager, it wasn't unusual for me to come home from school to find Mom had made a new dress for me because she knew I had party to attend that night. Because of the unconditional, sacrificial love shown me by my earthly parents, I am able today to be secure in Christ's love.

I'm well aware that I have a background that some of you might not have had. Perhaps you read about my growing-up experience and felt angry, sad or depressed because your family life was hard. Because of your childhood experiences, you might find it difficult to know and understand the full extent of God's love for you.

Let your mind go back to your own childhood for a minute. What was it like in your home? Christian psychologists tell us that we usually view God with the same eyes as we view our earthly parents.

God tells us in His Word, "To whom much is given, much is required" (see Matt. 25:29, *KJV*). I knew, when I accepted Jesus at the age of 12, that He would require much from me because I had the privilege of growing up in a home full of love. I had many friends whose parents were divorced or abusive. I even had one friend who said she would never have children because of the childhood she had experienced.

No matter the kind of childhood we had, God desperately wants to come in and teach us about His kind of love.

PRAYER

Jesus, I ask You to come into my life as my Father today. Teach me what this "love that surpasses knowledge" is like.

Journal: Make a list of all the reasons you find it hard to trust God. Go over the list and ask Jesus to heal each one of these hurts from your past.

—Carole Lewis

DECEMBER 1

NO FAVORITES

Know this love that surpasses knowledge—that you may be filled to the measure of all the fullness of God

EPHESIANS 3:19

It's very easy to love some people. They're happy and caring—the perfect friends. Then there are those who rub us the wrong way. They're no fun to be around, and you'd just as soon avoid them. We all know people in both groups.

Do you suppose God sees people the same way we do? Not according to His Word. Christ is full of love and compassion for each person. He does not play favorites. If we want the fullness of God, we need to start practicing love toward all, regardless of race, color or creed.

God does not give us "cousins." We are all His children.

PRAYER

Loving Father, help us to love as You love. Help us to be willing to overlook others' faults and personalities and love them with a genuine love just as You do us. We know this will please You.

Journal: Make a list today of the people you find hard to love. Ask God every day to help you love each of these people. Send each one a note this week complimenting something they have done.

—Joe Ann Winkler

DECEMBER 2

PROTECTED BY LOVE

Know this love that surpasses knowledge—that you may be filled to the measure of all the fullness of God

EPHESIANS 3:19

God created in us the desire for a full life. It is the enemy who lies, telling us that with God there are limits, rules and restrictions—all meant to curb our fun and hold us back.

In First Place the nine commitments and the accountability can feel like a prison to some people. They'll often tell the leader which commitments they will and won't keep. I was one of those people.

When I first arrived, I made it clear I'd come only for the Bible study—even though I weighed 200 pounds and was very unhealthy.

In time I realized that the accountability was not a punishment or a restriction. It was like a fortress I could run to for protection from the great "roaring lion"—and even from my self. In John 14:21, Jesus tells us that if we have an obedience problem, we actually have a love problem. If we love Him and trust Him, we will want to obey Him. Second Peter 1:3-4 says, "His divine power has given us everything we need for life and godliness through our knowledge of him." We are given great and precious promises that through Christ we can have a life of divine possibilities and not be slaves to anything. Christ came so that we could have freedom!

As we walk with Christ every day through prayer and reading His Word, we will begin to grasp the meaning of the breadth, depth, length and height of Christ's love for us. We acquire a heart knowledge that will just blow our minds. It is a love beyond our understanding.

If we accept this love and run to it for protection, we find that God fills us with nothing less than the Spirit of Christ Himself.

PRAYER

Holy Spirit, illuminate the areas in my life in which I have not fully surrendered control to Christ. May I know that You love me with an everlasting love and that You draw me to You with loving-kindness. May my life of service and obedience be my gift of love back to You.

Journal: Are there any areas in your life that you have not surrendered to God?

—Becky Sirt

DECEMBER 3

Finally Satisfied

Know this love that surpasses knowledge—that you may be filled to the measure of all the fullness of God

EPHESIANS 3:19

First Place led me to a personal relationship with the Lord Jesus Christ. In awe of His amazing love for me, I willingly sat at His feet and began to drink in the knowledge of this love. In time, all the empty parts of my heart began to be filled to overflowing.

To sit at His feet and read Scripture was like a daily feast—with no calories! I had spent years trying to fill this void in my soul with excess food. All that did was make me excessively fat. As a result, I spent my days trying to fix my weight. I didn't know before First Place that it was God's love that I was seeking.

In truth, nothing in this world can satisfy the place reserved for God—not food and not even the perfect number on a scale. We may seek many things to fill us, but no matter where we go or how far we wander, God is waiting to do for us what nothing else can. God wants to fill us to the full measure with His love.

As we are filled with God and His love, we will naturally overflow with grace and love into the lives of others who need to know this love too. This is far more satisfying than going through the ups and downs of riding a scale and far more satisfying than craving food which could never satisfy.

PRAYER

Lord, forgive me for seeking other ways to fill my soul other than with Your amazing love. Thank You for waiting for me to find the truth. Thank You for satisfying me.

Journal: Do you believe the lie that more food, just one more bite will satisfy you? Do you believe the lie that if you only weighed a certain amount, you would be happy? Are you ready to turn to the Lord to fill you to the full measure of His love?

—Roberta Wasserman

DECEMBER 4

CHANGED FOR GOOD

You were taught, with regard to your former way of life, to put off your old self, . . . and to put on the new self, created to be like God in true righteousness and holiness.

EPHESIANS 4:22-24

Have you ever had fantasies of being someone else? This dream person would be the opposite of everything you dislike about yourself and your life.

Of course he or she would be thin, fit and self-assured. This person would have many friends and much influence. People would hang on every word that came from this person's mouth. This individual would have an adoring husband or wife and children who thought the person hung the moon.

Some fantasy, right?

God tells us in this verse that He wants to help us become someone else. He wants to come in and give us new bodies, friends, influence, words, mates and children. How in the world can He accomplish that?

In Evelyn Christenson's book *Lord Change Me,* she describes how God is able to turn our fantasies into fact. When God is given the power to come in and change me, He is then free to work on the circumstances that surround me. As I am able to put off my old self and put on the new self created to be like God, amazing things start to happen all around me.[3]

Many of us spend our entire life telling God that we will change—if only He will change our circumstances. God wants to change us *in order* to change our circumstances.

PRAYER

Jesus, change me so that You are free to change my circumstances.

Journal: Ask God to show you the areas of your life that need changing. Sit quietly before Him until He speaks.

—Carole Lewis

RIGHT THINKING

You were taught, with regard to your former way of life, to put off your old self, . . . and to put on the new self, created to be like God in true righteousness and holiness.

EPHESIANS 4:22-24

Through First Place I learned what it means to put off my old self.

For me this was essential—probably even life-saving. I learned to stop the bingeing and self-destructive dieting and weight-loss methods. I learned to say no to the desires that raged within for more and more sweets and junk food.

Beneath it all, I was out of control. One bite was never enough. I always wanted more. Even when my body was stuffed, I wanted and craved more. These were deceitful desires. These desires deceived me into thinking that I would be satisfied. I was never satisfied with more. If anything, I was less satisfied with my body, my appearance and my weight.

My mind had to be renewed. I learned that I was created to be like God, and as that truth sank in, I just could not imagine Jesus bingeing on junk food. In fact, I imagined Him eating healthy foods, in limited amounts. I imagined Him eating when hungry and stopping when full. The more I focused on my Lord and what He would do, the less I walked in my old ways.

It took time, but I learned new ways of eating. Today I feel great when I think about my choices. I believe God has blessed my obedience to Him in this area of my life.

PRAYER

Lord, thank You for saving me from deceitful desires. Thank You for renewing my mind and showing me just what Jesus would do.

Journal: Do you desire good things or bad things? Would you be willing to invite Jesus to your next meal? Are you ready to make healthy choices with your food?

—Roberta Wasserman

December 6

Making Space

You were taught, with regard to your former way of life, to put off your old self, . . . and to put on the new self, created to be like God in true righteousness and holiness.

Ephesians 4:22-24

For the longest time, my computer and I had a love-hate relationship. I am very fond of all a computer can do, but I struggled with the difficult process of learning this modern technological tool.

During this learning process, my emotions have traveled from agonizing tears to hysterical laughter.

Just as I began to understand and enjoy the wonders of saving and deleting files, formatting documents, automatic page-numbering and much more, a special new message dashed across my computer screen one day. It said simply that I had no more space to store information and I should delete unneeded documents in order to give the computer the number of bytes required for storing more.

Easier said than done.

I learned that day that permanently deleting anything from a computer is not simple. After much new frustration and counsel from a wise computer professor, I met my waste bin. Aghast at the amount of stored "garbage" there, I used new knowledge to empty it. As I pushed the right button for the final time, I watched the cartoonlike illustration showing the waste bin emptying. A clean screen appeared.

As I watched this, a truth from God sank in. A sluggish, overstuffed computer is the picture of my life when I choose to hang on to the former self like so much garbage. The clean screen is the new self God desires for me when I allow Him to work in me regularly.

My computer is no longer a "love and hate" place. It is a "love and learn" place where God works too.

Prayer

Father, You are the author of truth. You are Truth. Help me empty the waste bin often and maintain a healthy "love and learn" place with You.

Journal: What must you delete from your life today so that you are open to the truth God wants you to see? What frustrations, fears and habits can you list right now and then throw away, so you can be a renewed, joyful learner?

—Nan Olmstead

DECEMBER 7

PAINT THAT STICKS

You were taught, with regard to your former way of life, to put off your old self, . . . and to put on the new self, created to be like God in true righteousness and holiness.

EPHESIANS 4:22-24

The Message renders these verses: "Since, then, we do not have the excuse of ignorance, everything—and I do mean everything—connected with that old way of life has to go. It's rotten through and through. Get rid of it! And then take on an entirely new way of life—a God-fashioned life, a life renewed from the inside and working itself into your conduct as God accurately reproduces his character in you."

Have you ever painted a wall? Paint can cover up some pretty awful things and make the dingiest room look bright and new. But if you want your paint to stick and the job to last, you need to clean the walls with soap and water before you start to paint.

In much the same way, you must put down, or lay aside your old self, so you can then allow God to renew the spirit of your mind. You can then put on your new self.

You won't get the same results in painting if you don't clean the wall before you paint. Some of the old stuff could seep through and mar the appearance of the wall. In the same way, you can't change your life until you put aside the dirt that is ruling your life, allow God to renew you and then put on your new self.

We must take off the old dingy rags and allow the Lord to give us a bath. Then, best of all, we can put on the clothes that will make us look like our heavenly Father!

PRAYER

Father, I'm taking off the old habits of turning to food for comfort and I'm standing still, so You can give me a bath. I look forward to wearing the new outfit that will make me look just like You!

Journal: What in your life do you need to remodel?

—June-Marie Avery

DECEMBER 8

IN WITH THE NEW

You were taught, with regard to your former way of life, to put off your old self, . . . and to put on the new self, created to be like God in true righteousness and holiness.

EPHESIANS 4:22-24

To be like God, righteous and holy, we must discard our old habits. And this means *change*. Many of us have something in common—we're old friends with various diets that didn't work. First Place has meant many changes for us.

In the Gospels I read about the woman who had hemorrhaged for 12 years. What impressed me most was that she alone out of everyone in a huge crowd was healed by Jesus—and that came about because she simply reached out and touched His robe.

First Place gave me a spirit of courage I'd never had before. I came to believe that if I approached God boldly every day in my quiet time, He would surely recognize my heart's desire to be healed—and He would notice me. I began to expect Him to make First Place a healthy way of life instead of "just another diet."

That's where the reaching out to touch Him came in. I became willing to make necessary adjustments in my old self to accommodate His work. I claimed His words to the sick woman: "Daughter, you took a risk of faith, and now you're healed and whole. Live well, live blessed. Be healed of your plague" (see Matt. 9:22).

A gamut of changes definitely began for me. The changes God asked me to make took me outside my old self and put me on an entirely new level—I was never to return to some of my old ways.

From time to time, I still find myself struggling. I know more changes lie ahead. And I look forward to the healing He has yet to bring to my life.

PRAYER

Lord, thank You that First Place allows You to make necessary changes in my life. Thank You that with Your help I am able to put off my old self and put on the new self You created for me. Make me mindful and open my heart to Your teachings of righteousness and holiness, applying these qualities to my life today.

Journal: What changes do you need to make in order to reach out to God? Choose one, and write down what you need to do about it today.

—Judy Marshall

DECEMBER 9

LIVING LOVE

Live a life of love, just as Christ loved us and gave himself up for us as a fragrant offering and sacrifice to God.

EPHESIANS 5:2

After I die, I would love for people to say that I lived a life of love. If they said this about it me, it would mean that God had done the loving through me, since God is love. Living in this earthly body, though, I am incapable of loving people the way God loves them. My love will always have a condition: If you will do this or that, then I will love you.

How thankful I am for the supreme example of selfless love we have in Christ. Jesus died so that I might spend eternity with Him. He also died so that He might live a life of love in and through me. This means He wants to love that rebellious teenager through me. He wants to use me to love that mean husband or wife. He wants to love that coworker or church member so much that every time a person looks at me, it is His love that is seen.

Jesus desires for our lives to have the sweet fragrance of Him. That won't happen until we give Him permission to do what we are incapable of doing. When He is allowed to love the unlovely through us, those very people start to smell His sweet fragrance and want it for themselves.

PRAYER

Jesus, I want to live a life characterized by love. Help me today to show Your love to everyone who comes my way.

Journal: Write the names of the unlovable people in your life. Ask God to start loving these people through you today.

—Carole Lewis

DECEMBER 10

COMFORTING LOVE

Live a life of love, just as Christ loved us and gave himself up for us as a fragrant offering and sacrifice to God.

EPHESIANS 5:2

Do you ever thank the Lord for a rainy day? It is so tempting to grumble and complain about another rainy day, especially if it's been raining day after day. Complaining about things over which we have no control is especially tempting.

What if we took another approach? What if we decided to listen to the gentle dripping of the rain as it hits the green grass or blossoming flowers? What if we took a walk to smell the fresh air after it has rained?

What I am saying is that we can come to love God more if we learn to love the small joys in life that He provides.

Today I want to thank Him for the out-of-my-control circumstances that feel like days of rain in my own life. I know that He has allowed them all. I take comfort that these rainy days are allowed in love. Because of this, I can grab an umbrella and live a life of love, just as Christ loved me and gave Himself up for me as a fragrant offering and sacrifice to God.

I praise the Lord for rain, because it reminds me that God can refresh my spirit—no matter what's happening in my life.

PRAYER

Lord, help me to live wisely this day and make good choices to enjoy Your love whatever the outside or inside weather.

Journal: What are three loving things you can do today as a fragrant offering to God?

—Carol Moore

LOVE'S FRAGRANCE

Live a life of love, just as Christ loved us and gave himself up for us as a fragrant offering and sacrifice to God.

EPHESIANS 5:2

The sense of smell can sometimes warn us of danger. It can also touch emotions and move our hearts. It makes happy memories come back to life, and it enhances the flavor of foods.

Why did God create us with a sense of smell? Sometimes while watching my weight, I've thought of this ability as a curse.

But just think what we would have missed if we had not been able to smell flowers, rain, babies after a bath, or the ocean. Would our lives have been as full? Here we see a great example of God thinking of the little things to bless people for abundant living every day.

The sacrifice of Christ was a life of perfect obedience to God and of perfect love for men. His obedience was so absolute and His love was so deep that He accepted the cross and endured all the shame. Because of His love, Christ's life became a fragrant offering to God.

In 2 Corinthians 2:15, Paul says that we Christians bear the sweet aroma of Christ. When we imitate God's attitude of love, kindness, forgiveness and mercy in our behavior—when we're following Christ—there is a kind of scent that other people pick up. We are not like others.

We are called to love people with the same sacrificial love that characterizes Jesus' love for them. We are called to bear with them and forgive them in love, as Christ has done.

If Christ lives in our hearts, our hearts will be full of a sweet, precious perfume. Every life we touch will smell the perfume as we pass by. Every word, every action, every thought we have will leave behind a lingering aroma.

PRAYER

My Savior and friend, fill my heart with the perfume of Your sweet love. Help me to take the time to be a sweet aroma for someone who needs a blessing today. Live through my life with Your love and power.

Journal: Are you delighting in the little things that make life special? What does your aroma smell like? Is that aroma a sweet smell of Christ or is it a cheap imitation?

—Becky Sirt

DECEMBER 12

WILLING TO SACRIFICE

Live a life of love, just as Christ loved us and gave himself up for us as a fragrant offering and sacrifice to God.

EPHESIANS 5:2

When I began First Place, I weighed almost 300 pounds. I really wanted to make this program work in my life, so I searched the Scriptures and came to several conclusions that transformed my life and created the lifestyle changes that have enabled me through Jesus Christ to maintain my goal weight for four years.

One problem I used to have concerned my lunch. When I was at my largest, after I ate, all I wanted to do was sleep. When I began First Place, I knew that my lunch break had to consist of two sections. The first was my food and the second was exercise. I came to the conclusion that Jesus is the best personal trainer I could ever have. Why do I say that?

As I read this Scripture—that Christ loved me and gave Himself up as a fragrant offering and sacrifice—I knew I must give up the thing I really wanted to do *first,* which was eat lunch. I knew that if I ate first, I would get sleepy and never exercise.

That meant the thing I really didn't want to do, I had to do first. But how could I get it to be a fragrant offering and sacrifice to God? I didn't *want* to exercise—I wanted to *eat.*

Here is what my heavenly personal trainer had me do: Each day, I gave to Him an exercise tithe offering. If I had an hour lunch break, before I put a bite of food in my mouth, I gave to Him a 10-minute walk.

Before too long, that "exercise tithe" began to be a fragrant offering and sacrifice not only to Jesus but also to me.

Now I look forward to whatever He asks me to do for Him each day. In His own way, by His love, He has changed me from within.

PRAYER

Father, as I exercise, give me a new joy and excitement that I can move for You. Bless this tithe of movement I give to You each day.

Journal: Ask the Lord to show you a plan and offer it to Him as a fragrant offering and sacrifice.

—Beverly Henson

DECEMBER 13

MORE THAN WORDS

Live a life of love, just as Christ loved us and gave himself up for us as a fragrant offering and sacrifice to God.

EPHESIANS 5:2

Jesus Christ gave up His life for me. He went to the cross and suffered and sacrificed everything for me.

But what did that have to do with my weight problem?

This Scripture made me realize the depth of what Jesus had done for me. What was I willing to do for Him in expression of my gratitude? Was it truly too much for Him to ask me to give up that piece of dessert? Was it really too much for Him to ask me to give up that second helping of food? How much did I appreciate what the Lord had done for me? How much did I truly love Jesus Christ? Did I love Him more than what the pantry offered me?

All these thoughts went through my mind as I considered the command in this Scripture. Jesus did not just *say* He loved me. He died to show me *how much* He loves me. Was I willing to show Jesus how much I loved Him, by following through with repenting of my sinful eating habits and developing new and healthier choices?

Through the First Place program, I was given all that I needed to succeed. How grateful I am for one more evidence of His love—His ministry to me through First Place.

PRAYER

Lord, thank You for loving me so much that You died on the cross for my sins. Forgive me for loving so many other things more than I have loved You.

Journal: Have you accepted the truth that Jesus Christ gave up everything for you? Are you willing to express your gratitude to Him? Are you willing to give up the excess food?

—Roberta Wasserman

DECEMBER 14

WALKING LIGHTS

You were once darkness, but now you are light in the Lord. Live as children of light.

EPHESIANS 5:8

Today, I read in the newspaper about a precious 17-year-old girl who died in a plane crash. I wept as I read that she died on her mother's 44th birthday. After recently losing one my own daughters, I can identify with the pain of parents who lose children.

This young woman was the daughter of a local pastor, and it was apparent that even in her short life she had learned what it meant to live as a child of light. The article told about the mission trips this young woman took and how she led prayers in worship services. She was shining for Christ in a dark world.

Two men who were staff members of the church also died in the crash. One had just moved here from another state and the other was the youth minister. The article stated that the church's youth program went from stagnant to turbo-charged under his direction.

One church lost three living lights for Christ when that plane crashed. Each time the light of another believer dies, those of us who remain must shine even brighter.

I was saddened that the story was tucked way back in the newspaper, because it should have been on the front page. Every true follower of Christ is a miracle walking around in an earthly body that, instead of walking in darkness, God has filled with light. The lost world desperately needs to know this light-giving person named Jesus.

Since we do not know how many days we have to serve God faithfully here, may each of us live as children of light in our dark world today.

PRAYER

Dear Jesus, shine through me today in every word I say and everything I do.

Journal: Write about areas of your life that still have dark places of sin or unbelief. Ask Jesus to shine His light into every dark corner.

—Carole Lewis

DECEMBER 15

STAYING IN THE LIGHT

You were once darkness, but now you are light in the Lord. Live as children of light.

EPHESIANS 5:8

Every time I read this verse I think of the song we'd sing as small children: "This little light of mine, I'm going to let it shine." Yet how often did I fail to shine because I was overweight and self-conscious.

I know from being a First Place leader that a person who is overweight will more than likely be the last person to feel comfortable speaking in a crowd. I can remember when I was younger, I would make up excuses for not going to the altar when the Holy Spirit would convict me. I used to think, *I am not going down there; I can pray just fine from here.*

Actually, I had a fear that I would get down and need help getting up. I would tell myself that people would make fun of me or feel sorry for me, so I would not allow the light of holy conviction to be seen in me and be a witness to others.

But Christ does not want us to hide our light. He wants us to let it shine. We cannot do that from our seat. We have to make that first step.

When I was lost and searching for Christ, my grandfather, who is a Baptist minister, would say, "The first step is the hardest. After that, God will carry you." I found out at the age of 13 that what my grandfather had said was true. I remember my fear of conviction, but I also remember never looking back after that first step. That is a day I will always treasure, the day I asked Christ into my heart.

But I *did* hide my light—mostly out of shame for my size. I felt ashamed that I could not control my eating. Then I was introduced to First Place and that changed my thoughts. I began to read God's Word and realized that I need only please Him, not others. Christ saved me at age 13 and changed my heart—but it took until I was age 30 for Christ and the world to see my light shine.

PRAYER

I want to let my light shine for You, Lord. I don't want to hide it. I know that the world may see me in a different light, but I need only to trust You with a childlike faith and I will never walk in darkness alone again.

Journal: What are some changes you need to make to let your light shine for Christ?

—Tanya McClanahan

DECEMBER 16

REFLECTING HIS LIGHT

You were once darkness, but now you are light in the Lord. Live as children of light.

EPHESIANS 5:8

I recently read somewhere that only when God has found us are we able to think or see straight. Once we meet Jesus and He touches our lives with His glory, He is able to give our lives new meaning. Then our minds take on a new light—God's light. Everything is affected. His light influences the way we think about our lives, our relationships and the world—even the way we eat. It is our choice to allow His light to reflect in our lives and shine on others.

When my sons were young Halley's comet became visible from Earth. Since it returns every 77 years, this ancient comet might be able to be seen by my sons twice in their lifetimes. So the first time it became visible, we searched the dark sky and finally saw what we had so diligently waited for. Several nights with binoculars we observed the main part of the comet—a simple soft ball of light that flowed away from the sun into a very long trail of light.

As Christians, we should resemble Halley's comet. The core of our lives should be a true, simple reflection of Christ's light. And as we pass through others' lives, we should leave a long trail of His light streaming away from us—a lighted path for others to follow in order to find the Son who pierces the darkness around them.

PRAYER

Lord, thank You for piercing my darkness and illuminating my life with Your light.
Keep shining ON and IN me so that my thoughts and actions reflect Your light.
May I live as a child of light and help others find You in their darkness.

Journal: Do you have any shady areas or darkness in your life that need God's light today? Because you are light in the Lord, what changes can you make to better reflect His light? Who needs to see a brighter reflection of Christ in you today?

—Judy Marshall

December 17

Radiant Light

You were once darkness, but now you are light in the Lord. Live as children of light.

Ephesians 5:8

My years of struggling with overeating were a long period of darkness for me.

I spent most of my time isolated from others and hiding my secret indulgence in food. Hours were spent bingeing on food to numb the pain of living, and then more time was spent trying to cure the consequences of excess weight.

When the Lord touched this painful area of my life, slowly the light of His presence was revealed. He came into the dark recesses of my heart and mind to deal with the destructive areas of my life. His truth brought light to me, and I began to radiate those truths. I radiated His love through my renewed attitude and the new choices I made, which eventually became healthier habits.

Over time, people saw the difference in me. I spent less time hiding and more time reflecting Jesus to others. The longer I walk in His light, the less I desire to ever return to that period of darkness. It has become easier and easier to walk away from the foods that used to tempt me.

Today I know the truth and am not deceived by the same foods and habits that kept me in the dark. I am very grateful, and I shine now for His name's sake.

Prayer

Lord, thank You for bringing light to my life. Thank You for setting me free from the power of darkness that controlled me for so long.

Journal: What are you trying to hide? Are you tired of doing the same thing over and over, expecting the consequences to be different? Are you ready to have God's light shine on your life so that you can walk out of darkness?

—Roberta Wasserman

DECEMBER 18

PEACEMAKERS

Make every effort to keep the unity of the Spirit through the bond of peace.

EPHESIANS 4:3

Most of us know that unless we can learn to live and work in unity with others, there will be no peace. As children in kindergarten, we learned not to bite or hit. As adults, we are more subtle because we have learned to bite with our words and hit others with our bad attitude. It is imperative that all of us learn what it means to "make every effort" to be united in Christ with every other believer through the bond of peace.

One of my friends is a really nice lady. She loves the Lord and has many talents that she uses for Him. One of her spiritual gifts is service, and she serves others with passion and love. The one lesson she still needs to learn, however, is how "to keep the unity of the Spirit through the bond of peace."

Every time she has any kind of problem, she feels it's her right to unload her frustration on everyone around her. After she does this, she feels so much better. "I just needed to vent" is her common refrain.

But what about those of us who are the recipients of the garbage she dumps? Our peace can be shattered, all because she hasn't learned that she has an obligation always "to make every effort to keep the unity of the Spirit through the bond of peace."

Unloading frustration onto others is one form of unity smashing—but what about gossip or criticism? These practices also rob believers of the unity and peace that should be the outstanding characteristics of people who belong to the family of God.

PRAYER

Lord, teach me how to "keep the unity of [Your] Spirit through the bond of peace."

Journal: Ask God to search your heart today, to see if there are any practices in your life that disturb the peace of others and the unity of the Body of Christ. Who are the people in your life with whom you need to live in "the bond of peace"? Write their names in your journal and pray that God will use you in their lives.

—Carole Lewis

DECEMBER 19

Bonds of Peace

Make every effort to keep the unity of the Spirit through the bond of peace.

EPHESIANS 4:3

A few months after the death of my husband, my grandson, Tyler Matthew, was born. After holding this new little one in my arms, knowing that he and his precious mother were fine, I left the hospital to drive to a high school reunion in another state.

Shortly after my arrival, I received a call from my son telling me that Tyler had developed a very rare problem with his lungs and the doctor's prognosis was not optimistic for his survival. I immediately rushed home, and we spent many days at the hospital praying for his recovery. During this time, God gave us many promises from His Word. Each one offered comfort and assurance that He was at work on our behalf.

In the meantime, Thanksgiving was looming and none of us was eager to celebrate without all of our family together. A friend had told me earlier that I needed to do something different that year. I guess God also thought it was a good idea because we were soon making plans to celebrate Thanksgiving at Luby's—a restaurant in the medical center! We had a wonderful day that culminated with the news that Tyler was being moved out of ICU and was on his way to recovery. I can tell you for sure that God is concerned about the smallest details of our lives. He allowed us "to keep the unity of the Spirit through the bond of peace" as we celebrated this holiday season together, rejoicing with the knowledge that God had come through the trial with us and our precious baby would soon be going home.

PRAYER

Lord, You care about us down to the minutest details of our lives.
Thank You for Your love and Your Word that sustain us in every trial we face,
assuring us of Your faithfulness to us.

Journal: Are you giving God just the big problems in your life, thinking you can handle the details? Write in your journal all the little details that you are trying to handle and give them to God today and He will give you His peace.

—Pat Lewis

DECEMBER 20

DRAWING OTHERS CLOSE

Make every effort to keep the unity of the Spirit through the bond of peace.

EPHESIANS 4:3

The New York Subway doesn't waste any time. People enter, a bell sounds, the door closes and the train takes off—*quickly*. My "mother's heart" still beats wildly when I remember an incident that took place on the subway when my daughter was seven.

Going to New York City was part of a wonderful summer vacation. We went from place to place on the subway. While boarding subway cars in the midst of the jostling crowds, we made every effort to bind ourselves together as each of us hung on to someone else. One time as we boarded a car during the afternoon, my seven-year-old daughter was still outside the door when the subway bell sounded. I gave a mighty yank, trying to pull her through as the doors closed upon her. I felt weak kneed as I pondered what could have happened if she had been left standing alone in the subway in downtown New York—if we had not been bonded together by a strong grip.

As believers, we should make the same effort to create and maintain unity among ourselves. This can only be done through the Holy Spirit, as we allow Him to build the bond of peace among us. Only then can we avoid leaving someone outside and alone. Only then can we avoid dissension over trivial matters within the Church.

How about it—are you willing to let God work through you to keep the unity of the Spirit?

PRAYER

Lord, am I in a state of disunity with someone? Teach me, through Your Spirit, to build a bond of peace. Teach me what it means to live in unity with all people.

Journal: What part does God want you to play in building unity with others?

—Helen McCormack

DECEMBER 21

KEEPING RIGHT ORDER

Make every effort to keep the unity of the Spirit through the bond of peace.

EPHESIANS 4:3

During a move, I lost something that was dear to me—something from an inherited set of silverware that had belonged to my grandmother.

When I unpacked my kitchen, I found that I had misplaced a fork from the set. When you lose part of a set or a collection, the entire set loses its value. I found I couldn't have peace in my life until I found that missing piece. I looked everywhere and would not be satisfied until the entire set was back together.

When I was overweight, I felt like a set that had lost a piece. Nothing in my life would ever line up. I was out of order. I had no peace. I was constantly seeking to be thin, rather than seeking first the kingdom of God and His righteousness. Through First Place I learned to seek first the Kingdom, rather than seek first to be thin. When I began to seek the Kingdom, I found that missing piece of my life. I felt as if I finally had unity in my own life through the Spirit of the Lord.

That's when I remembered what it was like to find the missing piece I'd lost from my grandmother's valuable silverware. Once the unity of the Spirit began to take hold in my life, I felt like a complete set of silver. What binds your life is the peace you find through the unity of the Spirit.

Once the Father restores wholeness to your soul, you never want to misplace a piece of it. You strive to keep your life in holy order.

PRAYER

Father, there are days when I feel like all the pieces of my life are out of place. I feel like a set with a missing piece. Jesus, bring that unifying peace as You fill the gaps in my life.

Journal: What do you feel is missing from your life? Ask God to begin to work to restore your sense of completeness.

—Beverly Henson

DECEMBER 22

WORKING FOR UNITY

Make every effort to keep the unity of the Spirit through the bond of peace.

EPHESIANS 4:3

By the shelf that held a display of turkey bacon in the grocery store, I was asked by two women about the different brands being offered. They were beginning a diet and wanted to know about low-fat foods. I told them I had lost 147 pounds and was something of an expert on turkey bacon!

Their eyes sparkled. "Which diet are you on?!" they asked excitedly. Their faces showed disillusionment, however, when I told them I had lost my weight by participating in the First Place program. They said, "Oh, we've tried that diet. It doesn't work."

I wanted to tell them that they were right to think that as a "diet," First Place doesn't work. In First Place *you* work! Anything worth having is worth working for. We have to "make every effort." In 1 Corithians 3:9, Paul tells us we are laborers together with God. He is going to do His part for sure, but we have to do our part as well.

First Place is a way of living that God gave to us as a tool. A shovel is a tool that will never dig a hole until we take hold of it and do the work.

To those of you working hard at this program, make every effort to use this tool the Lord has given you to labor with Him. You will find the unity of the Spirit of the Lord and a bond of peace with God like you've never experienced before.

PRAYER

Father, I thank You that You trust me to labor together with You. I know You will do Your part, but help me, Father, to be faithful with my part of the labor.

Journal: Ask the Lord to help you realize that First Place is a useful tool the Lord has given you to labor with Him. It is not a diet but a lifestyle change that will bring you closer to Jesus.

—Beverly Henson

DECEMBER 23

Staying in the Truth

Our struggle is not against flesh and blood, but against the rulers, against the authorities, against the powers of this dark world and against the spiritual forces of evil in the heavenly realms.

EPHESIANS 6:12

Sometimes, I have to be right in the middle of an anxiety attack before I realize that the worry I'm feeling has nothing to do with my situation. The devil has a lot of power in this world, and he is able to stir up lots of trouble trying to defeat believers. When will we learn that he only has the power to defeat us *if* we give it to him?

As you've gathered by now, my mom is suffering from dementia. Because she has always been such a warm, funny, outgoing person, we find ourselves fretting and anxious because we can't fix her problem. She sincerely believes that we need to take her home, even though she has lived with us for more than two years. Some days she repeatedly asks to go home.

I have realized that the reason I get anxious is because she will never be the mom of my youth again. God has shown me that it is okay to grieve this loss but it is not okay to let this loss rob me of my joy in Him. If I ever let the enemy get his foot into the door of my mind, a bulldozer is seemingly needed to retrieve me from the ditch!

My struggle should never be with God, and I am learning the hard way to run into His arms to receive the help I need. God always comes through in power and helps me—if I remember to stop and pray when I sense the anxiety starting to mount.

PRAYER

Lord, I want to praise You for having the power to calm my anxious heart. Help me to keep my eyes on You, not the evil ruler of this world.

Journal: Write down the anxiety-causing circumstances in your life. Ask God for His help in dealing with each one.

—Carole Lewis

DECEMBER 24

LIONS OR KITTENS?

Our struggle is not against flesh and blood, but against the rulers, against the authorities, against the powers of this dark world and against the spiritual forces of evil in the heavenly realms.

EPHESIANS 6:12

Some ladies in our church were recently invited to another church to provide music and a message for a luncheon.

As I was preparing the message God had given me, I had a mental picture of several lions prowling around the luncheon tables. I knew I had to bring in more prayer power!

I asked the leader of our Unceasing Prayer Ministry to get her team on their knees. Interestingly enough, she told me she was trying to envision these lions, but all she could see was kitty cats. I begged, "Keep praying!"

We had bathed this luncheon in so much prayer that it seemed to drip off our elbows, and the afternoon turned out to be a spiritual success. We saw the glory of God.

Well after the luncheon was over and we had returned home, we remembered one of the table decorations had been kittens! God is good—and he has a sense of humor too. He turned my fear into faith!

PRAYER

Lord, cause me to see where the battlefield lies. Lord, open my spiritual eyes to see Your glory. Cause me to recognize the fear in my life and turn it over to You. Thank You for the gift of laughter and my holy weapon of prayer.

Journal: From what does your fear stem? Is your life different from the way it was six months ago or even six weeks ago? Ask Him to open the eyes of your heart.

—Denise Peters

DECEMBER 25

ON THE WINNING SIDE

Our struggle is not against flesh and blood, but against the rulers, against the authorities, against the powers of this dark world and against the spiritual forces of evil in the heavenly realms.

EPHESIANS 6:12

In my past attempts to lose my excess weight before I joined First Place, obstacles never failed to block my path. Almost every time I'd start a weight-loss program, with the very best intentions, the celebrations would start: Someone would have a birthday, and of course I couldn't pass up a piece of cake. Someone else would have a party, and I just had to try everything served that evening. A holiday would approach, and I just couldn't resist the traditional foods.

These obstacles were just enough to break down my good intentions.

Then First Place led me to the Word of God—and this particular Scripture helped me to realize that my battle was not being waged just against forces of this world. There were spiritual forces out there trying to set me up to fail. Temptation lies in wait around every corner.

God's Word brought me so much comfort, knowing that He was on my side. I learned that He was cheering for me and would be there to lead me through the temptations and toward victory.

God did this very thing for me—He gave me victory! Today I am led more by the Holy Spirit and less by the desires of my flesh.

PRAYER

Lord, forgive me for the years that I gave in to my flesh. Thank You for leading me to First Place and to Your Holy Word where I am taught the truth.

Journal: How many times have you fallen off your diet program due to a celebration involving food? Are you ready to be led by the Word of God and the Holy Spirit to be victorious in this area?

—Roberta Wasserman

DECEMBER 26

READ THE INSTRUCTION BOOK

Our struggle is not against flesh and blood, but against the rulers, against the authorities, against the powers of this dark world and against the spiritual forces of evil in the heavenly realms.

EPHESIANS 6:12

My son, Ben, and I decided it was time to hang some doors in our new home. We only had three to hang; and, fortunately for us, the previous owner left the hinges and the doors that we needed.

We screwed in the hinges to the frame for the first door and had it up in 10 minutes. What a piece of cake! Only two to go.

After an hour or so of screwing in the hinges every possible way and not being able to get the door to hang properly—too much room at the bottom or at the top or the door didn't swing the right way—we were beside ourselves. What went so wrong after our first attempt went so right?

Now that everything had failed, we decided we needed to check the directions in a carpentry book. Once we read the expert advice, we knew where we'd gone wrong, and we had the other two doors up in no time.

Isn't that what this verse is trying to say to those of us who want to live a spiritual life—that we need God's wisdom and tactics to replace our own understanding? Sure, we may get it right once in a while, the way a blind squirrel is sure to find a nut on occasion. But the darkness ultimately prevails, unless we walk in the true light and power of Jesus.

PRAYER

Father, fill me with the confidence to trust in Your wisdom and to see Your way in all things.

Journal: What isn't going right for you at home or at work and how can you look to God for direction today?

—Bruce Barbour

DECEMBER 27

COVERED BY HIS PRAYER

Pray in the Spirit on all occasions with all kinds of prayers and requests.

EPHESIANS 6:18

I think the greatest legacy Jesus left us is the promise that His Spirit comes to live inside us the instant we become His children. Then, as we grow in Christ, we learn what it means to "pray in the Spirit on all occasions with all kinds of prayers and requests."

Sometimes I pray when I know what I need. Other times I don't have a clue what I need. That's when I'm thankful the Holy Spirit of God takes over and prays for me. Either way, I'm covered at all times. The only requirement is for me to keep a clean slate with God. This means that I don't let sin build up to the point that my sin forms a wall between God and me.

One time, I had a clear sense of something God wanted me to do. Each morning as I would try to pray, the Holy Spirit would quietly tell my spirit what God was asking of me. I ignored His still small voice for almost six weeks before I finally gave in and did what God wanted. During this six-week period, because of my stubborn refusal to do what God had directed, I didn't have quality time with Him. I would still show up for my quiet time, but God seemed to be silent and distant.

What solved the problem? God hadn't moved. I had.

I always feel such joy and peace after God wins a war. After all, He's God and I'm not!

PRAYER

Father, I want You to be free to answer when I call. Show me if there is anything You want me to do or not to do.

Journal: Has something or someone come between you and God? Write God a letter asking for His forgiveness. Ask Him to help you. He will!

—Carole Lewis

DECEMBER 28

SPIRIT-LED PRAYER

Pray in the Spirit on all occasions with all kinds of prayers and requests.

EPHESIANS 6:18

A friend of mine is a Christian songwriter and singer in Salt Lake City. He is one of the few Christian artists in that predominantly Mormon city. One evening, I was attending a small home Bible study in Houston, and we talked about Mormonism. I mentioned my friend to the group and asked for prayer on his behalf.

As we prayed, the burden for him became greater. It was clear that the Holy Spirit was directing us in how to pray. Once we finished, I realized that we had fervently prayed for him for 20 minutes.

When I talked to him a week later, I told him that our group had prayed for him. He was amazed! He said that same night at exactly the same time, he had been invited to the home of a Mormon family. When he arrived, there were several other Mormon families there. His first thought was that they were going to try to convert him to their religion. But as they sat down for the meal, the owner of the house spoke up and said that all the families there that night were disillusioned with Mormonism—they wanted to know about true Christianity.

He spent the next few hours sharing Christ with them, and several of them gave their lives to Christ that very night.

It was obvious to me that we had "prayed in the Spirit" on that occasion and seen results.

In Romans 8:26, the apostle Paul tells us that we don't know what to pray for, but the Holy Spirit prays through us if we allow Him. Our requests of the Lord are never a burden to Him. He delights in our continually asking, seeking and knocking.

PRAYER

Lord, help me to pray in the Spirit according to Your will. Let me make a difference in Your kingdom on my knees. Let me be faithful to "stand in the gap" for Your purposes.

Journal: Write down instances when you prayed in the Spirit and then tell how the Lord answered those prayers.

—Jeff Nelson

DECEMBER 29

ALL KINDS OF PRAYER

Pray in the Spirit on all occasions with all kinds of prayers and requests.

EPHESIANS 6:18

Have you ever called tech-support when your computer crashed? Conversation with them was direct and clear, wasn't it? You tell them, " My computer is down and I need immediate assistance!" and you get help. When you do that with God, that's prayer.

Some time ago, when I went through the ordeal of losing my voice and my ministry, I prayed all kinds of prayers.

My first prayer was for immediate healing and liberation from the condition. "After all, God," I prayed, "You called me to ministry, You afforded me my education, You furnished me with communication skills, and now I can't talk. What's up with that?" In technical terms, my "computer was down" and I needed *immediate* assistance.

By the time my restoration came, a long time later, my prayers had changed significantly. I rarely prayed for healing; rather, I prayed for insight. My physical condition mattered less than being useful in the Kingdom. I hadn't given up on God's power, but my priorities were reordered to more closely resemble His.

Here's the thing: My prayers, at various times, expressed frustration, disappointment, thankfulness, anger, anxiety and hope. My requests were for myself, my family and my friends who were praying for me without seeing *results*, and for strength to stay the course. And God heard them all!

Learning to pray all kinds of prayers candidly is incredibly freeing. Try it! God is big enough to handle your hurts, your impatience—all of it!

PRAYER

Lord, You know where I am broken, where I hurt, where I'm discouraged, where I am weak. Give me the courage to pray honestly and the grace to follow You wherever You may lead.

Journal: What frustrations and hurts have you hidden and been afraid to admit to God? For what have you prayed without considering His will? Do you know someone who is struggling and needs your prayer support? How will you pray for that person?

—Duane A. Miller

DECEMBER 30

A Big God

Pray in the Spirit on all occasions with all kinds of prayers and requests.

EPHESIANS 6:18

Through First Place, I realized that God was only a prayer away every moment of my day. As long as I followed the plan to the best of my ability, His Holy Spirit led me and I felt His presence. Whenever I overate or indulged in binge foods, I felt separated from God.

As time went on, I totally disliked this separation. It was far more satisfying to have the Lord's presence than to indulge in one bite of a favorite food. The closer I walked with the Lord, the more I depended upon Him and prayed over this area of my life. At first I thought it was very insignificant to ask this magnificent God to help me with my eating choices. Then I realized I had Him in a very tiny box. God is *huge*, and He is able. He is able to handle *all* that concerns me, even the little details of my life. He loves me with an everlasting love. What I eat at every meal concerns Him.

He has provided healthy food for me to eat so that my body functions at its absolute best. The Holy Spirit has taught me and led me to a deep, abiding relationship with this trustworthy God. I have learned to pray at all times, for all things—even for my very next bite.

PRAYER

Lord, forgive me for keeping You in a tiny box and believing that You were too big to care. Thank You for showing how deeply You do care for me.

Journal: How big is God to you? Do you keep Him in a box? Through prayer, do you give Him all your concerns—even the little ones?

—Roberta Wasserman

DECEMBER 31

OUT OF THE MOUTHS OF BABES

Pray in the Spirit on all occasions with all kinds of prayers and requests.

EPHESIANS 6:18

I used to tell my kids that when they heard a ringing in their ears, it was God's way of reminding them I was praying for them.

One day we were out driving and heard a siren coming up from behind us. It was an ambulance, and we pulled out of the way just as it raced by with lights flashing, sirens screaming. A second car followed right behind it, also with its lights flashing.

Amid all the excitement, Matt, my oldest son, who was about seven at the time, said, "Daddy, let's pray for the people in the ambulance and the car following them." Out of the mouths of babes!

Now every time any one of us sees an ambulance or hears one coming, we pray for God's comfort and presence to prevail over pain and fear. We may not know exactly what to pray for, but God promises His Spirit will lead our hearts to the need. Our call is to be watchful and sensitive to what's happening in the lives of loved ones, friends, coworkers and all those around us.

Yes, God brings needs and people to mind throughout the day; and our response should always mirror Matt's: "Let's pray for them."

PRAYER

Lord, open my ears to hear Your voice as You bring particular people and their needs to mind today.

Journal: When you think of who you can pray for, who comes to mind? Make a list and be diligent in listening for God's still small voice.

—Bruce Barbour

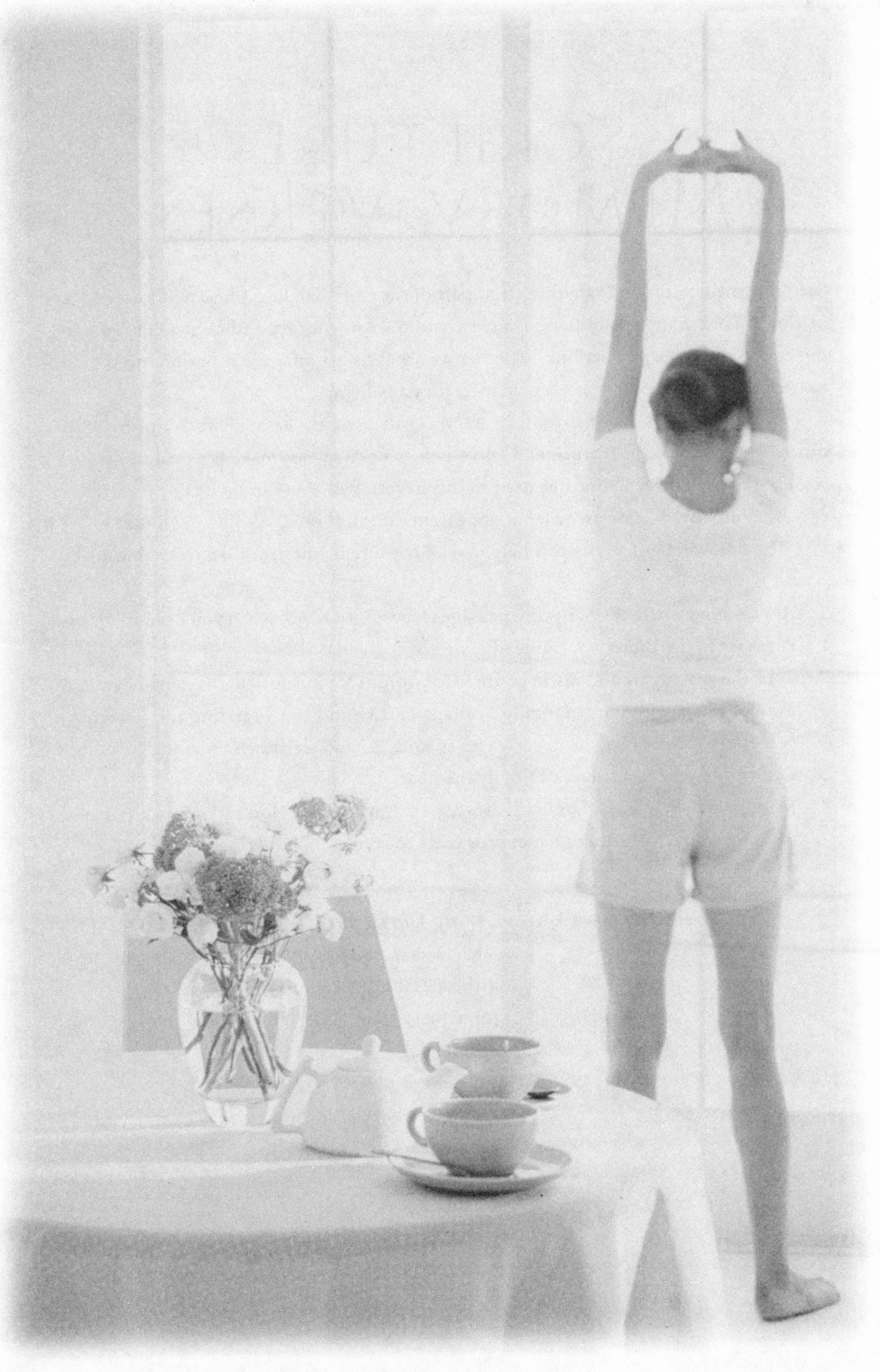

Scripture Memory Verses

Scripture memorization is an important part of the Christian life. A heartfelt knowledge of God's Word equips us to handle any situation we might face and allows His light to direct our decisions and actions—whether we are facing a difficult situation, need help to overcome temptation or need guidance for daily living.

By hiding God's Word in your heart, you will also be able to share Scripture with others who need words of truth and encouragement. Why not make it a goal to memorize each of the 80 key Scriptures used in this devotional? You can do it! For your reference, they are listed below in order of appearance in this book.

The following guidelines will help make Scripture memorization a reachable goal:

1. Always state where the Scripture passage is found. This way when you need to locate the verse in the Bible, you can readily do so.
2. Take the verse apart and insert pictures for words that are difficult to remember. For example, if you were memorizing Romans 15:13 and kept forgetting the reference, you might think of two teenagers, ages 15 and 13, who are always "roamin'" around.
3. Quote the verse to a friend or family member.
4. Memorize the verse as a family. This is a great way to share God's Word together and will be a source of encouragement for years to come.

Section One: *Giving Christ First Place*

Matthew 6:33

Matthew 21:22

John 14:21

Psalm 69:5

1 Corinthians 10:13

Matthew 4:4

Romans 12:2

1 Corinthians 6:19-20

Proverbs 16:3

John 13:34-35

Section Two: ***Everyday Victory for Everyday People***

Deuteronomy 30:11

Ecclesiastes 5:5

1 Peter 5:8

2 Corinthians 10:4

Jeremiah 33:3

2 Corinthians 5:9

Acts 20:24

Zechariah 4:6

Romans 8:1

Psalm 9:10

Section Three: ***Life Under Control***

Psalm 51:12

Romans 15:13

Philippians 4:8

Galatians 2:20

Philippians 4:12-13

Romans 12:3

James 1:26

Luke 9:23

Hebrews 10:24-25

1 Thessalonians 5:23

Section Four: ***Life That Wins***

Romans 5:8

Jeremiah 29:11

Hebrews 11:6

Galatians 5:22-23

Nehemiah 8:10

Philippians 4:7

Galatians 6:9

Colossians 3:12

Matthew 11:29

Galatians 5:16

Section Five: ***Seeking God's Best***

John 6:35

Malachi 3:7

1 Thessalonians 5:18

Titus 2:13-14

1 Samuel 16:7

James 4:7

Philippians 4:19

Joshua 3:5

1 Corinthians 15:58

Psalm 23:5-6

Section Six: ***Pressing On to the Prize***

Philippians 3:14

Hebrews 11:8

Mark 4:19

Colossians 3:14

1 Timothy 6:11

1 Corinthians 9:24

1 Peter 5:4

Hebrews 12:1

Hebrews 12:2

Hebrews 12:15

Section Seven: ***Pathway to Success***

Proverbs 29:18

Psalm 20:4

Deuteronomy 6:5

Ephesians 6:11

2 Peter 1:3

Psalm 139:23-24

1 John 5:4-5

Isaiah 30:21

2 Timothy 1:14

1 Peter 2:9

Section Eight: ***Living the Legacy***

Ephesians 1:4

Ephesians 2:8-9

Ephesians 2:14-15

Ephesians 3:19

Ephesians 4:22-24

Ephesians 5:2

Ephesians 5:8

Ephesians 4:3

Ephesians 6:12

Ephesians 6:18

ENDNOTES

Section One

1. Oswald Chambers, "January 20: Are You Fresh for Everything?" *My Utmost for His Highest* (Westwood, NJ: Barbour and Company, Inc., 1963), p. 20.
2. Ibid.
3. Ibid.
4. Zig Ziglar, *See You at the Top* (New York: Pelican Publishing Company, 1975), n.p.

Section Two

1. Oswald Chambers, "August 18: Have You Ever Been Expressionless with Sorrow?" *My Utmost for His Highest* (Westwood, NJ: Barbour and Company, Inc., 1963), p. 231.

Section Three

1. Florence Littauer, *Personality Plus: How to Understand Others by Understanding Yourself* (Grand Rapids, MI: Revell, 1992), n.p.
2. C. S. Lewis, *The Weight of Glory* (San Francisco, CA: Harper San Francisco, 2001), n.p.
3. Trent C. Butler, ed. *The Holman Bible Dictionary* (Nashville, TN: Broadman and Holman Publishers, 1991), s.v. "crucifixion."
4. Henry Blackaby, *Experiencing God: Knowing and Doing the Will of God* (Nashville, TN: LifeWay Press, 1990), p. 15.

Section Four

1. James Strong, *The New Exhaustive Concordance of the Bible* (Nashville, TN: Thomas Nelson Publishers, 1984), s.v. "na'am."
2. Ibid., s.v. "apokrinomai."
3. Oswald Chambers, quoted in Beth Moore, *Jesus, the One and Only* (Nashville, TN: LifeWay Press, 2000), p. 132.

Section Five

1. Oswald Chambers, "January 9: Intercessory Introspection," *My Utmost for His Highest* (Westwood, NJ: Barbour and Company, Inc., 1963), p. 9.

Section Eight

1. Frederick Faber, quoted in William Barclay, *The Letters to the Galatians and Ephesians* (Philadelphia, PA: The Westminster Press, 1958), p. 86.
2. James Strong, *The New Exhaustive Concordance of the Bible* (Nashville, TN: Thomas Nelson Publishers, 1984), s.v. "charis."
3. Evelyn Christenson, *Lord Change Me* (Colorado Springs, CO: Chariot Victor Publishing, 1993), n.p.

Contributors

June-Marie Avery
First Place Member
Artesia, New Mexico

Bruce Barbour
First Place Consultant
Thompson's Station, Tennessee

Irene Bonner
First Place Leader
Dunwoody, Georgia

June Chapko
First Place Leader
San Antonio, Texas

Anita Clayton
Lenoir City, Tennessee

Jim Clayton
Pastor/First Place Leader
Lenoir City, Tennessee

Luane Clemmer
First Place Member
North Augusta, South Carolina

Rick Crawford
Songwriter
Montgomery, Texas

Betha Jean Cunningham
First Place Member
San Angelo, Texas

Elisa Davis
First Place Member
Glendale, Arizona

Karen Duffy
First Place Member
Pataskala, Ohio

Danna Gilmore
First Place Member
San Antonio, Texas

Jeannie Gramly
First Place Leader
Sand Springs, Oklahoma

Vicki Harnly
First Place Member
Mountville, Pennsylvania

Laura Hartness
First Place Leader
Kernersville, North Carolina

Rob Heath
Pastor
Hanahan, South Carolina

Vicki Heath
Hanahan, South Carolina

Beverly Henson
First Place Leader
Meridian, Mississippi

Bill Heston
Senior Vice President
Howard Payne University
Brownwood, Texas

Kathy Hickey
First Place Member
Clarksville, Arkansas

Pauline Hines
First Place Networking Leader
New Orleans, Louisiana

Mary Etta Jackson
First Place Leader
Houston, Texas

Jill Jamieson
First Place Networking Leader
Cassville, Missouri

Jan Jarrett
First Place Leader
Hendersonville, North Carolina

Rick Jones
First Place Leader
Houston, Texas

Janet Kirkhart
First Place Networking Leader
Mt. Orab, Ohio

Bonnie Ler
First Place Member
Minot, North Dakota

Carole Lewis
First Place National Director
Houston, Texas

Pat Lewis
First Place Staff Member
Houston, Texas

Anne Marenko
First Place Member
Daleville, Mississippi

Judy Marshall
First Place Leader
Gilmer, Texas

Tanya McClanahan
First Place Networking Leader
Maryville, Tennessee

Helen McCormack
First Place Member
Minot, North Dakota

Duane Miller
Pastor
First Place Conference Speaker
Houston, Texas

Carol Moore
First Place Networking Leader
Meridian, Mississippi

Marie Muller
First Place Member
Silver Spring, Maryland

Jeff Nelson
Songwriter/Producer
First Place Scripture Memory Music
Franklin, Tennessee

Martha Norsworthy
First Place Leader
Murray, Kentucky

Nan Olmsted
First Place Leader
Springfield, Missouri

Carolyn O'Neal
First Place Leader
Houston, Texas

Carolyn Owen
First Place Leader
Charlotte Court House, Virginia

Pattie Perry
First Place Networking Leader
Norfolk, Virginia

Denise Peters
First Place Leader
Loveland, Ohio

Karen Rhodus
First Place Leader
West College Corner, Indiana

Terri Richardson
First Place Leader
Vega, Texas

Diana Robinson
First Place Networking Leader
Lithonia, Georgia

Martha Rogers
First Place Leader
Houston, Texas

Kathy Runion
First Place Networking Leader
Greer, South Carolina

David Self
Associate Pastor
Houston, Texas

Wanda Shadle
First Place Member
Houston, Texas

Becky Sirt
First Place Leader
The Woodlands, Texas

Kay Smith
First Place Associate Director
Roscoe, Texas

Tina Smith
First Place Member
Beaufort, South Carolina

Ben Steelman
First Place Member
Hattiesburg, Mississippi

Dee Brewer Strickland
First Place Member
Austin, Texas

Tarena Sullivan
First Place Leader
Fort Wayne, Indiana

Nancy Taylor
First Place Leadership Training Director
Houston, Texas

Carol Van Atta
First Place Leader
Troutdale, Oregon

Roberta Wasserman
First Place Leader
Riva, Maryland

Shelley Wilburn
First Place Member
West Frankfort, Illinois

Eva Williamson
First Place Leader
Houston, Texas

Scott Wilson
First Place Food Consultant
Cumming, Georgia

Joe Ann Winkler
First Place Member
Overland Park, Kansas